www.bma.org.uk/library

PAIN MANAGEMENT

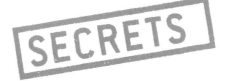

WITHDRAWN
FROM LIBRARY

BRITISH MEDICAL ASSOCIATION

0942476

ACQUISITION

PAIN MANAGEMENT

SECRETS

Third Edition

Charles E. Argoff, MD
Professor of Neurology
Albany Medical College
Director, Comprehensive Pain Program
Albany Medical Center
Albany, New York

and

Gary McCleane, MD
Consultant in Pain Management
Rampark Pain Centre
Lurgan, United Kingdom
Consultant Anaesthetist
Lagan Valley Hospital
Lisburn, United Kingdom

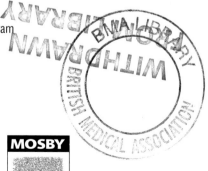

MOSBY

ELSEVIER

WITHDRAWN
BMA LIBRARY
BRITISH MEDICAL ASSOCIATION

MOSBY
ELSEVIER

1600 John F. Kennedy Blvd.
Ste 1800
Philadelphia, PA 19103-2899

PAIN MANAGEMENT SECRETS   ISBN: 978-0-323-04019-8

Copyright © 2009, 2003 by Mosby, Inc., an affiliate of Elsevier Inc.

No part of this publication may be reproduced or transmitted in any form or by any means, electronic
or mechanical, including photocopying, recording, or any information storage and retrieval system,
without permission in writing from the publisher. Permissions may be sought directly from Elsevier's
Rights Department: phone: (+1) 215 239 3804 (US) or (+44) 1865 843830 (UK); fax: (+44) 1865
853333; e-mail: healthpermissions@elsevier.com. You may also complete your request on-line via the
Elsevier website at http://www.elsevier.com/permissions.

NOTICE

Knowledge and best practice in this field are constantly changing. As new research and experience
broaden our knowledge, changes in practice, treatment and drug therapy may become necessary
or appropriate. Readers are advised to check the most current information provided (i) on
procedures featured or (ii) by the manufacturer of each product to be administered, to verify the
recommended dose or formula, the method and duration of administration, and contraindications.
It is the responsibility of the practitioner, relying on their own experience and knowledge of the
patient, to make diagnoses, to determine dosages and the best treatment for each individual
patient, and to take all appropriate safety precautions. To the fullest extent of the law, neither the
Publisher nor the Editors assume any liability for any injury and/or damage to persons or property
arising out of or related to any use of the material contained in this book.

The Publisher

Library of Congress Cataloging-in-Publication Data

Pain management secrets. – 3rd ed. / [edited by] Charles E. Argoff,
Gary McCleane.
   p. ; cm.
  Includes bibliographical references and index.
  ISBN 978-0-323-04019-8
1. Pain–Miscellanea. 2. Analgesia–Miscellanea. I. Argoff, Charles
E. II. McCleane, Gary.
  [DNLM: 1. Pain–therapy–Examination Questions. WL 18.2 P144 2010]
  RB127.P33239 2010
  616′.0472–dc22

2008038141

Acquisitions Editor: Jim Merritt
Developmental Editor: Nicole DiCicco
Project Manager: Mary Stermel
Marketing Manager: Allan McKeown

Working together to grow
libraries in developing countries

www.elsevier.com | www.bookaid.org | www.sabre.org

ELSEVIER   BOOK AID International   Sabre Foundation

Printed in China

Last digit is the print number: 9   8   7   6   5   4   3   2   1

CONTENTS

CONTRIBUTORS

Charles E. Argoff, MD
Professor of Neurology, Albany Medical College; Director, Comprehensive Pain Program, Albany Medical Center, Albany, New York

Zahid H. Bajwa, MD
Assistant Professor of Anesthesia and Neurology, Harvard Medical School; Director, Clinical Pain Research, Department of Anesthesia and Critical Care, Beth Israel Deaconess Medical Center, Boston, Massachusetts

Allan I. Basbaum, PhD
Professor and Chair, Department of Anatomy and William Keck Foundation Center for Integrative Neuroscience, University of California, San Francisco, California

Martin R. Boorin, DMD
Department of Dental Medicine, Long Island Jewish Medical Center, New Hyde Park, New York

Stephen C. Brown, MD, FRCP
Director, Chronic Pain Program, Department of Anaesthesia, The Hospital for Sick Children; Assistant Professor, Department of Anaesthesia, University of Toronto, Toronto, Ontario, Canada

James N. Campbell, MD

Meir Chernofsky, MD
Associate Professor, Department of Internal Medicine/Gastroenterology, University of Medicine and Dentistry–New Jersey Medical College, Newark, New Jersey

Sita S. Chokhavatia, MD
Associate Professor, Department of Internal Medicine/Gastroenterology, University of Medicine and Dentistry–New Jersey Medical College, Newark, New Jersey

Susanne Bennett Clark, PhD
Associate Professor of Medicine and Physiology (Retired), Biophysics Institute, Boston University Medical Center, Boston, Massachusetts

W. Crawford Clark, PhD
Professor of Medical Psychology, Department of Psychiatry, College of Physicians and Surgeons, Columbia University; Research Scientist VI, Department of Biopsychology, New York State Psychiatric Institute, New York, New York

Stephen A. Cohen, MD, MBA
Instructor of Anesthesia and Critical Care, Harvard Medical School; Director, Industry Relations, Department of Anesthesia and Critical Care, Beth Israel Deaconess Medical Center, Boston, Massachusetts

Ellen Cooper, MS
Administrator, Department of Neurology, Long Island Jewish Medical Center, New Hyde Park, New York

Ricardo Cruciani, MD, PhD

Robert A. Duarte, MD
Co-Director, Pain and Headache Treatment Center, Long Island Jewish Medical Center; Assistant Professor, Department of Neurology, Albert Einstein College of Medicine, Bronx, New York

Andrew Dubin, MD

Brad Galer, MD

Gilbert R. Gonzales, MD
Associate Member, Department of Neurology, Section of Pain and Palliative Care, Memorial Sloan-Kettering Cancer Center, New York, New York

Helen Greco, MD
Assistant Professor, Department of Obstetrics and Gynecology, Albert Einstein College of Medicine, Bronx, New York; Chief, Benign Gynecology, Long Island Jewish Medical Center, New Hyde Park, New York

Ronald Greenberg, MD
Associate Professor of Clinical Medicine, Division of Gastroenterology, Albert Einstein College of Medicine, Bronx, New York; Long Island Jewish Medical Center, New Hyde Park, New York

Michael M. Hanania, MD
Assistant Professor of Anesthesiology, Division of Pain Management, Albert Einstein College of Medicine, New Hyde Park, New York

Nelson Hendler, MD, MS

Ronald Kanner, MD, FAAN, FACP
Chairman, Department of Neurology, North Shore–Long Island Jewish Medical Center, New Hyde Park, New York

Abbas Kashani, MD
Attending Physician, Department of Otolaryngology/Head and Neck Surgery, Beth Israel Medical Center; Attending Physician, Wyckoff Heights Medical Center, New York, New York

Richard B. Lipton, MD
Professor and Vice-Chair of Neurology; Professor of Epidemiology and Social Medicine, Albert Einstein College of Medicine, Bronx, New York

Gary McCleane, MD
Consultant in Pain Management, Rampark Pain Centre, Lurgan, United Kingdom; Consultant Anaesthetist, Lagan Valley Hospital, Lisburn, United Kingdom

Patricia A. McGrath, PhD
Scientific Director, Chronic Pain Program, Department of Anaesthesia, The Hospital for Sick Children; Professor, Department of Anaesthesia, University of Toronto, Toronto, Ontario, Canada

Jeffrey S. Meyers, MD, LAc
Medical Director, Delaware Curative Physical Therapy and Rehabilitation, Wilmington, Delaware

Lawrence C. Newman, MD
Associate Professor, Department of Neurology, Albert Einstein College of Medicine, Bronx, New York; Director, The Headache Institute, St. Luke's-Roosevelt Hospital Center, New York, New York

Bryan J. O'Young, MD
Clinical Associate Professor, Department of Rehabilitation Medicine, New York University School of Medicine; Attending Physician, Rusk Institute of Rehabilitation Medicine, New York, New York

David S. Pisetsky, MD, PhD
Professor of Medicine and Immunology, and Chief of Rheumatology, Division of Rheumatology, Allergy, and Clinical Immunology, Duke University Medical Center; Staff Physician, Veterans Administration Medical Center, Durham, North Carolina

Russell K. Portenoy, MD
Professor, Department of Neurology, Albert Einstein College of Medicine, Bronx, New York; Chair, Department of Pain Medicine and Palliative Care, Beth Israel Medical Center, New York, New York

Jason E. Silvers, BS

Howard S. Smith, MD, FACP
Academic Director of Pain Management, Department of Anesthesiology, Associate Professor of Anesthesiology, Internal Medicine and Physical Medicine and Rehabilitation, Albany Medical College, Albany, New York

Steven A. Stiens, MD, MS
Associate Professor, Department of Rehabilitation Medicine, University of Washington School of Medicine; Attending Physician, Spinal Cord Injury Unit, Veterans Affairs Puget Sound Health Care System, Seattle, Washington

Brian Thiessen, MD
Private Practice, Neurology and Neuro-oncology, Vancouver, British Columbia, Canada

Mark A. Thomas, MD
Associate Professor, Department of Rehabilitation Medicine, Albert Einstein College of Medicine; Program Director, Physical Medicine and Rehabilitation, Montefiore Medical Center, Bronx, New York

Dennis R. Thornton, PhD
Assistant Professor, Departments of Psychiatry/Psychology and Neurology, Albert Einstein College of Medicine, Bronx, New York

Carol A. Warfield, MD
Professor of Anesthesia and Critical Care, Harvard Medical School; Chair, Department of Anesthesia and Critical Care, Beth Israel Deaconess Medical Center, Boston, Massachusetts

Mark A. Young, MD
Chair, Department of Physical Medicine and Rehabilitation, The Maryland Rehabilitation Center, State of Maryland Department of Education; Faculty, Johns Hopkins University School of Medicine; Faculty, University of Maryland School of Medicine, Baltimore, Maryland

PREFACE

Inspection of the "pain" section of any bookstore will reveal a wide and diverse range of texts that address everything from the basic science that underpins our understanding of pain all the way through to the clinical treatment of specific conditions. We are spoiled with choices. These books largely use scientific evidence to validate the propositions that they make and provide an invaluable resource for anyone interested in pain and its treatment, although deciding which book best fits the individual's requirement can be problematical.

The third edition of *Pain Secrets* differs from most of these books. It contains a refreshing mixture of scientifically robust information combined with a more anecdotal nature. It has become fashionable to discredit opinion unless it is based on the results of rigorously performed studies, and yet by ignoring the combined wealth of knowledge possessed by experienced practitioners based on years of involvement in their field, we risk having a less complete knowledge of our field of interest than would otherwise be the case. *Pain Secrets* is liberally seeded with little "pearls of wisdom," which many will find interesting, thought provoking, and hopefully useful. Some of these you may know already, but almost certainly others will be new. They have the potential for transforming the practitioner from being knowledgeable and widely read to being even more effective in his or her practice than before. These useful pieces of knowledge have a value that is timeless, and they are not a representation of a current fashion in our thinking about pain. As such, they can provide the reader with an insight that normally is acquired only by long years of practical experience.

Perhaps one of the other distinguishing features of *Pain Secrets* is that it can be used when a specific answer to a specific question is needed. Each chapter concentrates on one facet of pain management. Contained in each chapter are a series of individual questions for which an answer is provided. Alternatively, the book can be read chapter by chapter to give a more comprehensive insight into the subject being considered. Given the style used and the content of each chapter, this book should be of interest, indeed value, to anyone involved in pain management, whether they are fully qualified or still in training. It should also be of use to those in whom pain management is an incidental requirement rather than a primary focus of interest.

Charles E. Argoff
Gary McCleane

TOP 100 SECRETS

1. Pain is defined by the International Association for the Study of Pain as "an unpleasant sensory and emotional experience associated with actual or potential tissue damage, or described in terms of such damage."

2. In primary pain syndromes, the pain itself is the disease. Examples include migraine, trigeminal neuralgia, and cluster headache.

3. Secondary pain syndrome is due to an underlying structural cause, such as trigeminal neuralgia due to a tumor pressing on the cranial nerve.

4. The key element in taking the clinical history of a patient with pain is to evaluate the complaint of pain. Important factors are location, radiation, intensity, characteristics/quality, temporal aspects, exacerbating/triggering and relieving factors, circumstances surrounding the onset of pain, and potential mechanisms of injury.

5. Pain classification provides the clinician with invaluable information about the possible origin of the pain. More importantly, it directs the health care practitioner toward a proper pharmacologic treatment plan.

6. There are a number of different measurements for pain intensity. Think about treating pain as analogous to treating hypertension: you would never use antihypertensive medications without measuring the patient's blood pressure on each visit. The same is true of pain.

7. Pain assessment is a multidimensional approach to the evaluation of pain attributes, which include the intensity, duration, and location of pain and its somatosensory and emotional qualities.

8. There are ample studies that suggest that pain is treated less aggressively in women and in ethnic minorities, and the reasons for this are multifactorial.

9. Brief Pain Inventory (BPI) measures both the intensity of the pain (sensory component), as well as the interference of the pain in the patient's life.

10. The essential element of a good pain evaluation is to believe that the pain is real!

11. The most common conceptual mistake that the examining clinician makes is trying to conceptualize pain as either organic or psychological ("psychosomatic").

12. The Axial Loading Test, a pain amplification test, has the patient stand while pressure is applied over the skull.

13. The Rotation Test, a pain amplification test, has the patient stand with his or her feet together, and the shoulders and hips are rotated in the same plane.

14. Hoover's Test, a pain amplification test, has the patient lie supine with the weak leg elevated while the examiner keeps a hand under each of the heels.

15. Provocative testing is often the most helpful examination element in determining the cause of pain (the "pain generator").

16. Anterior flexion of the head opens the neuroforamina. As the head turns from side to side or tilts from side to side, the ipsilateral intervertebral foramen closes.

17. Clinically, a root lesion can be differentiated from injury to a peripheral nerve by noticing that a number of muscles may be innervated by the same root, but through different nerves.

18. Visceral pain tends to be poorly localized and felt in the midline, and it is often experienced as a dull soreness that fluctuates in severity.

19. Somatic pain is typically more acute, intense, sharp, localized, and aggravated by movement.

20. Referred pain combines features of both visceral and somatic pain and is well localized in areas distant from the precipitating stimulus.

21. Carnett's Test can help distinguish chronic abdominal pain due to disease of the abdominal wall from that of intraabdominal origin.

22. Pelvic congestion syndrome is due to pelvic vascular engorgement, which presents as heaviness and pain.

23. Irritable bowel syndrome (IBS) is characterized by bouts of abdominal cramping and frequent bowel movements, and pain due to IBS may be aggravated in the luteal phase of the menstrual cycle.

24. Tricyclic antidepressants are widely used drugs for the treatment of fibromyalgia and myofascial pain syndrome.

25. Exercise can be helpful in the treatment of fibromyalgia and myofascial pain syndrome, as the best outcome appears to result from conditioning or aerobic exercise.

26. The youngest age for which patient-controlled analgesia is appropriate is 7 years old; those aged 5 to 6 have variable success.

27. The side effect of pruritus with opioid use can be treated with an antihistamine such as diphenhydramine or a low-dose intravenous infusion of naloxone (1-3 mg/kg/hr). Oral naltrexone and propofol also have been reported to relieve pruritus.

28. Breast cancer treated with mastectomy and radiation of the brachial plexus region may develop ipsilateral pain with arm and hand weakness (a brachial plexopathy) after treatments, but if the symptoms are referable to the lower brachial plexus (i.e., lower trunk), it is most likely due to tumor recurrence.

29. Steroid pseudorheumatism is characterized by arthralgias, diffuse myalgias, muscle and joint tenderness on palpation, and diffuse malaise without objective inflammatory signs on examination.

30. Codeine has no intrinsic analgesic effect but requires a metabolic step to occur (which converts it to morphine) for analgesia to be produced.

31. Duration of action of the local anesthetics depends on a number of factors, including the agent in question, the vascularity of the tissue into which it is injected, and with some of the local anesthetics, the coadministration of epinephrine.

32. Steroids have a number of effects on neural function that may enhance local anesthetic action that include antiinflammatory and membrane stabilizing effects.

33. Neurolysis should be regarded as an irreversible and potentially permanent procedure to be considered only when other treatment modalities have failed and is nowadays almost exclusively reserved for the treatment of intractable cancer pain.

34. Radiofrequency neurolysis uses high-frequency waves to produce thermal coagulation of the nerves in which a probe is inserted percutaneously, and correct position is confirmed by fluoroscopy and motor and/or sensory stimulation.

35. Treatment of CRPS type I becomes less satisfactory in the later stages of disease, and when the condition is neglected, it may progress to a disability that dominates the life of the patient.

36. Celiac plexus block may be performed with fluoroscopic or computed tomographic guidance, which is necessary when the anatomy is distorted by disease or body habitus.

37. Intraspinal administration presents a high concentration of opioids directly to the dorsal horn and modulates nociceptive input in the acute situation.

38. All opioids are not created equal. Opioids can be divided into two classes: lipophilic (lipid-soluble) and hydrophilic (lipid-insoluble).

39. Conditions that may respond to spinal cord stimulation are radicular pain from failed back surgery, ischemic pain from peripheral vascular disease, pain from peripheral nerve injury, phantom limb pain or stump pain, and complex regional pain syndrome (reflex sympathetic dystrophy, causalgia).

40. Conditions that usually do not respond to spinal cord stimulation are postherpetic neuralgia, pain from spinal cord injury, and axial pain in failed back syndrome.

41. Microvascular decompression requires a craniotomy, which is the open procedure that can be used to treat trigeminal neuralgia.

42. A well-run multidisciplinary pain treatment center requires that a single health care provider function as the leader of the team with the responsibility for coordinating all of the medical efforts, laboratory studies, ancillary therapies, and medications and should be available during all hours that the center is open to provide continuity of care.

43. Primary afferent nociceptors contain a variety of neurotransmitters, including the excitatory amino acid glutamate and a variety of neuropeptides, such as substance P and calcitonin gene–related peptide.

44. Pain in cognitively impaired patients and young children can be estimated by their responses to a scale consisting of a series of faces whose expressions range from smiling to discomfort to desperate crying.

45. The most common form of primary headache is tension-type headache (TTH).

46. The treatment of TTH, like the treatment of migraine, can be divided into two major categories: nonpharmacologic and pharmacologic therapies. The pharmacologic therapies are divided into acute (abortive) and preventive (prophylactic).

47. Virtually any medication can cause rebound headache; therefore, it is important to limit the dose of all acute medications.

48. Migraine is a major public health problem by almost any standard. It is a highly prevalent disorder that affects 11% of the U.S. population and produces enormous suffering for individuals and their families.

49. The gradual evolution of symptom includes the mix of positive and negative features, and the temporal association with headache helps identify migraine aura or differentiate from other kinds of focal episodes of neurologic dysfunction. The patient's age and risk factor profile may also point the clinician in one diagnostic direction or another.

50. Migraine is considered a neurologic disease because changes in the brain give rise to inflammatory changes in cranial and meningeal blood vessels that in turn produce pain.

51. Acute treatments of migraine should be matched to the overall severity of the patient's illness, the severity of the patient's attack, the profile of associated symptoms, and the patient's treatment preferences.

52. For the patient who awakens with severe, full-blown attacks of migraine with prominent nausea and vomiting, nonoral therapy may be the only effective option.

53. For patients who have attacks of migraine that begin gradually or who are unsure if the attack will be mild or severe, it is best to begin with oral agents and escalate therapy if the attack increases in severity.

54. For a patient with both moderate and severe attacks of migraine, treatment may begin with an NSAID (plus metoclopramide), and a triptan can be used either as an "escape medication" or for the more severe attacks.

55. The major groups of medication used for migraine prophylaxis include the beta blockers, antidepressants, serotonin antagonists, anticonvulsants, and calcium channel blockers.

56. Cluster headaches are characterized by attacks of excruciatingly severe, unilateral head pain in which attacks last 15 to 180 minutes and recur from once every other day up to eight times daily.

57. A very small minority of cluster sufferers report that typical migraine triggers induce their headaches.

58. Cluster patients pace, sit upright in a chair, or bang their heads against a wall.

59. Migraineurs lie quietly in a dark room and attempt to sleep.

60. There are headaches with features of both migraine and cluster that cannot be adequately categorized in either group. These patients often have an intermediate disorder referred to as *cluster-migraine variant*.

61. The paroxysmal hemicranias are a group of rare, benign headache disorders that resemble cluster headache in most ways but do not respond to anticluster medications.

62. The differential diagnosis between clusters or paroxysmal hemicranias is exceptionally important, as the paroxysmal hemicranias are often resistant to the medications that typically prevent cluster headaches.

63. The paroxysmal hemicranias exhibit unique responsiveness to indomethacin but not to other nonsteroidal antiinflammatory agents. Initial therapy consists of indomethacin 25 mg three times a day.

64. The pain of subarachnoid hemorrhage is often severe and may require potent analgesics.

65. The most important differentiating factor between a benign tension-type headache and a brain tumor headache is probably the time course. A new-onset headache that progresses over days to weeks is much more suspect of representing a space-occupying lesion than is a chronic headache that has been stable over a long period.

66. While the pathology of the brain tumor is not important in determining the clinical presentation, the location of the tumor may be.

67. Systemic hypertension does not usually cause an increased intracranial pressure headache.

68. The reason is unclear, but the most common predisposing factor in benign intracranial hypertension is that most patients with pseudotumor cerebri are obese women.

69. Primary and metastatic brain tumors are among the most common intracranial causes of increased intracranial pressure.

70. When evaluating the patient with a complaint of headache, elevated sedimentation rate, advanced age, jaw claudication, and diplopia have the best positive predictive value for TA.

71. As soon as the diagnosis for giant cell arteritis is suspected, initiate prednisone therapy.

72. While headache is one of the most common pain complaints for which patients seek medical help, it is uncommonly associated with a serious systemic illness.

73. The first-line agent for trigeminal neuralgia remains carbamazepine.

74. In occipital neuralgia, a sharp pain originates at the base of the skull and shoots up the back of the head. It may go as far forward as the coronal suture.

75. Some patients who had clearly defined causes for back pain continue to suffer from the same pain even after the causative agent is eliminated, because there are synaptic changes and there may be neuronal hyperactivity, expression of new genes, and other central phenomena that perpetuate the perception of pain.

76. Straight leg raising is used to diagnose nerve root compression from disc disease. It is most commonly used to look for lower lumbar root pathology.

77. The term *sciatica* has come into rather broad usage, and usually refers to any sharp pain that radiates down the posterior aspect of the leg.

78. You can approach the patient with chronic idiopathic pelvic pain with psychologic and pharmacologic approaches.

79. Neuropathic pain is suggested when patients use terms to describe their pain that are consistent with a dysesthesia, which is defined as an abnormal pain complaint.

80. Most patients experiencing chronic pain report depressive symptoms at some point during the course of their condition.

81. Newborn infants are more sensitive to painful stimuli than adults, and children report stronger pain for stimuli that evoke moderate tissue damage in comparison with adults.

82. Generally, patients with mild to moderate cognitive impairment can still complete some short self-assessment scales.

83. Physical dependence is a state in which rapid discontinuation of a drug or administration of an antagonist produces an abstinence syndrome.

84. Physical dependence can develop entirely separate from addiction.

85. Addiction is a primary, chronic, neurobiologic disease with genetic, psychosocial, and environmental factors influencing its development and manifestations.

86. The five main characteristics of addiction are chronicity, impaired control, compulsive use, continued use despite harm, and craving (the five Cs).

87. Adjuvant analgesics are drugs that have primary indications other than pain but are analgesic in some painful conditions.

88. Traditional Chinese Medicine holds that the mechanism of action for acupuncture analgesia is release of stagnation of qi (the vital force).

89. Physical modalities refer to any therapeutic medium that utilizes the transmission of energy to or through the patient.

90. Topiceuticals can be safely added to an existing pain treatment plan without worry about drug-drug interactions with other body-wide (systemic) analgesics.

91. Transdermal preparations are formulated to deliver medication across the skin and into the bloodstream; the bloodstream carries the medication throughout the body for a body-wide or systemic effect.

92. The clinical implications of the pharmacokinetic changes seen in the older patient are given diminished volume of distribution, longer half-life, and reduced clearance; it follows that plasma levels will be elevated for a longer period after a given dose.

93. Headaches are the seventh leading reason for outpatient visits in the United States and account for 2% to 4% of all emergency room visits.

94. Psychoanalytic theory divides the psyche into three functions: the id—unconscious source of primitive sexual, dependency, and aggressive impulses; the superego—subconsciously

interjects societal mores, setting standards to live by; and the ego—represents a sense of self and mediates between realities of the moment and psychic needs and conflicts.

95. The concept of a pain-prone personality evolved from psychodynamic theory. The dynamic was created to codify the process by which intrapsychic conflicts predisposed the individual to seek expression for repressed feelings in the form of somatic, particularly painful, complaints.

96. Most surveys show that about 40% of the U.S. populace uses some type of complementary medicine during a given year.

97. The National Center for Complementary and Alternative Medicine (NCCAM) categorized complementary and alternative medicine into five categories: alternative medicine systems, mind-body interventions, biologically based techniques, manipulative and body-based methods, and energy therapies.

98. Acupuncture is one of the oldest forms of recorded medical therapy, with documented cases going back more than 4000 years.

99. There are different types of acupunctue stimulation including manual, application of heat, electrical stimulation, moxa (gum wort), or laser.

100. It is unclear that any specific type of acupuncture is superior to another, although anecdotal evidence suggests that electroacupuncture may be useful for myofascial pain syndromes, and auriculotherapy for drug addiction.

I. OVERVIEW

CHAPTER 1

DEFINITIONS

Ronald Kanner, MD, FAAN, FACP

1. **What is pain?**
   The International Association for the Study of Pain defines pain as: "An unpleasant sensory and emotional experience associated with actual or potential tissue damage, or described in terms of such damage." Some dictionaries define pain as: "An unpleasant sensation, occurring in varying degrees of severity as a consequence of injury, disease, or emotional disorder." Inherent in both definitions is the concept that pain always has a subjective component. It is both a physiologic sensation and an emotional reaction to that sensation. In some cases, there may be no tissue injury, but the pain is no less "real." In clinical terms, Margo McCaffrey (an internationally regarded expert on pain) has defined pain most succinctly and appropriately: "Whatever the patient says hurts."

2. **What is the difference between pain and suffering?**
   Pain is a sensation plus a reaction to that sensation. *Suffering* is a more global concept—an overall negative feeling that impairs the sufferer's quality of life. Both physical and psychological issues are actively involved with suffering, and the pain itself may be only a small component. In some instances, pain may be an expression of suffering (see "Somatoform Disorders" in Chapter 29, Psychological Syndromes).

3. **What is the difference between impairment and disability?**
   Impairment is a medical concept; *disability* is a legal or societal concept. Impairment is any loss or abnormality of psychological, physiologic, or anatomic structure or function. According to the World Health Organization (WHO) definition, disability results from impairment; it is any restriction or lack of ability to perform an activity in the manner or within the range considered normal for a human. In governmental terms, disability is sometimes called a functional limitation. Another definition of disability is a disadvantage (resulting from an impairment or functional limitation) that limits or prevents the fulfillment of a role that is normal for an individual (depending on age, sex, and social and cultural factors). This definition corresponds to the WHO classification of handicap.

4. **What is meant by inferred pathophysiology?**
   We can rarely define with certainty the pathophysiologic mechanisms underlying a specific pain syndrome. However, a specific set of symptoms may lead us to believe that a pain syndrome is more likely due to nerve injury (neuropathic pain), lesions of muscle or bone (somatic nociceptive pain), or disease of the internal organs (visceral nociceptive pain). This *inferred pathophysiology* implies that we understand the basic mechanisms underlying a pain syndrome, and leads to the pathophysiologic classification of pain syndromes (see Chapter 2, Classification of Pain). This pathophysiologic classification may be overly self-serving, because we can only infer, and rarely verify, the true mechanism.

5. **What is the definition of nociception?**
   Nociception is the activation of a nociceptor by a potentially tissue-damaging (noxious) stimulus. It is the first step in the pain pathway.

6. **What is a nociceptor?**

A nociceptor is a specialized, neurologic receptor that is capable of differentiating between innocuous and noxious stimuli. In humans, nociceptors are the undifferentiated terminals of A-delta fibers and C fibers, which are the thinnest myelinated and unmyelinated fibers, respectively. A-delta fibers are also called high-threshold mechanoreceptors. They respond primarily to mechanical stimuli of noxious intensity.

7. **What is the difference between pain threshold and pain tolerance?**

Pain threshold refers to the lowest intensity at which a given stimulus is perceived as painful; it is relatively constant across subjects for a given stimulus. For example, most subjects will define a thermal stimulus as painful when it reaches about 50° C. Similarly, barring disease states, mechanical pressure produces pain at approximately the same amount of pressure across subjects. Pain threshold as it relates to sensitivity to pressure is measured with an algometer.

Pain tolerance, on the other hand, is the greatest level of pain that a subject is prepared to endure. Tolerance varies much more widely across subjects and depends on prescribed medications. Clinically, pain tolerance is of much more importance than pain threshold. (More detailed discussions of threshold and tolerance are found in Chapter 6, Pain Measurement.)

8. **You touch an apparently normal area of skin and the patient jumps with pain. Why?**

This reaction is an example of allodynia, an abnormal circumstance in which an innocuous stimulus is perceived as painful. It is common in many neuropathic pain conditions, such as postherpetic neuralgia, complex regional pain syndrome, and certain other neuropathies. Two different types of allodynia are described: thermal and mechanical. In thermal allodynia, an innocuous warm or cold breeze may be perceived as painful. With mechanical allodynia, a very light touch (such as the clothes rubbing against the skin) may be extremely painful, while firmer pressure is not.

In cases of allodynia resulting from neurological injury, the skin surface may appear normal. Allodynia is also present in skin sensitized by a burn or inflammation, but in these patients the affected skin is visibly abnormal.

9. **What is meant by analgesia?**

Analgesia is the absence of pain despite the presence of a normally painful stimulus. Analgesia can be produced peripherally (at the site of tissue damage, receptor, or nerve) or centrally (in the spinal cord or brain). In general, the nonsteroidal antiinflammatory drugs and other minor analgesics act primarily at the site of tissue damage, whereas opioids and so-called adjuvant drugs act primarily at the spinal cord or cerebral level.

10. **What is the difference between analgesia and anesthesia?**

Anesthesia implies loss of many sensory modalities, leaving the area "insensate." *Analgesia* refers specifically to the easing of painful sensation.

11. **What is meant by paresthesia?**

A paresthesia is **any** abnormal sensation. It may be spontaneous or evoked. The most common paresthesia is the sense that a limb "falls asleep" when a nerve in the limb is compressed; also known as "pins and needles." Paresthesias are not always painful.

12. **What is a dysesthesia?**

A dysesthesia is a painful paresthesia. By definition, the sensation is unpleasant. Examples include the burning feet that may be felt in alcoholic peripheral neuropathy or the spontaneous pain in the thigh felt in diabetic amyotrophy.

13. **What is hypoesthesia?**

Hypoesthesia is decreased sensitivity to stimulation. Essentially, it is an area of relative numbness and may be due to any kind of nerve injury. Areas of hypoesthesia are created intentionally by local infiltrations of anesthetics.

14. **What is formication?**

Formication is a form of paresthesia in which the patient feels as though bugs are crawling on his or her body. It is a common hallucinatory sensation in patients with delirium tremens. The term derives from the Latin word *formicae*, which means "ants."

15. **What is anesthesia dolorosa, and what is an example?**

Anesthesia dolorosa is a syndrome in which pain is felt in an area that is otherwise numb or desensitized. It commonly occurs after partial nerve lesions and is a typical complication of radiofrequency coagulation of the trigeminal nerve.

Patients with intractable trigeminal neuralgia are sometimes treated by percutaneous radiofrequency lesioning of the nerve (see Chapter 18, Trigeminal Neuralgia). In a certain percentage of patients, the original trigeminal neuralgia pain is replaced by spontaneous pain in a now denervated area. The paradox is that an otherwise insensitive area is painful.

16. **What is meant by neuralgia?**

Neuralgia is a clinically descriptive term that refers to pain in the distribution of a nerve or nerves. The condition described as "sciatica" may be due to the injury of the sciatic nerve but is more commonly due to spinal nerve root compression (at L5 or S1 vertebra); pain is felt in the distribution of the sciatic nerve (radiating down the posterior aspect of the leg). Trigeminal neuralgia, one of the most common primary neuralgias, is characterized by a jabbing pain in one or more of the distributions of the trigeminal nerve. Neuralgic pain is fairly characteristic: it is an electrical, shocklike pain.

17. **What is hyperpathia?**

The term hyperpathia refers to an abnormally intense pain response to repetitive stimuli. Usually the hyperpathic area of skin is not sensitive to a simple stimulus but overresponds to multiple stimuli. For example, a single pin prick may not be felt, but repetitive pin pricks produce intense pain. Hyperpathia is sometimes called summation dysesthesia.

18. **What are algogenic substances?**

Algogenic substances, when released from injured tissues or injected subcutaneously, activate or sensitize nociceptors (*algos* = pain). Histamines, substance P, potassium, and prostaglandins are examples of algogenic substances.

19. **What is meant by sensitization?**

Sensitization is a state in which a peripheral receptor or a central neuron either responds to stimuli in a more intense fashion than it would under baseline conditions or responds to a stimulus to which it is normally insensitive. Sensitization occurs both at the level of the nociceptor in the periphery and at the level of the second-order neuron in the spinal cord (see Chapter 3, Basic Mechanisms).

In the periphery, tissue injury may convert a high-threshold mechanoreceptor (which normally would respond only to noxious mechanical stimuli) into a receptor that responds to gentle stimuli as though they were noxious. Centrally, the second-order neurons (those on which the primary afferents synapse) also may become hyperexcitable. When spinal cord neurons are hyperexcitable, they may fire spontaneously, giving rise to spontaneous pain. This is typically the case after deafferentation (see Question 21).

20. What is a "lancinating" pain? What does its presence imply?
Lancinating literally means "cutting." It is a sharp, stabbing pain that is often associated with neuropathic syndromes. The word is virtually never used by patients but is frequently used by pain specialists.

21. Define deafferentation.
Deafferentation implies the loss of normal input from primary sensory neurons. It may occur after any type of peripheral nerve injury. Deafferentation is particularly common in postherpetic neuralgia and in traumatic nerve injuries. The central neuron on which the primary afferent was to synapse may become hyperexcitable.

22. Describe the gate control theory of pain.
The basic premises of the gate control theory of pain are that activity in large (nonnociceptive) fibers can inhibit the perception of activity in small (nociceptive) fibers and that descending activity from the brain also can inhibit that perception. Given this construct, it is easy to understand why deafferentation may cause pain. If the large fibers are preferentially injured, the normal inhibition of pain perception does not occur.

23. What is meant by "breakthrough" pain?
If a patient has good pain control on a stable analgesic regimen and suddenly develops an acute exacerbation of pain, this is referred to as breakthrough pain. It often occurs toward the end of a dosing interval because of a drop in analgesic levels. "Incident" pain is a type of breakthrough pain that occurs either with a maneuver that would normally exacerbate pain (weight bearing on an extremity with a bone metastasis) or with sudden disease exacerbation (hemorrhage, fracture, or expansion of a hollow viscus).

 Pain resulting from falling analgesic levels is best controlled by increasing the dose or shortening the intervals between doses. Incident pain, on the other hand, is usually best handled by administering an extra dose of an analgesic before the exacerbating activity.

24. What is tabetic pain?
Tabetic pain was first described in tabes dorsalis, a complication of syphilis. It is a sharp, lightning type of pain. Also called lancinating pain, it is one of the more common neuropathic pains.

25. True or false: central pain arises only when the original insult was central.
False. The term central pain is applied when the generator of the pain is believed to be in the spinal cord or the brain. The original insult may have been peripheral (nerve injury or postherpetic neuralgia), but the pain is sustained by central mechanisms. The basic process may be central sensitization. Central pain also may occur after central injuries, such as strokes or spinal cord injuries. The pain tends to be poorly localized and of a burning nature.

26. What is meant by referred pain?
Pain in an area removed from the site of tissue injury is called referred pain. The most common examples are pain in the shoulder from myocardial infarction, pain in the back from pancreatic disease, and pain in the right shoulder from gallbladder disease. The presumed mechanism is that afferent fibers from the site of tissue injury enter the spinal cord at a similar level to afferents from the point to which the pain is referred. This conjoint area in the spinal cord results in the mistaken perception that the pain arises from the referral site.

27. Describe phantom pain.
Phantom pain is pain felt in a part of the body that has been surgically removed. It is common for patients to have phantom sensation postoperatively; that is, after limb amputation, the patient feels as though the limb is still present. This sensation occurs in nearly all patients

undergoing amputation. It usually subsides over days to weeks. A small percentage of patients develop true phantom limb pain, which may be extraordinarily persistent and resistant to treatment.

28. **What is meralgia paresthetica?**
Meralgia paresthetica is a syndrome of tingling discomfort (dysesthesias) in an area of nerve injury, most commonly the lateral femoral cutaneous nerve. It is characterized by a patch of decreased sensation over the lateral thigh; this area is dysesthetic. Meralgia paresthetica may be caused by more proximal nerve compression.

29. **What is the difference between fast pain and slow pain?**
Fast pain is a relatively localized, well-defined pain that is carried in the neospinothalamic tract. Slow pain is more diffuse and poorly localized and presumed to be carried in the paleospinothalamic tract. In the periphery, C fibers generally subserve slow pain and A-delta fibers subserve fast pain.

30. **What is the difference between primary and secondary pain syndromes?**
In primary pain syndromes, the pain itself is the disease. Examples include migraine, trigeminal neuralgia, and cluster headache. A secondary pain syndrome is due to an underlying structural cause—for example, trigeminal neuralgia due to a tumor pressing on the cranial nerve. One of the major diagnostic issues in any primary pain syndrome is to exclude an underlying destructive cause (tumor or infection).

31. **What is meant by palliative care?**
The WHO defines palliative care as "the active total care of patients, controlling pain and minimizing emotional, social, and spiritual problems at a time when disease is not responsive to active treatment." In a broader sense, it is usually taken to mean the alleviation of symptoms when the primary disease cannot be controlled. The concept is now being extended to include symptom management at earlier stages of terminal diseases.

32. **What are some of the published definitions of addiction?**
According to the American Psychiatric Association's *Diagnostic and Statistical Manual of Mental Disorders (DSM-IV)*, addiction is "a primary, chronic neurobiologic disease, with genetic, psychosocial, and environmental factors influencing its development and manifestations. It is characterized by behaviors that include one or more of the following: impaired control over drug use, compulsive use, continued use despite harm, and craving."
    According to the WHO, addiction is "a state, psychic and sometimes also physical, resulting from the interaction between a living organism and a drug, characterized by behavioral and other responses that always include a compulsion to take the drug on a continuous or periodic basis in order to experience its psychic effects, and sometimes to avoid the discomfort of its absence. Tolerance may or may not be present."

33. **What is the definition of physical dependence?**
Physical dependence is a state of adaptation that is manifested by a drug class–specific withdrawal syndrome that can be produced by abrupt cessation, rapid dose reduction, decreasing blood level of the drug, and/or administration of an antagonist.

34. **What is the definition of drug tolerance?**
Drug tolerance is a state of adaptation in which exposure to a drug induces changes that result in a diminution of one or more of the drug's effects over time.

35. **What is the definition of pseudoaddiction?**

    Pseudoaddiction is an iatrogenic syndrome of abnormal behavior developing as a direct consequence of inadequate pain management. Treatment strategies include establishing trust between the patient and the health care team and providing appropriate and timely analgesics to control the patient's level of pain.

KEY POINTS

1. It is imperative that the differences among nociception, pain, and suffering be recognized so that patients can be appropriately evaluated and treated.

2. Paresthesias may or may not be painful.

3. An understanding of breakthrough pain is important to providing a patient with optimal pain control.

4. Recognizing the differences among addiction, pseudoaddiction, physical dependence, and tolerance are essential to effectively prescribing analgesics to patients with chronic pain.

BIBLIOGRAPHY

1. Heit HA: Addiction, physical dependence, and tolerance: precise definitions to help clinicians evaluate and treat chronic pain patients, *Journal of Pain and Palliative Care Pharmacotherapy* 17(1):15-29, 2003.

2. Merskey N, Bogduk N, editors: *Classification of chronic pain: task force on taxonomy*, 2nd ed, Seattle, 1994, International Association for the Study of Pain Press.

3. Nicholson B: Taxonomy of pain, *Clin J Pain* 16:S114-S117, 2000.

4. Portenoy RK, Kanner RM: Definition and assessment of pain. In Portenoy RK, Kanner RM, editors: *Pain management: theory and practice*, Philadelphia, 1996, F.A. Davis, pp 3-18.

CHAPTER 2

CLASSIFICATION OF PAIN

Robert A. Duarte, MD, and Charles E. Argoff, MD

1. **List the bases for the most widely used classifications of pain.**
   Pain is a subjective experience that does not lend itself to the usual classifications. On a practical basis, pain classifications depend on the following:
   - Inferred pathophysiology (nociceptive vs. nonnociceptive)
   - Time course (acute vs. chronic)
   - Location (painful region)
   - Etiology (e.g., cancer, arthritis)

2. **What is the neurophysiologic classification of pain?**
   The neurophysiologic classification is based on the inferred mechanism for pain. There are essentially two types: (1) nociceptive, which is due to injury in pain-sensitive structures, and (2) nonnociceptive, which is neuropathic and psychogenic. Nociceptive pain can be subdivided into somatic and visceral (depending on which set of nociceptors is activated). Neuropathic pain can be subdivided into peripheral and central (depending on the site of injury in the nervous system believed responsible for maintaining the pain).

3. **What is nociceptive pain?**
   Nociceptive pain results from the activation of nociceptors (A-delta fibers and C fibers) by noxious stimuli that may be mechanical, thermal, or chemical. Nociceptors may be sensitized by endogenous chemical stimuli (algogenic substances) such as serotonin, substance P, bradykinin, prostaglandin, and histamine. Somatic pain is transmitted along sensory fibers. Visceral pain, in comparison, is transmitted along autonomic fibers; the nervous system is intact and perceives noxious stimuli appropriately.

4. **How do patients describe pain of somatic nociceptive origin?**
   Somatic nociceptive pain may be sharp or dull and is often aching in nature. It is a type of pain that is familiar to the patient, much like a toothache. It may be exacerbated by movement (incident pain) and relieved upon rest. It is well localized and consonant with the underlying lesion. Examples of somatic nociceptive pain include metastatic bone pain, postsurgical pain, musculoskeletal pain, and arthritic pain. These pains tend to respond well to the primary analgesics, such as nonsteroidal antiinflammatory drugs (NSAIDs) and opioids.

5. **How do patients describe pain of visceral nociceptive origin?**
   Visceral nociceptive pain arises from distention of a hollow organ. This type of pain is usually poorly localized, deep, squeezing, and crampy. It is often associated with autonomic sensations including nausea, vomiting, and diaphoresis. There are often cutaneous referral sites (e.g., heart to the shoulder or jaw, gallbladder to the scapula, and pancreas to the back). Examples of visceral nociceptive pain include pancreatic cancer, intestinal obstruction, and intraperitoneal metastasis.

6. **How do patients describe pain of neuropathic origin?**
   Patients often have difficulty describing pain of neuropathic origin because it is an unfamiliar sensation. Words used include *burning, electrical,* and *numbing.* Innocuous stimuli may be

perceived as painful (allodynia). Patients often complain of paroxysms of electrical sensations (lancinating or lightning pains). Examples of neuropathic pain include trigeminal neuralgia, postherpetic neuralgia, and painful peripheral neuropathy.

7. **Clinically, how do you distinguish between paresthesia and dysesthesia?**
   Paresthesia is described simply as a nonpainful altered sensation, e.g., numbness. Dysesthesia is an altered sensation that is painful, e.g., painful numbness.

8. **What are examples of deafferentation pain?**
   Deafferentation pain is a subdivision of neuropathic pain that may complicate virtually any type of injury to the somatosensory system at any point along its course. Examples include well-defined syndromes precipitated by peripheral (phantom-limb) or central (thalamic pain) lesions. In all of these conditions, pain usually occurs in a region of clinical sensory loss. With phantom-limb pain, the pain is actually felt in an area that no longer exists. Patients with thalamic pain, also known as Dejerine-Roussy syndrome, report pain in all or part of the region of clinical sensory loss.

9. **What is the difference between complex regional pain syndromes I and II?**
   According to the International Association for the Study of Pain (IASP), complex regional pain syndrome I (CRPS I; formerly known as reflex sympathetic dystrophy) is defined as "continuous pain in a portion of an extremity after trauma, which may include fracture but does not involve a major nerve, associated with sympathetic hyperactivity." The IASP defines CRPS II (formerly known as causalgia) as "burning pain, allodynia, and hyperpathia, usually in the foot or hand, after partial injury of a nerve or one of its major branches."

10. **Describe "phantom limb" phenomena.**
    A phantom limb sensation is a nonpainful perception of the continued presence of an amputated limb. It is part of a deafferentation syndrome, in which there is loss of sensory input secondary to amputation. Phantom limb pain describes painful sensations that are perceived in the missing limb. Phantom limb sensation is more frequent than phantom limb pain, occurring in nearly all patients who undergo amputation. However, the sensation is time-limited and usually dissipates over days to weeks. On occasion, these sensations may be confused with stump pain, which is pain at the site of the amputation. Thoroughly examine the stump of any patient complaining of persistent phantom limb pain to rule out infection and neuroma.

11. **How is the multidimensional pain inventory used to classify chronic pain patients?**
    The Multidimensional Pain Inventory is a self-report questionnaire designed to assess chronic pain patients' adaptation to their symptoms and behavioral responses by significant others. Section 1 includes five scales that describe pain severity and cognitive-affective responses to pain. Section 2 assesses the patient's perceptions of how his or her significant others respond to pain complaints. Section 3 examines various activities, such as those undertaken in the household, in society, and outdoors.

12. **What is meant by psychogenic pain?**
    Psychogenic pain is presumed to exist when no nociceptive or neuropathic mechanism can be identified and there are sufficient psychologic symptoms to meet criteria for somatoform pain disorder, depression, or another *Diagnostic and Statistical Manual of Mental Disorders (DSM-IV)* diagnostic category commonly associated with complaints of pain. Psychogenic pain is rarely pure. More commonly, psychological issues complicate a chronic pain syndrome or vice versa.

13. **What is the World Health Organization (WHO) ladder?**

In the 1980s, WHO published guidelines for the control of pain in cancer patients. These guidelines correlate intensity of pain to pharmacologic intervention: Mild pain (step 1) requires nonopioid analgesics with or without adjuvant medications. If the patient does not respond to treatment or the pain increases, the guideline suggests moving to step 2 by adding a mild opioid to the previous therapy. If the pain continues or increases in severity, then the clinician goes to step 3 and adds a strong opioid to the prior therapy. This algorithm has also been used in patients with non–cancer-related pain.

14. **What is myofascial pain syndrome?**

Myofascial pain syndrome is defined as a regional pain syndrome characterized by the presence of trigger points and localized areas of deep muscle tenderness in a taut band of muscle. Pressure on a trigger point reproduces the pain. In comparison, fibromyalgia is a systemic pain disorder associated with tender points in all four quadrants of the body for at least 3 months' duration, often with associated sleep disturbance, irritable bowel syndrome, and depression. In myofascial pain syndrome, these associated features are significantly less frequent.

15. **What is the advantage of classifying pain?**

Classification provides the clinician with invaluable information about the possible origin of the pain. More important, it directs the health care practitioner toward a proper pharmacologic treatment plan. For example, neuropathic pain syndromes generally respond to adjuvant medications such as tricyclic antidepressants and to anticonvulsants. In nociceptive pain states, the implementation of NSAIDs alone or in combination with opioids is the mainstay of treatment.

16. **Describe the temporal classification of pain. What is its shortcoming?**

The temporal classification of pain is based on the time course of symptoms and is usually divided into acute, chronic, and recurrent. The major shortcoming is that the division between acute and chronic is arbitrary.

17. **How is acute pain defined?**

Acute pain is temporally related to injury and resolves during the appropriate healing period. There is usually no secondary gain on the patient's part, but social, cultural, and personality factors may play some role. Acute pain often responds to treatment with analgesic medications and treatment of the precipitating cause. Delay or improper therapy can lead to chronic pain.

18. **How is chronic pain defined?**

Chronic pain is often defined as pain that persists for more than 3 months or that outlasts the usual healing process. However, the cognitive-behavioral aspect, not duration, is probably the essential criterion of the chronic nonmalignant pain syndrome. Chronic non–cancer-related pain serves no useful biologic purpose.

19. **How is chronic pain classified in patients with cancer?**

Chronic pain in patients with cancer is categorized according to whether it is tumor-related, treatment-related, or unrelated to the cancer. Tumor-related pain may occur at the site of the primary tumor or at a site of metastasis. Treatment-related pain can be secondary to the use of chemotherapeutic agents (peripheral neuropathy), radiation therapy (radiation plexitis, myelopathy, or secondary tumors), or surgery (postmastectomy syndrome, radical neck syndrome, postthoracotomy syndrome). Approximately 10% to 15% of the pain syndromes that occur in cancer patients are unrelated to the underlying cancer and cancer treatment.

20. **What is meant by an etiologic classification?**

An etiologic classification pays more attention to the primary disease process in which pain occurs, rather than to the pathophysiology or temporal pattern. Examples include cancer pain, arthritis pain, and pain in sickle cell disease. Therapeutically, it is less useful than a pathophysiologic classification.

21. **What is the basis of the regional classification of pain?**

The regional classification of pain is strictly topographic and does not infer pathophysiology or etiology. It is defined by the part of the body affected, then subdivided into acute and chronic.

KEY POINTS

1. Pain can be classified according to inferred pathophysiology, time course, location, or etiology.

2. Proper pain classification may aid in the proper treatment of the pain problem.

3. Chronic non–cancer-related pain significantly differs from acute pain in that chronic non–cancer-related pain serves no useful biologic purpose.

BIBLIOGRAPHY

1. Bruehl S, et al: External validation of IASP diagnostic criteria for Complex Regional Pain Syndrome and proposed research diagnostic criteria, *Pain* 81:147-154, 1999.

2. Donaldson CC, et al: The neural plasticity model of fibromyalgia, *Pract Pain Manag* 12-16, July/August, 2001.

3. Merskey H, Bogduk N, editors: *Classification of chronic pain: task force on taxonomy*, 2nd ed, Seattle, 1994, International Association for the Study of Pain Press.

4. Nicholson B: Taxonomy of pain, *Clin J Pain* 16:S114-S117, 2000.

5. Okifuji A, Turk DC, Eveleight DJ: Improving the rate of classification of patients with the Multidimensional Pain Inventory: classifying the meaning of "significant other," *Clin J Pain* 15:290-296, 1999.

6. Simons DG, et al: Origins of low back pain. Part 1 and Part 2. *Postgrad Med* 73:66-108, 1983.

7. Twycross R, et al: Cancer pain classification. Part 1 of 2. *Acta Anesthesiol Scand* 41:141-145, 1997.

8. World Health Organization: *Cancer pain relief*, 2nd ed, Geneva, 1996, WHO.

CHAPTER 3

BASIC MECHANISMS

Allan I. Basbaum, PhD

1. **What are nociceptors?**
   Nociceptors are neurons that respond to noxious thermal, mechanical, or chemical stimulation. The term is used for both peripheral and central neurons; however, because the receptor is located in the periphery, the term is best associated with small myelinated (A-delta) and unmyelinated (C) fiber primary afferent neurons. In the central nervous system, neurons that respond to noxious stimulation are considered nociresponsive. These are the "higher-order" neurons.

2. **What properties characterize A-delta and C fibers?**
   A-delta fibers are small-diameter (1 to 6 μm), myelinated primary afferent fibers; C fibers are smaller-diameter (1.0 μm) unmyelinated primary afferents. The A-delta fibers conduct at velocities between 5 and 25 milliseconds; C fibers conduct at 1.0 μm/sec. A major component of the C fibers are polymodal nociceptors, which respond to thermal, mechanical, and chemical noxious stimulation. These express primary afferent nociceptors respond more selectively to noxious thermal or mechanical stimulation. It is unclear whether there are specific neurotransmitters associated with the modality subtypes of A-delta and C fibers.

3. **Distinguish between first and second pain.**
   First and second pain refers to the immediate and delayed pain responses to noxious stimulation. Other terms that denote these pains are fast and slow pain or sharp/pricking and dull/burning pain. The stimuli that generate first pain are transmitted by A-delta, small, myelinated afferents. Second pain results from activation of C fibers, which conduct impulses much more slowly, thus accounting for the time difference.

4. **What are some of the molecules that are unique to the nociceptor?**
   All nociceptors use glutamate as their primary excitatory neurotransmitter. However, several other transmitters coexist with glutamate, and the differences in transmitters define the two major classes of nociceptors: The peptidergic class contains calcitonin gene–related peptide and substance P. The nonpeptide class is characterized by its binding of a unique lectin (IB4) and the fact that many of these neurons express the P2X3 purinergic receptor, which responds to adenosine triphosphate (ATP). Whether these classes mediate different types of pain remains to be determined; however, recent tracing studies indicate that the different subsets of nociceptors engage different circuits in the spinal cord and different ascending pathways.

   A molecule that is present only in C-fiber nociceptors and that is relevant to the transmission of nociceptive messages is a possible therapeutic drug target. This is because the side-effect profile of such a drug would be limited by the fact that it is less likely to bind to unwanted sites in the central or peripheral nervous system. The cell bodies of small-diameter neurons in the dorsal root ganglion (which are the cell bodies of C fibers) contain several unique molecules, including the following:

   - A tetrodotoxin-resistant Na channel (TTX-R)
   - The vanilloid receptor (TRPV1), which is targeted by capsaicin, the active ingredient in hot peppers

- The P2X3 subtype of purinergic receptor, which is targeted by ATP
- A special type of dorsal root ganglion (D) specific acid-sensing ion channel (DRASIC)

Most recently, a class of G protein–linked receptors has been shown to be uniquely expressed in the dorsal root ganglion.

5. What are TRP channels?

TRP channels are a large family of transient receptor potential channels that allow ions to flow in response to a variety of stimuli, including temperature, many plant-derived compounds, and endogenous molecules. Different TRP channels cover the range of temperatures sensed by afferent fibers. For example, the threshold for TRPV1 is around 43-45° C, which is close to the threshold for evoking heat pain. TRPV2 has a higher threshold. TRPV3 responds to warm temperatures. TRPM8 responds to cooling.

Capsaicin is the exogenous stimulus that binds TRPV1. Camphor binds TRPV3; wasabi, mustard oil, garlic, and cinnamaldehyde bind TRPA1. With the exception of TRPV1, we still do not have information on the endogenous chemical ligands that activate these channels. However, there is considerable evidence that bradykinin, via an action at the B2 subtype of G protein–coupled receptor, regulates the properties of the TRPV1 and TRPA1 receptors.

Importantly, the properties of the channels are altered in the setting of injury. For example, TRPV1 not only responds to capsaicin and noxious heat but is regulated by pH. In the setting of tissue injury, where pH is lowered, the threshold for opening the channel is reduced sufficiently so that normally innocuous temperatures can evoke action potentials in nociceptors that express TRPV1. Studies in animals indicate that the pain of bone metastasis is significantly attenuated in animals in which TRPV1 is deleted genetically.

6. How are nociceptors altered by tissue injury?

When there is tissue injury (e.g., an arthritic joint), the nociceptor is exposed to an inflammatory "soup" containing a host of molecules that influence the properties of the nociceptor. These molecules include prostaglandin products of arachidonic acid metabolism, bradykinin, cytokines, serotonin, and growth factors (notably nerve growth factor [NGF]). This all occurs in the setting of lowered pH. Together these molecules contribute to peripheral sensitization, that process through which the threshold for firing of the nociceptor is lowered. The most direct way to treat peripheral sensitization is with nonsteroidal antiinflammatory drugs, which block the cyclooxygenase enzyme.

7. Where do nociceptive fibers enter the spinal cord?

Nociceptive primary afferent fibers have their cell bodies in dorsal root ganglia. The central branches of these afferents enter the spinal cord through the dorsal root and ascend or descend a few segments in the tract of Lissauer. The central branches terminate predominantly in the superficial laminae of the dorsal horn, including lamina I, the marginal zone, and lamina II, the substantia gelatinosa. Some A-delta primary afferent nociceptors also terminate more ventrally in the region of lamina V and around the central canal.

The fact that the level of analgesia observed following anterolateral cordotomy may be up to two segments below the segment at which the cordotomy was performed is presumed to reflect the anatomical course of axons in Lissauer's tract. Some small-diameter primary afferents ascend the spinal cord one to two segments in the Lissauer's tract, ipsilaterally, before entering the spinal cord and synapsing upon dorsal horn neurons, including cells at the origin of the spinothalamic and spinoreticular pathways.

8. Where is the first synapse in the spinal cord?

There is a differential projection of small-diameter and large-diameter primary afferent fibers to the spinal cord dorsal horn. The largest diameter Ia primary afferents arise from muscle spindles and make monosynaptic connection with motoneurons in the ventral horn.

Large-diameter, nonnociceptive primary afferents synapse on neurons in lamina III and lamina IV that are at the origin of the spinocervical tract and on wide dynamic range neurons (see Question 7) in lamina V. Small-diameter nociceptive A-delta and C fibers arborize most densely in the superficial dorsal horn. The C fibers predominantly synapse with neurons in lamina I; they also synapse upon dorsally directed dendrites of neurons located more ventrally (e.g., in lamina V). In addition, there are connections with interneurons in the substantia gelatinosa. Many A-delta nociceptors terminate in lamina V.

9. **What is meant by a second-order neuron?**
Second-order refers to all of the spinal cord neurons that receive input from the primary afferent fibers, including interneurons and projection neurons. Second-order neurons are also located in the dorsal column nuclei; these receive input from large primary afferent fibers that ascend to the medulla via the dorsal and posterior columns. Note that many second-order neurons receive convergent input from small-diameter nociceptive primary afferents and from large-diameter nonnociceptive primary afferent fibers.

10. **What is a wide dynamic range neuron?**
Wide dynamic range refers to neurons in the spinal cord that respond to a broad range of intensity of stimulation. For example, there are neurons in lamina V that respond to nonnoxious brushing of the cell's receptive field, as well as to intense mechanical stimulation and to noxious heat. Many wide dynamic range neurons also receive a visceral afferent input. By contrast, nociceptive-specific neurons respond exclusively to stimulus intensities in the noxious range.

Importantly, all primary afferent fibers are excitatory. Thus, any inhibitory effect that results from stimulation of large-diameter fibers (e.g., by vibration) results from an indirect mechanism involving inhibitory interneurons that influence the firing of the wide dynamic range neuron.

11. **Describe the major ascending pathways that transmit nociceptive information.**
The two major pathways of nociceptive information are the spinothalamic tract and the spinoreticular tract. The cell origin of the spinothalamic tract is in the dorsal horn and intermediate gray matter of the spinal cord. Axons of these neurons cross to the anterolateral quadrant and ascend to the thalamus, where they synapse on neurons in the lateral thalamus and in the intralaminar nuclei, located more medially. An additional ascending pathway, recently described, arises from neurons in the most superficial lamina of the dorsal horn, lamina I. These neurons project via pathways in the dorsal part of the lateral funiculus and terminate in the rostral brainstem, including the parabrachial nuclei. The output of these neurons would not be cut by the traditional spinothalamic tractotomy/anterolateral cordotomy, which in part may account for the failure of cordotomy and for the return of pain that often occurs.

The spinoreticular pathway parallels the spinothalamic tract. Neurons at the origin of the spinoreticular pathway are abundant in the deeper parts of the dorsal horn and in the ventral horn (laminae VII and VIII). The axons of these neurons project bilaterally to reticular formations at all levels of the brainstem. The output of the reticular neurons is predominantly to intralaminar thalamic nuclei and to the hypothalamus, thus, the origin of the term *spinoreticulothalamic pathway*.

The spinoparabrachio-amygdala pathway is more recently described. The axons in this pathway, which arise from neurons in the dorsal horn, target neurons of the parabrachial nucleus located in the dorsolateral region of the pons. The parabrachial neurons, in turn, project to the amygdala, which is a major component of the limbic system and is involved in emotions. This indicates that there is a relatively direct input from the spinal cord to regions of the brain involved in the affective component of the pain experience. There are other ascending pathways, including one that projects directly from the spinal cord to the hypothalamus. Very recently, a visceral "pain" pathway that courses in the dorsal columns of the spinal cord was described.

12. **What are the major neurotransmitters involved in nociception?**

Primary afferent nociceptors contain a variety of neurotransmitters, including the excitatory amino acid glutamate and a variety of neuropeptides, such as substance P and calcitonin gene–related peptide. Glutamate acts upon several subtypes of receptors, including AMPA receptors that mediate a rapid depolarization of dorsal horn neurons, via influx of sodium and efflux of potassium. The NMDA receptor, which gates calcium (in addition to sodium and potassium), is involved in long-term changes in dorsal horn processing that are produced by noxious stimulation. Substance P activates subpopulations of dorsal horn neurons and also contributes to some of the long-term changes produced by persistent injury.

13. **What are the major neurotransmitters involved in antinociceptive functions?**

Dorsal horn nociception can be regulated by both local inhibitory interneurons and descending inhibitory pathways that arise in the brainstem. The majority of inhibitory interneurons use the neurotransmitters gamma-aminobutyric acid or glycine. These inhibit the firing of dorsal horn nociceptive neurons by both presynaptic and postsynaptic controls. Other interneurons contain one of the endorphin peptides: enkephalin or dynorphin. These increase potassium conductance, thereby hyperpolarizing neurons. In some cases, they presynaptically block the release of neurotransmitters from primary afferent fibers by decreasing calcium conductance. The major descending inhibitory pathways use either serotonin or norepinephrine. Consistent with the presence of these diverse inhibitory neurotransmitter mechanisms, intrathecal injection of a variety of compounds (e.g., opioids, clonidine) produces profound antinociceptive effects.

Another major approach to regulating nociceptive processing is to influence Ca^{2+} channel function on primary afferents. Reduction of voltage-gated Ca^{2+} channels will result in decreased transmitter release. This can be generated directly, via drugs that act on the channel. For example, gabapentin binds to the $\alpha\delta2$ subunit of a variety of Ca channels. Ziconotide, a cone snail–derived peptide approved for intrathecal use in the treatment of pain in patients who already carry an intrathecal pump, blocks the N-type calcium channel. Morphine and other opioids indirectly reduce Ca channel activity.

14. **What are the clinical and investigational roles of capsaicin?**

Capsaicin, the algogenic substance in hot peppers, selectively stimulates primary afferent C fibers. These C fibers express TRV1, capsaicin receptors that nonselectively gate cations, including sodium and calcium, which depolarize axons. Selective antagonists to capsaicin have been developed. These will hopefully reduce the contribution of this channel in conditions where the environment of injury (e.g., low pH) results in prolonged opening of the channel.

Capsaicin itself may help as an analgesic. When administered to neonatal animals, capsaicin destroys C fibers; when administered to adults, it produces a long-term desensitization of the C fibers, possibly by depletion of their peptide neurotransmitters, such as substance P. The desensitization is associated with a decreased response to noxious stimulation, which provides a rational basis for the therapeutic use of capsaicin in patients. To date, topical application of capsaicin has shown some promise in the treatment of postherpetic neuralgia pain and postmastectomy intercostal neuralgia. Both low-dose and high-dose approaches are being evaluated; the latter probably lead to transient destruction of C-fiber terminals.

15. **What is the laminar organization of the dorsal horn of the spinal cord?**

The dorsal horn of the spinal cord can be divided into distinct laminae on cytoarchitectural grounds, using traditional cell (Nissl) stains. This anatomical organization is paralleled by physiological laminar organization. Neurons in laminae I and II, the substantia gelatinosa, respond either exclusively to noxious stimulation or to both noxious and nonnoxious stimuli. Neurons in laminae III and IV, the nucleus proprius, predominantly respond to nonnoxious stimuli. The majority of neurons in lamina V are of the wide dynamic range type, i.e., they respond to both nonnoxious and noxious stimuli and have visceral afferent inputs. Neurons in lamina VI respond predominantly to nonnoxious manipulation of joints.

16. **What is substance P-saporin, and how might it be used to treat chronic pain?**
When substance P is released from primary afferent nociceptors, it binds to the neurokinin-1 (NK1) receptor that is located on large numbers of "pain" transmission neurons, many of which are located in lamina I of the superficial dorsal horn. Although antagonists of the NK1 receptors failed in clinical trials, perhaps because selective blockade of the contribution of substance P is insufficient, another approach that targets the NK1 receptor is showing promise. The idea is to ablate the neurons that receive the substance P input. To this end, substance P is conjugated to the plant-derived toxin saporin. When saporin enters cells it blocks protein synthesis, leading to the death of the cells. By itself saporin cannot enter cells. It requires a carrier, which in this case is substance P. The substance P-saporin conjugate binds to the NK1 receptor, which is then internalized into the neuron, carrying the toxin with it. Intrathecal injection of the conjugate in animals produces a significant reduction of tissue and nerve injury–induced pain (allodynia and hyperalgesia), but it does interfere with acute pain processing. The molecule is undergoing studies in larger animals with a view to eventually use in patients. This is an irreversible ablative procedure, but it is much more selective compared to, for example, anterolateral cordotomy.

17. **How is the spinal cord influenced by peripheral nerve injury?**
Peripheral nerve injury was originally thought to only functionally disconnect the periphery from the spinal cord. Because the dorsal root ganglion is not injured when the peripheral nerve is damaged, neither anatomical nor biochemical changes in the proximal limb of the dorsal root or in the dorsal horn were expected. In fact, we now know that there are changes in the dorsal root ganglia and in the spinal cord neurons with which they are connected.

  Among the changes is a significant decrease in the concentration of substance P message and substance P peptide in neurons of the dorsal root ganglia. Also, substance P levels are decreased in the terminals of primary afferent fibers in the dorsal horn. Significant changes in postsynaptic neurons include an upregulation of the opioid peptide, dynorphin, in dorsal horn neurons.

  The electrophysiologic consequences of peripheral nerve injury are also profound. A massive release of glutamate acts on NMDA receptors to produce long-term changes in the physiologic properties of the dorsal horn neurons. Central sensitization (i.e., hyperexcitability) of dorsal horn neurons in the setting of injury is particularly common and may contribute to postinjury pain states. Peripheral nerve injury may also induce a loss of inhibitory controls (secondary to the killing of GABAergic interneurons). This would produce an epileptic-like condition that may contribute to the ongoing burning pain and the allodynia and hyperalgesia in neuropathic pain conditions.

18. **Provide a plausible explanation for the phenomenon of referred pain.**
A very likely explanation for the phenomenon of referred pain relates to the convergence of visceral and somatic afferent input to wide dynamic range neurons of lamina V. Thus, increased activity of visceral afferent secondary to injury to viscera is interpreted by the brain as having arisen from the source of the convergent somatic input. It is thus "referred" to the somatic site. Indeed, local anesthetic injection of the site of reference can reduce referred pain even though the site of injury is clearly in the viscera.

19. **What is neurogenic inflammation?**
Neurogenic inflammation refers to the inflammation that is produced through the release of substances from the nervous system—in particular, from small-diameter primary afferent fibers. Although most studies emphasize the contribution of the primary afferent C fibers, there

is also evidence for a contribution of sympathetic postganglionic terminals. The primary afferents release peptides that act on postcapillary venules. These become leaky, resulting in plasmic extravasation and vasodilatation. Electrical stimulation of peripheral nerves that have been disconnected from the central nervous system can evoke neurogenic inflammation by antidromic activation of C fibers and the resultant release of neuropeptides in the periphery.

20. **How are substance P and CGRP implicated in the phenomenon of neurogenic inflammation?**
Cell bodies in the dorsal root ganglion synthesize substance P and calcitonin gene related peptide (CGRP) and transport these peptides by axoplasmic transport both to the central and peripheral terminals of the primary afferents. The peptides are stored in the periphery and can be released when the terminals are depolarized as a result of injury. The targets of substance P in the periphery include mast cells, blood vessels, and a variety of immunocompetent cells. In concert with the CGRP, which produces a profound vasodilatation, substance P significantly increases plasma extravasation from postcapillary venules. The extravasation of protein from vessels is accompanied by fluid, producing the characteristic swelling (tumor) of inflammation. The heat and redness (calor and rubor) of inflammation can be accounted for by the neurogenic vasodilatation.

Some groups believe that this process is critical to the pain associated with migraine and, indeed, triptans block neurogenic inflammation, via an action on 5HT-1B/D receptors located on the terminals of primary afferent nociceptors. Although antagonists of the NK1 receptor failed as a treatment for migraines in clinical trials, blockade of CGRP shows promise as a migraine treatment. Other investigators, however, believe that the triptans exert their antimigraine action by binding to receptors located in the central nervous system.

21. **Differentiate primary and secondary hyperalgesia.**
Primary hyperalgesia refers to a sensitization process that enhances "pain" transmission via a peripheral mechanism. For example, in the setting of inflammation, there is synthesis of arachidonic acid, which is acted upon to produce prostaglandins. These lipid mediators in turn act on the terminals of primary afferent nociceptors and lower their threshold for firing. The nociceptors are sensitized. All of this occurs via a peripheral mechanism.

Secondary hyperalgesia refers to the sensitization that occurs because of changes in spinal cord processing. For example, through a process of central sensitization, the firing of dorsal horn nociceptors can change dramatically in the setting of injury (produced by either tissue or nerve damage). The threshold for activation of dorsal horn "pain" transmission neurons drops, their receptive field size increases, and they may become spontaneously active. Pain can now be produced by activation of low threshold mechanoreceptive (A-beta) afferents.

22. **What is the contribution of the NMDA receptor to the production of pain?**
Glutamate that is released from primary afferent fibers acts upon two major receptor types in the dorsal horn: the AMPA and the NMDA receptors. Under normal conditions, the NMDA receptor is blocked by the presence of a magnesium ion in the channel. When neurons are depolarized via glutamate action at the AMPA receptor, the magnesium block is relieved, and glutamate action at the NMDA receptor is effective. This results in entry of calcium into the postsynaptic neuron, which in turn activates a variety of second-messenger systems that produce long-term biochemical and molecular changes in these neurons.

The physiologic consequence of these changes is a hyperexcitability of the dorsal horn neuron, i.e., central sensitization. This is manifested as an increase in the size of the receptive field of nociresponsive neurons, a decreased threshold, and a potential for spontaneous activity of the neuron. The allodynia (pain produced by nonnoxious stimuli) and hyperalgesia (exacerbated pain produced by noxious stimuli) associated with nerve injury may reflect NMDA-mediated long-term changes in dorsal horn neuronal processing.

23. **Describe the regions of the thalamus that have been implicated in the processing of nociceptive information.**
Two major regions of thalamus have been implicated in the processing of nociceptive information: (1) the lateral thalamus, including the ventral posterolateral (VPL) and ventral posteromedial nuclei (VPM), and (2) the intralaminar nuclei of the medial thalamus. The VPL receives input via the spinothalamic tract, as well as a major input from lemniscal pathways originating in the dorsal column nuclei. The VPM receives input via the nucleus caudalis and the principal trigeminal nucleus. Stimulation of the lateral thalamus in patients who are not experiencing pain does not produce significant pain. By contrast, in patients who have ongoing pain, electrical stimulation can reproduce pain, suggesting a reorganization of the nociceptive input to the thalamus under conditions of persistent injury.
   The output of the lateral thalamus is largely to the somatosensory cortex. However, connections with the limbic and insular cortex are probably necessary for the affective components of pain to be generated. As noted earlier, however, "pain" inputs can also engage the limbic system via connections from the spinal cord to the amygdala via the spinoparabrachio-amygdala pathway. The medial thalamus, including the intralaminar nuclei, receives direct spinothalamic and spinoreticular thalamic projections. Cells in this region have larger receptive fields and are thought to contribute to the diffuse character of pain perception. The cortical connections of the more medial regions of the thalamus are presumed to be involved in the affective component of the pain perception.

24. **Is there a cortical representation of pain?**
Yes, there is a cortical representation of pain. Traditional teaching suggested that the cortex was not necessary for the experience of pain. This was based on clinical studies wherein stimulation rarely produced pain and large lesions did not completely disrupt the pain experience. Imaging studies with positron emission tomography (PET) or functional magnetic resonance imaging (MRI) (largely in experimental settings), however, have identified several cortical regions that are activated when humans experience pain. Among these are the somatosensory cortex, the anterior cingulate gyrus, and the insular cortex. This distributed processing in the cortex clearly reflects the complex nature of the pain experience, which includes sensory discriminative, affective, and cognitive aspects. Lesions of any single region may thus not be sufficient to eliminate pain.

25. **What do we know about the cortical mechanism underlying the sensory and emotional components of the pain experience?**
The PET studies mentioned in Question 24 also examined what occurs during hypnotic analgesia. When subjects were hypnotized so as to decrease the unpleasantness generated by a heat stimulus, the "activity" generated in the anterior cingulate gyrus was dramatically decreased but without significant change in activity in the somatosensory cortex. These results suggest that the anterior cingulate gyrus processes information more related to the affective component of the pain experience than to the sensory discriminative component. These studies also illustrate that under hypnotic analgesia, the information does access cortical centers but that the nature of the perception reported is altered.

26. **What information do we have on the mechanism of placebo analgesia?**
Several years ago it was reported that the opiate antagonist naloxone can reverse the analgesia produced by a placebo. This led to the hypothesis that placebo analgesia involves release of endorphins and activation of an endogenous pain control circuit. This striking finding has received considerable support in recent studies in which regulators of endorphin processing have been shown to enhance the effect of a placebo. The new studies followed upon basic experimental evidence that the neuropeptide cholecystokinin (CCK) counteracts the effect of endogenous opioids. The new studies demonstrated that injection of a CCK receptor antagonist significantly increased the analgesic effect of a placebo. Furthermore, the enhancing effect and the original placebo effect were both blocked by naloxone, indicating that the circuit involves

release of endogenous opioids, which act at opioid receptors. Recent imaging studies demonstrated that placebo analgesia is associated with activation of areas involved in the endorphin-mediated descending control of pain processing, e.g., the periaqueductal gray region of the midbrain.

KEY POINTS

1. Nociceptors are neurons that respond to noxious thermal, mechanical, or chemical stimulation.

2. All nociceptors use glutamate as their primary excitatory neurotransmitter; however, several other transmitters coexist with glutamate and the differences in transmitters define the two major classes of nociceptors. The first major class of neurotransmitters includes the peptidergic neurotransmitters such as substance P and calcitonin gene–related peptide. The second major class is the nonpeptide class, characterized by its binding of a unique lectin and the fact that many of these neurons express the P2X3, purinergic receptor, which responds to ATP. It is not yet known how these are affected by different types of pain.

3. Glutamate that is released from primary afferent fibers acts upon two major receptor types in the dorsal horn: the AMPA and the NMDA receptors. The subsequent increased neuronal excitability that may follow such glutamate activity is often referred to as central sensitization.

BIBLIOGRAPHY

1. Apkarian AV, Bushnell MC, Treede RD, Zubieta JK: Human brain mechanisms of pain perception and regulation in health and disease, *Eur J Pain* 9:463-484, 2005.

2. Basbaum AI, Jessel T: The perception of pain. In Kandel ER, Schwartz J, and Jessel T, editors: *Principles of neuroscience*, New York, 2000, Appleton and Lange, pp 472-491.

3. Basbaum AI, Julius D: Toward better pain control, *Scientific Amer* 294:60-67, 2006.

4. Basbaum AI, Woolf CJ: Pain, *Current Biology* 9:R429-R431, 1999.

5. Casey KL: Concepts of pain mechanisms: the contribution of functional imaging of the brain, *Prog Brain Res* 129:277-287, 2000.

6. Craig AD, Bushnell MC, Zhang ET, Blomqvist A: A thalamic nucleus specific for pain and temperature sensation, *Nature* (Lond) 372:770-773, 1994.

7. Hökfelt T, Zhang X, Wiesenfeld HZ: Messenger plasticity in primary sensory neurons following axotomy and its functional implications, *Trends Neurosci* 17:22-30, 1994.

8. Julius D, Basbaum AI: Molecular mechanisms of nociception, *Nature* (Lond) 413:203-210, 2001.

9. Nichols ML, Allen BJ, Rogers SD, et al: Transmission of chronic nociception by spinal neurons expressing the substance P receptor, *Science* 286:1558-1561, 1999.

II. CLINICAL APPROACH

HISTORY TAKING IN THE PATIENT WITH PAIN

Howard S. Smith, MD, FACP, and Andrew Dubin, MD

1. **What are the key elements in taking the clinical history of a patient with a complaint of pain?**

    The first step in taking the clinical history of a patient with a complaint of pain is to evaluate the pain complaint. Important factors are location; radiation; intensity; characteristics and quality; temporal aspects; exacerbating, triggering, and relieving factors; circumstances surrounding the onset of pain; and potential mechanisms of injury. Additionally, the clinician should ascertain if the pain is constant and steady, intermittent or sporadic, or constant with exacerbating circumstances by gathering information regarding the occurrence and characteristics of any breakthrough pain. Furthermore, one should ascertain the patient's perception of why he or she has persistent pain, the duration of the pain, and changes in pain since its onset (e.g., any gradual or rapid progression in intensity or "spread" of location).

    The patient should specifically be asked about any perceived exacerbation of pain with innocuous light touch, with sheets or clothes on the painful body part(s), with the wind blowing on the pain, and with external temperature changes (e.g., is the pain worse in winter?). Patients should be asked about any specific clothing they wear, aides they use, or behaviors or activities they engage in to function optimally with the pain.

    The patient should be questioned about the function of the specific painful area and resultant changes in global physical functioning. Information should also be obtained regarding perceived restriction of range of motion; stiffness; swelling; muscle aches, cramps, or spasms, color or temperature changes; changes in sweating; changes in hair; nail growth; perceived changes in muscle strength; perceived positive (dysesthesias/itching) or negative (numbness) changes in sensation—including what may trigger these changes (if they are not constant) and when they are likely to occur.

    Many aspects of the patient's current life and perceived quality of life along with how this has changed because of pain should be questioned. Include the following:

    - Social functioning
    - Recreational functioning (e.g., how often the patient goes out to the movies, spectator sports, concerts, to play cards, etc.)
    - Emotional functioning
    - Mood/affect, anxiety
    - Identification of family members/significant others/friends and their relationships with the patient
    - Occupation (if any)—last time worked and why stopped

2. **If pain is a purely subjective phenomenon, how can its intensity be measured?**

    The only reliable measure of pain's intensity is the patient's report. Measures of pain intensity are not meant to compare one person's pain with another's; rather, they compare the intensity of one patient's pain at any given time with its intensity at another given time. Thus, physicians and patients can judge whether pain intensity is increasing or decreasing with time and treatment. It is sometimes helpful to have the patient compare the intensity of the current pain experience with prior experiences.

3. **How should pain intensity be recorded?**
   There are a number of different measurements for pain intensity (see Chapter 6, Pain Measurement), and it is not clear that any particular scale is universally better than any other. Some patients have greater ease with a verbal scale, some with a numerical, and some with a visual analog scale. It is, however, a good idea to use the same measure across time. Thus, verbal descriptors, such as "no pain, mild pain, moderate pain, severe pain, unbearable pain," or numerical scales can be graded on each visit.

4. **Can pain intensity be measured in children, the older person, and the cognitively impaired?**
   Once children reach an age of verbal skills, pain intensity can usually be quantified on a verbal scale. However, a number of scales work even for preverbal children (see Chapter 30, Pain in Children). Once children reach the preteen years, the same tools used in adults can be applied.
   The older person may present more difficult problems. If the patient is cognitively impaired, it is often difficult to assess pain intensity on a precise scale, and it becomes more valuable to judge the functional impairments resulting from pain. Furthermore, medications used to treat pain may increase cognitive impairment and make assessment even more difficult. Older patients may tend to be more stoic about pain and are reluctant to report high intensities. One of the most helpful factors when assessing pain in children, older patients, and/or cognitively impaired patients is eliciting from the caregivers any changes from the patient's baseline behavior.

5. **What information can be gathered from the character of the pain?**
   The McGill Pain Questionnaire contains numerous descriptors for pain. Certain words that patients choose may help to infer a specific pathophysiology. For example, a burning, dysesthetic, or electric shock–like pain usually implies neuropathic pain. An aching, cramping, waxing and waning pain in the abdomen usually indicates visceral, nociceptive pain.

6. **Why are the temporal characteristics of pain important?**
   The onset of pain is extremely important. The approach to pain of relatively recent onset should follow more closely the medical model, that is, a search for underlying cause. Acute pain usually indicates a new pathologic process, correction of which will relieve the pain. Chronic pain of long duration is less likely to be amenable to a standard medical model and requires a biopsychosocial approach (see Chapter 44, Physical Modalities: Adjunctive Treatments to Reduce Pain and Maximize Function). Chronic pain often outlives the initial cause and develops a life of its own; however, the events that initially resulted in the onset of pain may help guide potential therapeutic approaches to chronic pain.

7. **Why is the temporal course of the pain important?**
   Certain pain syndromes have classic temporal patterns. For example, cluster headaches may occur at the same time of the day, every day, during only certain months of the year. Rheumatoid arthritis is characteristically worse early in the morning on rising (morning stiffness). Similarly, chronic, daily abdominal pain that has persisted in an unchanging way for years is unlikely to have a clear medical cure, whereas episodic abdominal pain that allows long pain-free intervals punctured by severe bouts of pain is more likely to be due to focal pathology. The intensity of pain over time is also of significance. Acute, severe back pain that gradually improves probably should be followed expectantly, assuming that there are no signs of tumor or infection. On the other hand, pain that increases over days to weeks is of more concern.

8. **What is the best way to elicit the time course of a pain syndrome if the patient is having difficulty being specific?**
For the onset, ask the patient what he or she was doing when the pain started. If the patient can give a specific act or time of day, it is likely that the pain was of acute onset. To judge whether the pain is worsening or improving, look for functional signs; that is, ask the patient what he or she cannot do that he or she could do a few months ago. Also, ask what can they do. If functional ability is decreasing, the pain probably is increasing. The patient and clinician should attempt to construct a timeline of the pain, as well as precisely what patients did themselves in attempts to help the pain and any treatment designed by clinicians, including pharmacologic, interventional, neurophysical medicine techniques and modalities, behavioral medicine techniques, and neuromodulation techniques.

9. **What is the importance of ascertaining exacerbating and relieving factors?**
Specific pain syndromes have specific exacerbating and relieving factors. For example, tension headache is often relieved by alcohol, whereas cluster headache is characteristically exacerbated by alcohol intake. Back pain from a herniated disc is usually relieved by recumbency, whereas back pain from tumor or infection is either unrelieved or exacerbated by recumbency.

10. **A patient complains of back and leg pain but has trouble describing the exact distribution. What can you do to clarify the matter?**
Pain maps (body maps) are often useful for patients who have difficulty with verbal expression. A front and rear view of the body is presented on paper, and the patient simply pencils in the location of the pain. The patient may use different colors or different types of lines to describe different types of pain. This technique helps to define whether pain is in a nerve distribution or simply somatic. Also, having patients map out the pain distribution on their own body may be helpful for determining somatic versus nerve distributions.

11. **A patient has a rather nondescript headache that is getting worse over days to weeks. What should you consider?**
This patient's pain—a temporal pattern of vague onset with rapid acceleration in symptoms—should raise suspicion that a space-occupying lesion could be present. Even in patients with back pain, one should consider tumor or infection as a possibility.

12. **An 80-year-old woman complains of severe pain in the chest wall after having a rash in that area. You made the diagnosis of postherpetic neuralgia and plan to use a tricyclic antidepressant. What questions should you ask in the history?**
Before prescribing any medication, a careful history of prior medication use and prior medical illnesses is imperative. Particularly in an older person in whom we consider using a tricyclic antidepressant, these matters are of maximal importance. Tricyclic antidepressants have anticholinergic properties. Therefore, they can exacerbate glaucoma, cause urinary retention, and increase confusion (factors that are fairly common in the older person). Orthostatic hypotension and other anticholinergic side effects are also more common in older patients than in young patients.

13. **What specific questions should be asked about the medical history in patients with complaint of pain?**
Questions should be directed at ascertaining comorbid medical conditions, including at least the following three major factors: (1) Has the patient had other painful illnesses? The response to these illnesses helps to guide current therapy. (2) How has the patient responded to medications or treatments in the past? This information should include the following: how long it was tried and at what level/dose (e.g., celecoxib 200 mg for 3 weeks and then celecoxib 400 mg for 6 weeks); perceived effectiveness; perceived adverse side effects at various doses; and all testing/imaging and visits/evaluation by any health care professionals (with clinician

addresses and phone numbers). Attempts should be made to obtain all records from clinician offices, hospitals, imaging centers/laboratories, pharmacies, etc. The patient's current primary care physician and other involved health care specialists, along with current pharmacy/pharmacies, medication list (including complementary and alternative medications [e.g. herbal vitamins and over-the-counter agents]), and diet should be recorded. This information may limit the drugs that can be prescribed. For example, in patients with a history of hypersensitivity to a given medication, any medication in the same group should be avoided. If the patient has an aspirin allergy, nonsteroidal antiinflammatory drugs (NSAIDs) cannot be used without great caution. If patients tend to develop orthostatic hypotension or confusion easily, the tricyclics probably should be avoided. (3) Medical conditions that may limit treatment should be investigated. For example, glaucoma, benign prostatic hypertrophy, and cognitive impairment are relative contraindications to the use of tricyclic antidepressants because their anticholinergic properties may precipitate crises. In patients with a history of opioid abuse, the opioids may be used with great caution. In patients with active peptic ulcer disease, aspirin and NSAIDs may have limited utility. In patients with renal disease, NSAIDs and gabapentin may need to be "dose-adjusted" and used with caution. In patients with significant hepatic dysfunction, acetaminophen, NSAIDs, antiepileptic medications, antidepressants, opioids, and muscle relaxants should be used with caution.

14. **How does the family history affect a patient with pain?**
Aside from the obvious issue of familial diseases, role models are often found in the family. A careful history should be taken to determine whether either parent or older siblings have suffered from a chronic pain syndrome. In addition, the family's reaction to the pain syndrome should be noted.

15. **Is history of disability benefits of any importance?**
The issue has caused a great deal of argument in the literature, but there is no clear resolution. The general wisdom is that patients receiving significant compensation for illness are reinforced in their chronic pain. This has been called compensation neurosis. However, the evidence is somewhat tenuous at best, and such patients are probably best treated in the rehabilitative fashion.

16. **Are there any helpful clues in the history taking of a patient with ischial bursitis—"weaver's bottom"—that help support the diagnosis?**
The following clues, if uncovered during history taking, will help point to an ischial bursitis diagnosis: In patients with this condition (known as "weaver's bottom"), pain invariably occurs when they sit and always goes away when they stand up or lie on their side. However, when the patient resumes a seated position, the pain returns. They can point to the spot where it hurts and pressure reproduces their pain. Additionally, most patients with weaver's bottom are able to say "it hurts right here," and consistently point with their finger to the precise location of the painful spot.

17. **What are some elements that could help to determine residual function?**
   - Is the patient ambulatory? If yes, do they need an assist device? (e.g., cane, brace, walker, crutch)
   - How far can the patient ambulate?
     o Room distances
     o House distances
     o Limited community distances (150 to 200 feet)—able to walk length of driveway to mailbox
     o Community distances (e.g., mall walking)
   - How fast can the patient walk? (e.g., How long does it take the patient to get from the parking lot to your office? Compare this with your own time.)

- What capacity do the patients have to mobilize themselves in the community? (Know the environmental barriers they will encounter coming from parking lot to your office.)
- Is the patient able to dress himself/herself? Ask the following questions:
  - Can you put your own shoes and socks on with assist devices?
  - Do you use slip-on shoes?
  - Can you put a shirt on yourself?
  - Can you put on a pullover by yourself?
- For women with shoulder injuries:
  - If you wear a bra, are you able to put it on by yourself?
  - Do you fasten it in the back or do you fasten it in the front and then rotate it around?
- Are you able to do activities of daily living such as household duties and chores? (Can you brush your teeth? comb your hair?)
- Are you able to drive a car?
  - Can you get in and out of a car with relative ease in a reasonable time period?
- Are you able to get up and down from sitting on the toilet?
  - Do you have a sitting or standing or lying intolerance?
  - Are you able to bathe yourself?
  - Are you able to toilet yourself?

KEY POINTS

1. Taking an appropriate history is essential for the assessment and treatment of patients with acute and chronic pain.

2. Detailed history taking of non–pain-related issues may lead to more effective treatment of the pain by identifying potential adverse treatment interactions prior to their prescription.

3. Detailed history taking may also lead to improved functional outcome in patients with chronic pain by identifying more completely the true needs of the patient.

BIBLIOGRAPHY

1. Fields HL, editor: *Core curriculum for professional education in pain*, Seattle, 1995, International Association for the Study of Pain Press.
2. Pappagallo M, editor: *The neurological basis of pain*, New York, 2005, McGraw-Hill.
3. Portenoy RK, Kanner RM: Definition and assessment of pain. In Portenoy RK, Kanner RM, editors: *Pain management: theory and practice*, Philadelphia, 1996, F.A. Davis, pp 3-18.

SUGGESTED READINGS

1. Hord, ED, Haythornwaite JA, Raja SN: Comprehensive evaluation of the patient with chronic pain. In Pappagallo M, editor: *The neurological basis of pain*, New York, 2005, McGraw-Hill.
2. Horowitz SH: The diagnostic workup of patients with neuropathic pain. In Smith HS, editor: *The Medical Clinics of North America: pain management*, part I, vol. 91, Philadelphia, 2007, Elsevier, pp 21-30.

CHAPTER 5

PHYSICAL EXAMINATION OF THE PATIENT WITH PAIN

Howard S. Smith, MD, FACP, and Andrew Dubin, MD

1. **Which physical examination findings are the most reliable when evaluating the peripheral nervous system in a patient with chronic pain issues?**
   When evaluating the peripheral nervous system in a patient with chronic pain, sensory and motor findings are helpful but are of less utility than reflex testing because they can be affected by the patient. Alterations in reflexes are more reliable findings. Areflexia, hyperreflexia, or hyporeflexia usually are indicative of pathology.

2. **What is the medial hamstring reflex, and what are its implications?**
   When testing the medial hamstring reflex, the examiner has the patient sit on the examination table with knee flexed to 90 degrees. Then using outstretched fingers, the examiner compresses and stretches the medial hamstring tendons. Percussion over the fingers with the reflex hammer elicits the normal response of knee flexion. This is useful in determining whether the patient has an L5 radiculopathy (in this condition the patient has normal patellar tendon and Achilles tendon reflexes but an absent medial hamstring reflex).

3. **What is the axial compression test, and what are the implications of a positive test?**
   Axial compression involves compression of the cervical spine, directly caudad. A positive test occurs when pain is experienced, localized in the cervical region, or radiates distally.
   A positive test may indicate degenerative joint disease of the spine or nerve root impingement in the upper cervical spine.

4. **What is Spurling's test, and what are the implications of a positive test?**
   Spurling's test involves compression of the cervical spine while it is slightly extended, rotated, and tilted toward one side. In a positive test, pain radiates distally, usually in a radicular distribution, indicating nerve root compression in the mid to lower cervical region. The nerve compression is ipsilateral to the side that the neck is tilted.

5. **Under what circumstances is the chest expansion test used?**
   The chest expansion test may be used if ankylosing spondylitis is suspected. In normal subjects, the difference between the totally deflated and totally inflated chest is usually more than 4 cm. In ankylosing spondylitis, it is almost invariably less than 4 cm. The patient is asked to exhale fully, and the chest is measured. The patient is then asked to inhale fully, and the chest is measured again. The difference between the two measurements is the chest expansion and if less than 4 cm may indicate ankylosing spondylitis.

6. **What is the straight leg raising test and what are its implications?**
   Straight leg raising (SLR) is used to check for lower lumbar root irritation (radiculitis) or radiculopathy. In a supine position, the patient's leg is passively elevated from the ankle. The knee is kept straight. Normal patients can reach nearly 90 degrees without pain. In patients with lower lumbar nerve root irritation, SLR is relatively sensitive and produces pain radiating distally in a radicular distribution. Somewhat less sensitive but more specific is contralateral

SLR. In this case, the pain-free leg is elevated; in a positive test, pain is felt on the affected side (e.g., the side of the nerve roots involvement).

The straight leg raise is usually positive for sciatic pain going below the knee at 30 to 45 degrees, except in flexible dancers and athletes. Pain from tight hamstrings is localized to the muscle and tendons and may limit range of motion. If "true" sciatic pain radiating down the leg in a radicular distribution is experienced by the patient, then the examiner should bring down the leg 10 degrees until the pain subsides and plantarflex the foot, asking "does this make the pain worse?". If it does, this may indicate enhanced pain behavior. Then dorsiflex the foot. This tugs on the sciatic nerve and may worsen the pain of root irritation or impingement. If the examiner brings the leg down to where the pain gets better and then externally rotates the leg (hip), this should make the pain better, and internal rotation of the leg may make it worse. A more central herniation may yield pain in the affected leg on raising of the well leg.

7. **What is a sitting root test?**
   A sitting root test (SRT) is essentially the same as the SLR test, but the patient is sitting rather than supine. The implications are the same. Findings on straight leg raise and SRT should correlate. A positive SLR but negative SRT may indicate enhanced pain behaviors.

   In the Lasègue test, after the leg is extended from a sitting or supine position, the foot it dorsiflexed, which further stretches the root and causes or exacerbates pain.

8. **What is the FABER test, and how is it different from Patrick's maneuver?**
   FABER is an acronym for *f*lexion, *ab*duction, and *e*xternal *r*otation of both hips. When it produces low back pain on one side, it is indicative of sacroiliac joint dysfunction. When the same maneuver produces groin pain, it is called Patrick's maneuver and is indicative of hip joint pathology. Patrick's maneuver may be performed unilaterally, but the FABER test must be done bilaterally to avoid pelvic rotation.

9. **What is the tipped can test, and what are its implications?**
   In the tipped can test, patients attempt to assume the posture of holding a full cup in their hand with the shoulder abducted at 90 degrees and then horizontally adducted 45 degrees. They are then instructed to turn their hand over to empty out the cup. A positive test that correlates with a rotator cuff tear (or partial tear) would be pain and the arm dropping or inability to assume the test position secondary to pain and weakness. Minimal force applied by the examiners to the test arm may elicit a positive test in equivocal situations.

10. **How is the iliopsoas muscle evaluated?**
    The iliopsoas muscle originates from the transverse processes of vertebrae L2-L4 (or L1-3) and inserts into the lesser trochanteric tubercle. Iliopsoas pathology may present with paraspinal pain just off of midline and radiating to sacroiliac (SI) regions in the lower abdomen, groin, and or medial thigh. With the patient sitting on the table, resistive hip flexion reproduces the back and groin pain, and stretching the hip flexor will also reproduce the back pain and the groin pain. Iliopsoas spasm commonly occurs in patients with degenerative disc and/or joint disease.

11. **What is the scarf test, and what are its implications?**
    The patient abducts the affected upper extremity to 90 degrees at the shoulder and then horizontally adducts (actively or passively) the upper extremity across the chest to reach for the opposite shoulder. A positive test reproduces focal sharp pain at the acromioclavicular (AC) joint and may result in the patient dropping his or her arm to the side with abrupt complaint of pain. This may indicate AC pathology (e.g., arthritis) or AC joint separation.

12. **How is the piriformis syndrome evaluated?**
There are many approaches to evaluate the piriformis syndrome. With the patient sitting, the piriformis muscle is stretched by the examiner passively moving the hip into internal rotation with reproduction of radiating pain. The pain is relieved by the examiner passively moving the hip into external rotation. The patient then actively externally rotates the hip against resistance; reproduction of buttock pain may be indicative of piriformis pathology. If groin pain is experienced, this may be more indicative of hip pathology. Additionally, there is generally point tenderness on point palpation of the piriformis muscle.

13. **What is involved in the evaluation of chronic leg pain in the athlete?**
The patient with a recurring dull ache in the distal third of the tibia posteromedial aspect along with palpable tenderness in that area may have medial tibial stress syndrome ("shin splints"). Pain and tenderness (usually located above the distal third of the tibia but not necessarily) occasionally associated with erythema and/or localized swelling may be more indicative of a stress fracture. Using a tuning fork over the fracture site aids diagnosis of vibratory pain and is also common with stress fractures. Nerve entrapments may also cause leg pain over the distribution/location of the nerve(s) involved, which may be associated with Tinel's sign. Pain associated with common peroneal entrapment is often referred to the lateral aspect of the leg and foot. Pain associated with superficial peroneal nerve entrapment often involves the lateral calf or dorsum of the foot. Pain associated with saphenous nerve entrapment usually occurs just above the medial malleolus but may be referred to the medial aspect of the dorsum of the foot.

14. **What are the examination differences between popliteal artery entrapment syndrome and chronic exertional compartment syndrome?**
Symptoms of both popliteal artery entrapment syndrome and chronic exertional compartment syndrome may include pain, deep ache, cramping, and/or burning in the lower extremity occurring both with exercise and generally at rest. Therefore, in both of these conditions the physical examination should be performed after exercise.
In popliteal artery entrapment syndrome the examiner may appreciate exercise-induced swelling around the knee and/or exercise-induced tenderness in the posterior leg. Pulses should be palpated with the ankle in passive dorsiflexion or active plantar flexion with the knee in extension and a reduction in pulse indicative of popliteal artery entrapment syndrome. In chronic exertional compartment syndrome, after exercise the patient may note a sensation of increased fullness/sensory paresthesias to light touch after exercise. The examiner may appreciate diffuse palpable tenderness, focal muscle herniation, swelling, and/or muscle weakness.

15. **What is the jerk test, and what are its implications?**
The jerk test can be performed with the patient in a sitting position. The examiner holds and "stabilizes" the scapula with one hand. The patient's arm is abducted 90 degrees and internally rotated 90 degrees. An axial force is loaded with the examiner's other hand holding the patient's elbow, and a simultaneous horizontal adduction force is applied while the axial load is maintained. A positive test—a sharp pain with or without a posterior clunk or click—may indicate posterior and/or posteroinferior shoulder instability.

16. **What should the evaluation of a painful hypersensitive region of the body entail?**
Among other things the documentation of the painful area should include the presence and extent or absence of mechanical hyperalgesia (pinprick, light touch), thermal and/or mechanical allodynia, (punctuate, brush-evoked), autonomic or vasomotor disturbances, swelling, sudomotor disturbances, temperature or color changes, tremor, dystonia, trophic changes (hair, nails, skin), and other sensorimotor disturbances (e.g., weakness).

17. **How can you differentiate between an L4 and an L5 radiculopathy on physical exam?**

An L4 radiculopathy may manifest with an absent or attenuated patellar tendon reflex with weakness of quadriceps and tibialis anterior (TA) and maintained extensor hallicus longus (EHL) function, as both the quadriceps and TA share L4 innervation and the EHL is L5 innervation. An attenuated or absent medial hamstring reflex with weakness in EHL with maintained patellar tendon reflex and TA function would be consistent with an L5 radiculopathy.

18. **What is the most sensitive muscle on manual muscle testing to assess for an SI radiculopathy?**

The flexor hallicus longus (FHL) is the most sensitive muscle on manual muscle testing for SI radiculopathy because it allows for more discrete grading of SI motor function than the gastrocnemius. The manual muscle testing (MMT) of the FHL is performed by having the patient flex to great toe and the examiner tries to overpower the muscle using his or her hand.

TABLE 5-1. PHYSICAL EXAMINATION TECHNIQUES			
Region of Examination	Examination	Site/Technique	Positive Results & Implications
Spine **Cervical**			
	Axial Compression	Examiner puts hand on top of patient's head and directs pressure to compress cervical spine caudad.	Pain localized to neck or radiating distally (upper extremities [UEs]) may indicate DJD or cervical nerve root impingement.
	Spurling's	Examiner puts hand on top of patient's head with the cervical spine in slight extension, rotation, and side bent—direct pressure to compress cervical spine caudad.	Pain radiating from the neck distally (UEs) may indicate nerve root impingement.
Thoracic			
	Chest Expansion	Examiner measures the chest circumference after full exhalation and again after full inhalation.	Ankylosing spondylitis may be suspected if the difference between the two measurements is less than 4 cm.
DJD = degenerative joint disease.			

(Continued)

TABLE 5-1. PHYSICAL EXAMINATION TECHNIQUES (CONTINUED)			
Region of Examination	Examination	Site/Technique	Positive Results & Implications
Lumbar			
	Yeoman's	With patient prone, examiner stabilizes pelvis and extends each of patient's hips in turn with knees extended; then extends each leg with knee flexed.	Pain along lumbar spine may indicate pathologic process of discs, vertebrae, or the sacroiliac joint.
	FABER	In a supine position, examiner performs maneuvers with the patient's lower extremity involving flexion, abduction, and external rotation of the hip.	Pain in the lower back may be indicative of sacroiliac (SI) joint pathology/ dysfunction.
	Gaenslen's	With the patient in a supine position with one leg hanging off the table, the patient is asked to hip flex (provocative component can be done with downward pressure on the hanging thigh).	Pain in the lower back may be indicative of hip joint or SI joint pathology.
	Shober's	The examiner makes a mark at the level of S2 in midline and then 5 cm below and 10 cm above—the distance between the marks is measured with the spine fully erect and then flexed (forward).	An increase in the measurement between the marks from erect to flexed on less than 5 cm may be indicative of ankylosing spondylitis.

(Continued)

TABLE 5-1. PHYSICAL EXAMINATION TECHNIQUES (CONTINUED)

Region of Examination	Examination	Site/Technique	Positive Results & Implications
Extremities Shoulder			
	Supraspinatus	Examiner applies downward pressure to arms while patient holds arms abducted to 90 degrees in neutral position without rotation; then patient rotates and angles arm so thumb faces toward floor.	Pain or weakness may indicate tear of rotator supraspinatus muscle or tendon.
	Adson	Locate and palpate radial pulse while abducting, extending, and externally rotating patient's arm; ask patient to take a deep breath and turn head to arm being tested.	Marked decrease or absence of radial pulse could indicate presence of extra cervical rib, tightened neck muscle, or thoracic outlet syndrome.
	Yergason	With patient's elbow flexed to 90 degrees, examiner cups elbow in hand, then externally rotates arm with other hand on wrist and pulls down on elbow.	Pain may indicate that the biceps tendon has come out of its bicipital groove.
	Impingement	Examiner elevates patient's arm by force.	Pain under acromion may indicate supraspinatus tendonitis or impingement syndrome.

(Continued)

TABLE 5-1. PHYSICAL EXAMINATION TECHNIQUES (CONTINUED)

Region of Examination	Examination	Site/Technique	Positive Results & Implications
	Apprehension	Patient's arm is flexed, abducted, and then passively externally rotated.	A feeling of apprehension or instability with abduction and external rotation may indicate joint laxity due to inferior glenohumeral ligament complex.
	Painful Arc	Patient's arm is moved through flexed range of motion passively and then actively.	Shoulder pain between 120 and 180 degrees may indicate tachromioclavicular disease. (Shoulder pain between 60 and 120 degrees may indicate impingement syndrome.)
Elbow			
	Golfer's elbow	Examiner palpates medial epicondyle area while forearm is supinated and elbow and wrists are extended.	Pain is felt over medial epicondyle.
Wrist			
	Tinel's Sign	Examiner taps area between olecranon and medial condyle (for ulnar nerve) or taps volar surface at center of wrist (for median nerve).	Tingling along ulnar nerve pathway may indicate neuroma or ulnar tunnel syndrome. Tingling of fingers along median nerve pathway indicates carpal tunnel syndrome.
	Phalen's	Examiner has patient flex wrists tightly against each other at right angles and hold position for 1 min.	Numbness or tingling of thumb or fingers may indicate carpal tunnel syndrome.

(Continued)

TABLE 5-1. PHYSICAL EXAMINATION TECHNIQUES (CONTINUED)			
Region of Examination	Examination	Site/Technique	Positive Results & Implications
	Finkelstein's	Patient is asked to make fist with thumb inside; examiner grasps fist and deviates fist toward ulnar side while holding forearm stable.	Moderate to severe pain over abductor and extensor tendons of thumb may indicate tenosynovitis, also called deQuervain's or Hoffman's disease.
Hip	Gaenslen's	Patient lies on side with lower leg flexed to chest and upper leg hyperextended at hip; examiner stabilizes pelvis while extending upper leg (test leg). **or:** With patient supine and one leg flexed at knee to chest, patient extends other leg off edge of table; patient draws both legs up to chest, then slowly lowers test leg down into extension.	Pain may be noted in sacroiliac joints, which may be due to sacroiliac pathology, hip pathology, or L4 nerve root lesion.
	External Rotation Hip	The examiner passively externally rotates the lower leg.	Pain in hip may indicate hip pathology (e.g., arthritis).

(Continued)

TABLE 5-1. PHYSICAL EXAMINATION TECHNIQUES (CONTINUED)

Region of Examination	Examination	Site/Technique	Positive Results & Implications
Knee			
	Lachman	Patient lies supine; examiner holds patient's knee between full extension and 30 degrees flexion; femur is stabilized with one of examiner's hands while moving proximal aspect of the tibia forward with other hand.	As tibia is moved forward, there may be a soft, mushy feeling as opposed to the normal firmness, indicative of anterior or posterior cruciate ligament injury.
	McMurray	With patient supine, legs extended, examiner cups heel in hand and flexes leg fully and places other hand on knee joint with fingers on medial joint line and thumb on lateral joint line; leg is rotated internally and externally, then is gently extended as the examiner palpates medial joint line.	Click in knee joint may indicate tear of medial meniscus.
	Apley	Patient lies prone with knee flexed to 90 degrees. Examiner uses own knee to hold down patient's knee, then examiner rotates tibia medially and laterally, combined first with distension, then with compression.	If pain is greater with rotation and distraction than with compression, patient may have a ligament injury; if compression produces more pain meniscus may be torn.

(Continued)

TABLE 5-1. PHYSICAL EXAMINATION TECHNIQUES (CONTINUED)			
Region of Examination	Examination	Site/Technique	Positive Results & Implications
Ankle	Knee Anterior Drawer	Examiner sits on patient's foot for stability; then places hands around upper tibia and draws leg forward.	More than 6 mm forward movement with anterior cruciate ligament tears, or medial collateral ligament tears.
	Thompson	With patient lying prone or kneeling on chair with feet over edge of table or chair, examiner squeezes calf muscles.	Lack of or inability to plantar flex foot may indicate a ruptured Achilles tendon. (At times, even with rupture patient can plantar flex by action of long extensor leg muscles.)
	Ankle Anterior	With the patient in supine position, ankle in neutral position, and tibia stabilized, the examiner cups the heel and pulls it anteriorly.	If laxity is appreciated it may indicate injury to the deltoid or anterior talofibular.

KEY POINTS

1. Performing a comprehensive physical examination is vital to the appropriate evaluation of the patient with pain.

2. Numerous physical examination techniques may aid the examiner in making a specific pain diagnosis, as will considering patient symptom magnification.

3. The examiner should be extremely familiar with the anatomic localization information that can be obtained during a physical examination.

BIBLIOGRAPHY

1. Greenman P: *Principles of manual medicine*, Baltimore, 1989, Williams & Wilkins.
2. Hoppenfield S: *Physical examination of the spine and extremities*, Norwalk, Conn, 1976, Appleton-Century-Crofts.
3. Magee D: *Orthopedic physical assessment*, Philadelphia, 1992, W.B. Sanders.
4. Wadell G: Clinical assessment of lumbar impairment, *Clin Orthop Rehabil Res* 221:110, 1987.

CHAPTER 6

PAIN MEASUREMENT

W. Crawford Clark, PhD, Sita S. Chokhavatia, MD, Abbas Kashani, MD, and Susanne Bennett Clark, PhD

DIMENSIONS OF PAIN

1. **Name the five axes of pain according to the taxonomy devised by the International Association for the Study of Pain.**
   The taxonomy devised by the International Association for the Study of Pain lists the following five axes of pain:
   - Regions of the body
   - Systems affected
   - Temporal characteristics
   - Intensity and time since onset
   - Etiology

2. **Which major aspects or dimensions of pain and suffering must be considered when assessing pain? Define the dimensions.**
   Melzack and Casey argue for the following three dimensions of pain: (1) The sensory-discriminative dimension comprises the sensory aspects of pain, including intensity, location, and temporal aspects. (2) The affective-motivational dimension reflects the emotional and aversive aspects of pain and suffering. (3) The cognitive-evaluative dimension reflects the patient's evaluation of the meaning and possible consequences of the pain and illness or injury, including impact on quality of life and even death itself. This three-dimensional model is widely accepted because it integrates much of what is known about the physiology and psychology of pain and suffering.

PAIN SCALES

3. **Name three accepted types of scales for measuring the intensity of pain.**
   - Visual analogue scale
   - Numerical rating scale
   - Category rating scale

4. **Describe the analogue, numerical, and category scales. Which is most suitable for use with patients?**
   Visual analogue scales (VAS) are 10-cm lines anchored at the ends by words that define the bounds of various pain dimensions. The patient is asked to place a vertical mark on the scale to indicate the level of intensity of his or her pain, anxiety, depression, etc. The following are two VAS examples:

No Pain	Worst Possible Pain
No Anxiety	Worst Possible Anxiety

Numerical rating scales are similar to analogue scales except that numbers (e.g., 0 to 5) are entered along the scale.

With category scales, the patient is asked to circle the word that best describes his or her condition (e.g., for pain intensity: None, Moderate, Severe, Unbearable).

Each of the presented scales may be appropriate for patients.

5. **What is the "fifth vital sign" to be entered in the patient's chart?**
   The fifth vital sign is the rating score on a unidimensional pain scale. It is entered in the patient's chart along with respiration, blood pressure, heart rate, and temperature.

6. **What does a score obtained from the unidimensional pain scale mean?**
   The unidimensional pain scale score is supposed to reflect the intensity of the patient's physical (sensory) pain. However, it has been demonstrated that the score on a pain rating scale is not, as one might expect, related only to the intensity of somatosensory aspects of physical pain, but also to the intensity of emotional aspects of pain, including the patient's anxiety, fear, depression, and anger.

7. **What is the solution to the pain assessment problem described in question 6?**
   Scores on additional emotional scales related to anxiety, fear, depression, and anger must be obtained and factored into any decision about the level of the patient's pain.

8. **What is the difference between a rating scale and a questionnaire?**
   A rating scale represents a single dimension related to some aspect of pain or suffering; a questionnaire contains a large number of rating scales that encompass many dimensions of pain and related emotions.

PAIN ASSESSMENT BY QUESTIONNAIRES

9. **How is pain/emotion assessment accomplished? Why is it important?**
   Pain assessment is a multidimensional approach to the evaluation of pain attributes. These attributes include the intensity, duration, and location of pain and its somatosensory and emotional qualities. It is important because meticulous assessment is needed to tailor the patient's medication and dosage to his or her particular requirements; for example, to decide whether an analgesic should be supplemented with an anxiolytic, antidepressant, and/or psychotherapy. Careful evaluation also permits changes in medication to be monitored reliably.

10. **What is the most widely used pain questionnaire?**
    The McGill Pain Questionnaire, which has been translated into all major languages, was developed by Dr. Ronald Melzack of McGill University. It is a checklist of 87 descriptors of the sensory qualities of a patient's pain and related emotions, plus a line drawing of a body on which the patient sketches the location of the pain. The questionnaire also includes an overall intensity rating called the Present Pain Index.

11. **Describe the multidimensional affect and pain survey (MAPS).**
    The 101 descriptors of the Multidimensional Affect and Pain Survey (MAPS) questionnaire are grouped into 30 subclusters subordinated within three superclusters. Supercluster I, Sensory Pain, contains 57 descriptors of painful sensory qualities in 17 subclusters. Supercluster II, Emotional Pain (Suffering), contains 26 descriptors of negative emotional states in eight subclusters. Supercluster III, Well-Being, contains 18 descriptors of positive affect and health in five subclusters. The descriptors are placed in sentences to clarify their meaning. The patient rates these statements on a response scale that ranges from Not at All (0) to Very Much So (5).

Here are examples from each of the three MAPS superclusters:
  I. **Sensory Qualities Supercluster**
     The sensation and/or pain is BURNING   0 1 2 3 4 5
 II. **Suffering Supercluster**
     I feel DEPRESSED   0 1 2 3 4 5
III. **Well-Being Supercluster**
     I feel CALM   0 1 2 3 4 5

12. **Can administration of MAPS before surgery predict postoperative morphine consumption?**
    Yes, patients who before surgery anticipate greater pain and emotional distress actually consume more morphine postoperatively.

13. **What is the advantage of knowing the relative intensities of the sensory and emotional components that determine patients' ratings of "pain"?**
    If the relative strengths of the sensory and emotional components are known, medication (analgesics, anxiolytics, antidepressants) can be tailored more accurately to the patient's needs.

14. **Why is MAPS superior to other questionnaires?**
    The MAPS structure was determined objectively, by cluster analysis. The 101 items of MAPS were selected from an initial set of 270 descriptors by means of the pile-sort procedure. This procedure is based on pair-wise similarity judgments of the descriptors by healthy volunteers. The data were analyzed by the agglomerative, hierarchical clustering technique, using the average-linkage-between-groups algorithm. Descriptors that were highly similar according to cluster analysis, and descriptors that had different meanings (i.e., fell into different clusters) for female and male college students of Puerto Rican, Euro-American, and African-American background, were eliminated. Thus, the MAPS questionnaire was based on a dendrogram of 101 words that, unlike other questionnaires, is relatively free of gender and ethnocultural bias. These descriptors, clustered according to their location in the dendrogram, determine the structure of the MAPS.

15. **What are the three main advantages of MAPS?**
    The main advantages of MAPS over the McGill Pain Questionnaire are as follows:
    - The hierarchical organization of clusters within the three superclusters and of the pain descriptors within the subclusters is determined objectively from a large sample of volunteers, not subjectively from the diverse opinions of pain "experts."
    - The large number of words describing the emotional aspects of pain shortens test time by eliminating the need for additional psychologic questionnaires to probe the patient's emotional state.
    - The Well-Being Supercluster identifies an interesting subset of patients who say they are depressed and relaxed at the same time. Patients who respond in this manner may be those who are denying their pain because they fear that it may indicate a serious illness.

16. **What is the Brief Pain Inventory (BPI)?**
    The Brief Pain Inventory (BPI) measures both the intensity of the pain (sensory component) and the interference of the pain in the patient's life. Originally developed by a group focusing on cancer pain, the BPI is now one of the most commonly used pain assessment tools for all types of pain for both clinical and research purposes.

PAIN-RELATED QUESTIONNAIRES

17. **How is pain assessed in patients who, because of neurological or cognitive deficits, cannot communicate verbally?**
    Pain in cognitively impaired patients and young children can be estimated by their responses to a scale consisting of a series of faces whose expressions range from smiling to discomfort

to desperate crying. Patients indicate their pain by pointing to one of the faces. Recently, the Iowa Pain Thermometer has been developed to assess pain in younger patients, as well as in older adults. This scale is being increasingly used in practice.

18. **True or false: scores from questionnaires on emotional symptomatology (e.g., the Brief Symptom Inventory) can be relied upon when given to patients who are suffering pain.**
False. Scores from such questionnaires must be interpreted with caution. Test items that reflect depression in psychiatric patients (e.g., loss of appetite) may be due to a physical condition such as ulcers or may result from treatment, for example with narcotics, in medical patients. Accordingly, a medical patient with a high score on a test of psychologic status could be misdiagnosed as having a "psychological" problem.

19. **Which questionnaires are used to assess the general psychologic status of pain patients?**
The Derogatis Symptom Check List-90 (SCL-90) or its shorter version, the Brief Symptom Inventory (BSI), is often used to assess the psychologic status of pain patients. Patients use the lists to score how much they are bothered by a particular symptom. The Profile of Mood States (POMS) is also frequently used, because its questions do not allude to florid psychotic behavior.

20. **What is the effect on the physician-patient relationship when giving the patient a psychologic status questionnaire?**
Many patients resent being given a questionnaire that was obviously designed for psychiatric patients because it gives the impression that the physician does not believe that their pain is "real."

21. **Which standardized questionnaires can be used to assess physical function?**
Disability is assessed by the Health Assessment Questionnaire, the Sickness Impact Profile, and the Arthritis Impact Measurement Scale. Other scales measure social and work satisfaction, ambulation, and self-care. The Karnofsky scale is a behavioral scale widely used to assess the stages of disease progression in cancer patients. Many of these scales yield a score that locates the patient relative to population norms.

22. **What are the seven ways, quantified in the Coping Strategies Questionnaire, that patients use to cope with their pain? Can patients be taught these strategies?**
As quantified in the Coping Strategies Questionnaire, patients use the following seven strategies to cope with their pain: (1) diverting attention, (2) praying/hoping, (3) reinterpreting pain sensations, (4) avoidance of catastrophizing, (5) coping self-statements, (6) increased activity, and (7) ignoring sensations.
   Yes, patients can be taught to use these strategies to ameliorate their pain.

23. **What does the locus of control scale predict about the success of patients' pain coping strategies?**
Chronic pain patients who have high external locus of control scores (i.e., the course of their disease is in the hands of fate) exhibit more maladaptive pain coping strategies and greater psychologic distress than patients who score high on internal locus of control (i.e., have a sense that they can control the course of their illness).

24. **Which questionnaires are used to assess the behavioral/cognitive aspects of pain and suffering?**
Hypochondriasis, somatic concern, and denial behaviors are rated by the Illness Behavior Questionnaire developed by Pilowski. Other quantifiable measures of behavior include frequency of physician and/or hospital visits, number of surgeries for pain, constant changes in medication, sleep disturbances, and nonverbal pain behaviors such as limping, grimacing, or guarding.

25. **What is the Westhaven-Yale Multidimensional Pain Inventory?**
The Westhaven-Yale Multidimensional Pain Inventory is a standardized questionnaire used in patients with chronic pain. This inventory is aimed at measuring the sensory, medical, neurologic, cognitive, and psychologic aspects of pain, as well as the patient's capacity for enduring pain.

26. **Name a questionnaire that measures disability and suffering.**
The Sickness Impact Profile (SIP) provides a profile of patient disability; it includes questions about ambulation, body care, social interaction, alertness, sleep, work, and recreation.

27. **Which questionnaires evaluate in a general way the impact of chronic pain on the patient's psychosocial life?**
The Multidimensional Pain Inventory (MPI) and the Quality of Life Enjoyment and Satisfaction Questionnaire (Q-LES-Q) evaluate the impact of the patient's pain on his or her psychosocial life. The particular advantage of these questionnaires is that they distinguish overall severity of illness and severity of depression.

28. **Name a disease-specific quality-of-life questionnaire.**
The Irritable Bowel Syndrome Quality of Life (IBS-QOL) questionnaire is designed to monitor quality of life in patients with irritable bowel syndrome. A thorough review of questionnaires assessing quality of life in oncology patients has recently been published.

29. **What is a structured interview?**
A structured interview is an interview in which the interviewer asks a set of predetermined questions. In the more sophisticated versions, the set of questions asked (and those omitted) depend in part upon the patient's responses. Examples are the Interactive Microcomputer Patient Assessment Tool for Health (IMPATH) and the Behavioral Assessment of Pain (BAP) questionnaires.

30. **What additional scales are important in the assessment of chronic pain?**
Besides responding to a scale about their present pain, chronic pain patients communicate the breadth of their fluctuating symptoms by rating their pain over the past 1 or 2 weeks or during the period since their last visit on separate scales specifying "highest," "lowest," and "usual" pain. The average "lowest" and "usual" pain ratings give the best estimate; the "highest" rating tends to be erratic. A problem related to remembered pain is that when present pain is very intense, patients tend to overestimate their past pain.

31. **Is a scale that asks the patient to rate percentage of pain relief superior to a scale that compares pain ratings before and after separate treatments?**
Percentage of pain relief is generally considered a superior measurement tool when used to study analgesic effectiveness for acute pain. However, when the evaluation requires remembering the pain over a long treatment period, percentage of relief is a less sensitive measurement tool than comparison of changes in pain.

RELIABILITY AND VALIDITY

32. **What are the two essential characteristics of a rating scale or questionnaire?**
The two essential characteristics of a rating scale or questionnaire are reliability and validity.

33. **What is a reliable measure? Name three types of reliability tests.**
A reliable measure has the property of yielding consistent results. The following are the most common ways to assess reliability:
- By internal consistency, or split-half reliability
- By test-retest reliability
- By inter-rater reliability

For split-half reliability, similar items should receive similar scores. This requires questionnaires with two sets of similar items (e.g., Form A and Form B) that are usually, but not necessarily, administered on different occasions. The advantage is that two independent assessments of the patient's symptoms can be made on separate occasions. The questions are designed so that patients cannot intentionally or unintentionally base their second responses on their memories of the previous test.

Test-retest reliability indexes the consistency of the questionnaire. Patients should give the same answer to the same question if their medical status has not changed.

For questionnaires that may be answered by an outside observer (e.g., those concerning behavioral symptoms), inter-rater reliability is assessed by comparing the evaluations of the same patient by two or more raters.

34. **How is the reliability of a test quantified?**
Reliability is usually expressed numerically as a correlation coefficient, with 0.0 signifying total unreliability and 1.0 indicating perfect reliability. Reliability coefficients (Cronbach's alpha) above 0.85 are generally regarded as high and those between 0.65 and 0.85 as moderate.

35. **What is meant by the validity of a questionnaire?**
Validity means that the test measures what it is supposed to measure. To determine this, the scores on the measure are compared with various kinds of external standards; for example, the test score on a pain scale should be high in response to postoperative pain or to calibrated noxious stimuli.

36. **What is content, or face, validity?**
In this informal approach to measuring validity, a group of experts is simply asked to confirm the suitability, clarity, and organization of the questionnaire items.

37. **What is concurrent validity?**
A test is considered concurrently valid when responses to the new pain measure being investigated (predictor variable) correlate with results from a previous well-established (criterion variable) test.

38. **What is predictive validity?**
Predictive validity is examined through longitudinal or prospective studies. The predictor variable may be the score on a psychologic or pain questionnaire or a physiologic measure (e.g., hypertension). The criterion variable is an independently measured event (e.g., treatment outcome, such as intensity of postsurgical pain).

39. **What is discriminant validity?**
Discriminant validity is a statistical technique that validates a pain measure by evaluating each test item's ability to group patients according to an underlying shared characteristic; for example, how well each test item discriminates among patients with cluster, tension, and migraine headaches.

40. **What are the advantages of factor analyzing responses to a pain questionnaire?**
A pain questionnaire such as the McGill Pain Questionnaire may contain pain rating responses to 87 questions, making it difficult to interpret. By analyzing the intercorrelations among these responses, factor analysis determines a small number (three to five) of essential variables, or factors, that represent the important attributes of pain according to the test on a particular group of pain patients. For example, the response of low back pain patients to the McGill Pain Questionnaire were summarized by five factors: Immediate Anxiety, Perception of Harm, Somesthetic Pressure, Cutaneous Sensitivity, and Somatosensory Information.

PAIN MEMORY

41. How reliable are patients' reports of past pain?

In some studies, concordance between pain diaries and patients' later memories for the diaries' content has been fairly good. However, other studies have shown that remembrance of past pain is influenced by present pain intensity, anxiety, depression, and fear. Furthermore, one study of dental pain found that the pain intensity remembered 6 months later was more highly correlated with patients' expectation of pain recorded before surgery than with the pain they actually experienced, recorded after surgery. Also, it is quite likely that patients recall what they said in the past, not what they felt.

42. What is a pain diary?

A pain diary is a record of the patient's pain level, along with relevant variables such as emotional state, awake activity, sleep pattern, consumption of medication, and adverse side effects. The patient also notes events that may have caused the reported changes. Entries are made at specified times during the day such as upon awakening; at breakfast, lunch, and dinner; at bedtime; etc. More consistent and valid information is obtained if the patient responds to a checklist.

43. What is the value of a pain diary?

Pain diaries are important for optimal pain management. Retrospective analyses of pain diaries can suggest improved treatment strategies. They may also reveal exacerbating or ameliorating factors related to treatment that the patient and practitioner would otherwise overlook.

ASSESSMENT OF PAIN RESPONSES TO CALIBRATED NOXIOUS STIMULATION

44. What is "laboratory-induced" pain?

The expression "laboratory-induced" pain refers to sensory experiences induced by noxious stimuli that are precisely calibrated for intensity, duration, area, and location.

45. How is laboratory-induced pain used in research?

Laboratory-induced pain is used in research in the following ways:

- To study changes in threshold related to various diseases including schizophrenia, psychotic depression, bulimia, postherpetic and diabetic neuralgias, irritable bowel syndrome, sickle cell disease, lower back pain, poststroke central pain, fibromyalgia, etc.
- To study responses to stress (e.g., stress-induced analgesia)
- To determine whether there are gender, ethnocultural, age, and other differences in pain sensitivity
- In animals, to study neurosensory systems and responses to physiologic and pharmacologic interventions

46. Describe the method of limits, and define threshold.

In the method of limits procedure (also known as serial exploration), the subject responds to each of a series of brief, physically calibrated stimuli (thermal, cold, pressure, pinch, or electrical) that are increased stepwise in intensity. The threshold is identified as that intensity in the series at which the subject responds by saying, "Pain." Threshold is the inverse of sensitivity. A high threshold means that the subject is less sensitive to painful stimuli.

47. Define the pain sensitivity and tolerance thresholds.

The pain sensitivity threshold is the intensity at which the subject first reports pain. The pain tolerance threshold is the intensity at which the subject withdraws from the stimulus.

48. **What are the advantages and disadvantages of the method of limits procedure?**
    The method of limits procedure is useful for approximating the threshold in order to determine the intensities to be applied in more sophisticated and accurate procedures. Although thresholds were once thought to be pure measures of sensory function, it is now clear that they lack validity because they are heavily influenced by nonsensory, psychologic variables, such as the subject's expectations and attitudes. It is not possible, for example, to decide whether a diabetic patient with a high pain threshold to heat stimuli is simply stoical or is suffering from diabetic neuropathy.

49. **What is sensory decision theory?**
    Signal detection theory or sensory decision theory (SDT), like the medical decision-making model, is based on statistical decision theory and requires the subject to make decisions about which of two objectively definable events, A or B, has occurred. In the single interval rating procedure, the subject rates each presentation of calibrated stimuli of various intensities as being painful or not painful. From these responses, a 2-3-2 contingency table is created, and the hit and false alarm rates are computed.

	Response "Pain"	Response "Not Painful"
Higher intensity stimulus	Hits (sensitivity)	Misses
Lower intensity stimulus	False alarms	Correct rejections (specificity)

50. **What two indices of perceptual performance are obtained with sensory decision theory?**
    The discriminability index, d' or $P(A)$, reflects the functioning of the neurosensory system. High values suggest that neurosensory function is normal; low values suggest a sensory deficit caused, for example, by damage to sensory pathways (e.g., diabetic neuropathy). The discrimination index has also been shown to be decreased by analgesics such as morphine and by nerve blocks because they attenuate neural activity and therefore the amount of information reaching higher centers. Unlike the traditional pain threshold obtained by the method of limits, the SDT discrimination index is not influenced by psychologic variables such as expectation, stoicism, and mood.
    The other measure of perceptual performance, the report criterion, L_x or B, measures response bias—the willingness (low or liberal criterion) or reluctance (high or stoical criterion) to report pain. The report criterion is related to the subject's attitude toward reporting painful experiences. Attitudes depend on cultural factors such as stoicism or on personal emotional factors such as anxiety and depression.

51. **What has sensory decision theory analysis of responses to calibrated noxious stimuli revealed about the effects of analgesics and placebos on the pain threshold?**
    Many studies have used SDT to demonstrate the effects of attitudinal and emotional variables on the pain report. For example, a placebo described and accepted by the subjects as a powerful analgesic raised the traditional method of limits threshold—that is, it apparently decreased pain sensitivity. Analysis of the same data by SDT, however, demonstrated that only the report criterion had been raised (fewer pain reports); the discriminability index had not changed. Thus, the placebo-induced reduction in pain report was due not to an analgesic effect of the placebo, but to a criterion shift caused by the social demand characteristics of the experimental situation!

52. **Are there gender, ethnocultural, and age differences in pain thresholds?**
    Higher pain thresholds to calibrated noxious stimuli have been reported among northern Europeans compared to Mediterranean peoples and African-Americans. Irish Catholics and Yankee Protestants have been reported to have higher pain thresholds than Italians and Jews. These differences are probably caused by differences in stoicism (report criterion). The higher

pain threshold of older patients is probably due to a more stoical (high) report criterion as well as sensory loss (lower d′), compared with younger patients.

SDT has shown that the high method of limits threshold of Nepalese Sherpas compared to Western trekkers was due to a high (stoical) pain report criterion. The Sherpas' ability to discriminate among noxious electrical stimuli was the same as that of Westerners, suggesting that their nociceptive sensory systems were the same. The Sherpas were simply more stoical, probably as a result of their adaptation to a harsh climate.

It may be concluded that there is little evidence for ethnocultural differences in the discrimination of noxious stimuli, but there are significant cultural differences in the criterion for reporting pain. Probably most, if not all, of the differences in pain thresholds that have been reported among various groups are due to cultural differences in the criteria for reporting pain and not at all to differences in the sensory experience of pain itself.

53. **Are there ethnocultural differences in how patients and practitioners view which organ system is primarily responsible for pain?**
There are striking differences in the particular body organ that a culture focuses on as a source of pain. Germans are much more apt to complain of heart pain (and German cardiologists are more likely to read an electrocardiogram as abnormal). The French focus on the liver and even refer to a migraine headache as a "liver crisis." The English are most concerned about the gastrointestinal tract.

54. **Do physicians underestimate pain in certain ethnocultural groups?**
Studies in the United States have found that members of minority groups tend to be undermedicated for pain.

PHYSIOLOGIC MEASURES

55. **Are there any somatic measures that can be used as indicators of a patient's pain?**
With acute pain, heart rate initially increases, arterial oxygen tension decreases, and stress-related hormones are released. However, apprehension and anxiety alone produce similar changes. Also, baseline values vary widely diurnally and with age. Evoked potentials recorded from the scalp have been shown to be linked with the intensity of the noxious stimulus; however, an unexpected intense, but not painful, stimulus can produce similar evoked potential patterns. No single physiologic variable clearly distinguishes a painful from a nonpainful stimulus. In contrast to acute pain, there are no useful physiologic indicators of chronic, persistent pain.

56. **What have brain imaging studies revealed about the dimensions of pain?**
Brain imaging studies have demonstrated that noxious calibrated stimuli activate not only the primary and secondary somatosensory cortex, but many other regions of the brain including the anterior cingulate gyrus (which mediates emotions) and the prefrontal cortex (associated with cognitive processes). Other regions that respond to the intensity of noxious stimulation include the cerebellum, putamen, thalamus, and insula. These structures mediate the affective, motoric, attentional, and autonomic responses to pain and respond to gradations in the intensity of noxious stimuli. These regions are, of course, not solely pain-processing areas. Studies of patients suffering chronic pain and hypnotized subjects have revealed altered brain activity. The promise is there, but much work needs to be done before these complex brain activities can be fully understood and related to a patient's report of pain.

57. **Is it possible to measure the relative physiologic and psychologic contributions to treatment outcome; that is, to separate specific and nonspecific treatment effects?**
Yes. Specific effects of physiologically based procedures combine with nonspecific psychophysiologic effects to determine treatment outcome. In a study measuring the separate

contributions, there are two treatment conditions and two belief states (Table 6-1). The specific treatment is assumed to produce a real (i.e., physiologically based) therapeutic effect, and the sham treatment is assumed to be physiologically ineffective. In addition, the patient's belief as to whether he or she was in the real treatment or the sham treatment group is determined at the end of the study. The cell entries (A, B, C, D) in Table 6-1 are the numbers of patients rated as improved according to some objective criterion.

This approach yields the four-cell table into which patients with positive outcomes are placed on the basis of (1) physical treatment and (2) subjective opinion about which treatment they had received. A comparison of results according to the treatment the patients believed they had received, compared with what they actually received, permits comparison of how much of the group improvement was due to the specific effect of, say, an alternative-medicine treatment, and how much of the improvement was due to nonspecific psychophysiologic effects.

TABLE 6-1. SUCCESSFUL OUTCOME CONTINGENT ON TREATMENT AND BELIEF

	Patient's Belief in Treatment	
	Real Treatment	Sham Treatment
Specific Treatment*	A	B
Sham Treatment**	C	D

The cells A, B, C, and D represent the four possible objective and subjective treatment conditions. Based on research from National Institute of Dental and Craniofacial Research (NIDCR) 12725 and the Nathaniel Wharton Fund for Research and Education in Brain, Body and Behavior. The authors wish to thank John Kuhl, PhD, for his helpful suggestions.
* Accepted-site acupuncture, trial medication, transcutaneous electrical nerve stimulation (TENS), etc.
** Off-site acupuncture, standard medication, placebo, sham TENS, etc.

KEY POINTS

1. Numerous pain assessment tools are available to assist in the measurement of pain.

2. Pain assessment is a multidimensional approach to the evaluation of pain attributes that assists in the development of the most appropriate treatment plan for an individual patient.

3. Specialized pain assessment tools are available to be considered based on the particular condition, age, and abilities of the patient being evaluated.

BIBLIOGRAPHY

1. Clark WC: Pain and emotion. In Gonzales EG, Myers SJ, Edelstein JE, et al, editors: *Downey and Darling's physiological basis of rehabilitation medicine*, 3rd ed, Woburn, Mass, 2001, Butterworth, pp 815-848.

2. Clark WC: Pain, emotion, and drug-induced subjective states: analysis by multidimensional scaling. In Adelman G, Smith B, editors: *Encyclopedia of neuroscience*, 2nd ed, Amsterdam, 1999, Elsevier, pp 1561-1565. (Also available on CD-ROM.)

3. Clark WC: Pin and pang: research methodology for acupuncture and other "alternative medicine" therapies, *Am Pain Soc J Forum* 3:84-88, 1994.

4. Clark WC: Somatosensory and pain measurement by signal detection theory. In Adelman G, Smith B, editors: *Encyclopedia of neuroscience*, 2nd ed, Amsterdam, 1999, Elsevier, 1895-1898. (Also available on CD-ROM.)

5. Clark WC, Janal MN, Carroll JD: Multidimensional pain requires multidimensional scaling. In Loeser JD, Chapman CR, editors: *The measurement of pain*, New York, 1989, Raven Press.

6. Clark WC, Yang JC, Tsui SL, et al: Unidimensional pain rating scales: A Multidimensional Affect and Pain Survey (MAPS) analysis of what they really measure, *Pain*, 98(3):241-247, 2002.

7. Cleeland CS, Ryan KM: Pain assessment: global use of the Brief Pain Inventory, *Ann Acad Med Singapore*, 23 (2):129-128, 1994.

8. Drossman DA, Patrick DL, Whitehead WE, et al: Further validation of the IBS-QOL: a disease specific quality of life questionnaire, *Am J Gastroenterol* 95: 999-1013, 2000.

9. Endicott J, Nee J, Harrison W, Blumenthal R: Quality of life enjoyment and satisfaction questionnaire: a new measure, *Psychopharmacol Bull* 29:321-326, 1993.

10. Herr K, Spratt KF, Garand L, et al: Evaluation of the Iowa pain thermometer and other selected pain intensity scales in younger and older adult cohorts using controlled clinical pain: a preliminary study, *Pain Med*, 8 (7):585-600, 2007.

11. Kornblith AB, Holland JC: *Handbook of measures for psychological, social and physical function in cancer*, New York, 1994, Memorial Sloan-Kettering Center.

12. Melzack R, editor: *Pain measurement and assessment*, New York, 1983, Raven Press.

13. Mersky H, editor: Classification of chronic pain: descriptions of chronic pain syndromes and definitions of pain terms, *Pain* (Suppl 3):1-226, 1986.

14. Payer L: *Medicine and culture*, New York, 1988, Holt.

15. Sloan JA, Cella D, Frost M, et al: Assessing clinical significance in measuring oncology quality of life: introduction to the symposium, content overview and definition of terms, *Mayo Clin Proc* 77:367-370, 2002.

16. Turk DC, Melzack R, editors: *Handbook of pain assessment*, London, 1992, Guilford Press.

17. Yang JC, Clark WC, Tsui SL, et al: Preoperative Multidimensional Affect and Pain Survey (MAPS) scores predict post-colectomy analgesia requirement, *Clin J Pain* 16:314-320, 2000.

18. Zatzick DF, Dimsdale JE: Cultural variations in response to painful stimuli, *Psychosom Med* 52:544-557, 1990.

PSYCHOLOGICAL ASSESSMENT OF CHRONIC PAIN PATIENTS

Dennis R. Thornton, PhD, and Charles E. Argoff, MD

CHAPTER 7

1. **Why is a good psychological assessment essential?**

   The purpose of a psychological evaluation is to frame the pain experience in the context of a patient's life. Specifically, it evaluates the impact of pain on the patient's functioning and the role that the patient's psychological makeup has in the experience of pain. It is not designed to differentiate between organic and psychogenic pain. The evaluation should, however, assess the impact of anxiety, depression, and prior life experiences on pain. Assessing personality characteristics provides a means of helping the patient to maximize treatment efforts and minimize resistance.

2. **Does gender mediate an individual's response to pain?**

   Gender-related differences have been studied clinically and experimentally. Women are at greater risk of developing some specific chronic pain disorders and are more sensitive to experimentally induced pain than are men. Psychosocial factors, such as role beliefs, affective state, coping strategies, employment status, pain-related expectancies, hormonal effects, familial modeling, and intergenerational influences may exert a role in the observed differences.

3. **Do race and ethnicity exert an influence on the pain experience and response?**

   As with gender-related issues, the influence of ethnic background on the response to acute clinical, experimental, and chronic pain has been investigated extensively over the decades. Differences observed in a wide variety of settings have sometimes been confusing and contradictory. As with gender-related issues, the reader is encouraged to avoid overemphasis on any one article or research report and to survey the broad spectrum of literature to see the stated differences in context.

4. **What is the essential element of a good pain evaluation?**

   The essential element of a good pain evaluation is that the clinician believes that the pain is real! Whether or not an organic framework can be defined is somewhat less important in chronic pain than it is in acute pain. However, both physical and psychological issues must be addressed on the first visit.

5. **What data-collecting strategies can be employed to render a comprehensive assessment of the patient with chronic pain?**

   From the psychological perspective, patient involvement is essential to the pain assessment process. There are a number of tools available for self-reporting, including pain and activity diaries. These tools can provide an index of the following:
   - Pain intensity and characteristics
   - Onset and evolution of the pain syndrome
   - Patient attributions
   - Patient outlook on his or her condition
   - Personal and family background
   - Projected functional goals
   - Mood

Additionally, evaluation of behavioral responses from significant others can be enlightening. Whenever possible, collect naturalistic observations; they are invaluable. Try to observe the patient while he or she is engaged in routine activities and (ideally) unaware of your attention. Canvass secretaries and allied staff for their interactions with the patient.

6. **What methods can be used for the psychological assessment of patients with chronic pain?**
   The psychological interview can be supported by a number of "pencil-and-paper" indices. The interview should establish a conceptual framework, and the pencil-and-paper tests can be used to facilitate patient communication in order to quantify such issues as pain intensity, severity of mood disorder, and level of function.

7. **What factors commonly interfere with the accurate assessment of chronic pain?**
   Pain is an entirely subjective experience. Therefore, personal factors impact the process and accuracy of pain assessment. Cultural, ethnic, and linguistic patterns may influence both how the pain is expressed and how it is interpreted. Furthermore, clinicians are classically trained in the biomedical model, in which pain is believed to be due to a clearly identifiable point of tissue injury. In chronic pain, this may no longer be the case. A shift must occur to a biopsychosocial model, in which the complaint of pain is viewed in a more global framework.

8. **What is the most common conceptual mistake that the examining clinician makes?**
   Physicians often try to conceptualize pain as either organic or psychological ("psychosomatic"). This dichotomy is rarely absolute. True delusional pain is extraordinarily rare. Most commonly, psychological factors impact on the expression of pain, and pain has its impact on a patient's psychological well-being.

9. **How important are behavioral signs in assessing pain intensity in chronic pain?**
   The autonomic "flight-or-fight response" that we commonly associate with acute pain is often lacking in chronic pain. Therefore, tachycardia, diaphoresis, and agitation are often absent. Over time, patients adapt to chronic pain. This adaptation may be appropriate or inappropriate, given the circumstances. Similarly, signs of emotional distress may be replaced by a blunting of affect.

10. **Is there a specific format for interviewing patients with pain?**
    Interviews must be tailored to fit the situation. However, there is structure to the interview process. A biopsychosocial format is the most appropriate. It starts with the patient's complaint, which is clearly foremost in his or her mind. Aside from the usual questions regarding intensity, location, and character, the psychosocial variables to be addressed include the circumstances under which the pain began, its duration, the success or failure of various interventions, the patient's responses to these treatments and results, the impact of the pain on the patient's life, and the patient's expectations or goals of treatment.

11. **Why is determining the time of onset important?**
    The circumstances under which the pain arose may give some insight into the psychological phenomenon surrounding the pain syndrome. For example, traumatic injuries, such as motor vehicle accidents or major surgeries, may give rise to a posttraumatic stress disorder. Diseases with an insidious onset and an exacerbating-remitting course may provoke anxiety with each exacerbation of pain. If the pain syndrome was the result of a co-worker's negligence, poorly directed anger may be a significant component. Similarly, litigation and compensation surrounding an injury may be important factors.

12. **Describe psychological insights that can be gained from reviewing treatments that have failed.**
    Patterns of response and nonresponse may imply certain specific psychological syndromes. For example, patients who claim dramatic relief from certain treatments, only to fail a short while

after, may be engaging in idealization/demystification. This is typical of the hysterical personality disorder and may put the clinician at great risk for defeat. Similarly, patients who are unable to tolerate any medications, describing bad reactions to all, may be unconsciously sabotaging treatment. Thus, a careful history of all prior treatments, successful or otherwise, can be a guide to expectations of future interventions.

The same is true of the patient's perception of the prior treating clinicians. Much the same as a treatment can be rapidly valued and devalued, the same holds for a treating clinician.

13. **Is emotional distress a normal consequence of illness and pain? What does the absence of such a response imply?**
Serious illness, especially when accompanied by pain, raises numerous anxieties. Patients may fear very significant illness, incapacitation, or death. If they emphatically deny any anxiety or emotional impact, it is likely that these emotions are threatening to the patient and require further psychological evaluation. Patients may also intentionally minimize or deny psychological distress for fear that their complaints of pain will be interpreted as "psychosomatic" and they will be labeled as "crazy."

14. **What strategies can be employed to elicit the psychological impact of pain if a patient is unable to express it?**
The first step is to put the patient at ease by suggesting that psychological reactions to pain are quite normal. Cite some specific examples, such as posttraumatic stress disorder after war injuries, motor vehicle accidents, traumatic surgeries, and so on. Should this fail, it may be helpful to interview family members and significant others. They can describe pain behaviors, drug use patterns, altered functional roles, and mood changes. In addition, observing the interaction between the patient and significant others may provide useful insights into family dynamics and level of frustration.

15. **Why is the assessment of functioning and level of distress so important?**
Increasingly, clinical observation and research have highlighted functioning and level of distress because these factors are related to disability. More than pain intensity, performance difficulties and negative affect are statistically linked with greater disability. Difficulties in performing premorbid roles and activities erode self-esteem and hopefulness. The ensuing negative affect can foster a sense of giving up, which will help establish and perpetuate disability status.

16. **What specific areas of function should be addressed?**
Question the patient about his or her ability to work (both outside the house and in relation to the usual household duties) and the impact on social life, mood, sleep, sexual activity, and relationships with others.

17. **What specific work-related issues should be addressed?**
Determine what the patient's prior work status was and the feasibility of his or her returning to that type of work. Specifically, ask questions about the amount of skill required for the job, physical qualifications, and job satisfaction. The financial impact of working versus collecting disability payments should also be addressed. Also investigate the patient's work history with regard to relative job satisfaction, progress on the job, and time lost because of pain or illness.

18. **How can chronic pain affect social function?**
Chronic pain can impede a patient's ability to seek gainful employment. If the patient was originally the breadwinner, this role as head-of-household and power figure may diminish. Correspondingly, self-esteem may diminish, and the patient's interactions will necessarily change as a result. Pain may limit a patient's social sphere. In certain instances, this may actually serve a subconscious psychological function. Most commonly, patients complain that the pain strips them of their desire to interact with other people and that they feel "too tired to do anything."

19. **What are the normal affective reactions to chronic pain?**
It is probably more useful to define affective reactions as adaptive or maladaptive rather than normal or abnormal. Frustration and irritability are common affective reactions, but the emotional energy can be channeled into job rehabilitation—an adaptive use of those emotions. Reactions that lead to insomnia and social isolation are maladaptive.

20. **How can family members influence the patient's response to pain?**
In classic behavioral theory, certain behaviors are reinforced and others are discouraged. Although some degree of solicitousness on the part of a spouse or caretaker is appropriate for a patient in pain, excessive attention to the complaint may lead to infantilization and less adaptive behaviors by the patient. Directly question families about how they react to the patient's pain complaints or behaviors.

21. **Why should family dynamics be assessed?**
In certain circumstances, family interactions can serve to perpetuate pain. For example, if a couple has been at odds, they may unite to combat a common enemy (the pain). When this happens, they have an investment in maintaining the complaint of pain to shift focus away from their own problems.

22. **Why are questions about sexual activity important?**
Surveys of patients with chronic pain have shown that a high percentage of both men and women experience pain-related difficulties with sexual activity. Difficulty with position, exacerbation of pain, problems with arousal, performance worries, low self-esteem, and increased tension in the relationship were among the more commonly reported issues. Problems with sexual intimacy can contribute to increased risk for depression and interfere with the exchange of emotional support between patient and significant other.

23. **What are the recommended approaches for eliciting a family history?**
It is often advisable to have the spouse or other family members present for part of the initial interview. This will serve to substantiate the patient's complaints and give some insight into family interactions. The clinician can judge whether the family is supportive and whether they have a shared objective. Issues of interpersonal dependence can be brought out.
   Observe how the family interacts in the office. Ask both patients and family members to describe their daily routines. Ask the significant other how he or she knows that the spouse is in pain and what his or her response is.

24. **Name some adaptive and maladaptive coping mechanisms exhibited by patients with chronic pain.**
Adaptive
   - Seeking information
   - Demonstrating interdependence (appropriate reliance on family members)
   - Setting realistic goals
   - Successfully reallocating tasks and roles
Maladaptive
   - Overdependency on the partner
   - Unwillingness to undertake activities that promote independence
   - Personal and social isolation
   - Excessive anger

25. **What is meant by "pain behaviors"? How should they be assessed?**
Pain behaviors are the outward signs of pain and suffering. They may include simple verbal expressions of pain, or physical manifestations such as grimacing, posturing, and limping. More complex behaviors include functional limitations, changes in social interaction, or seeking health care.

26. **What is meant by "secondary gain"?**
Secondary gain is when the patient is reaping tangible benefits from having pain. The benefits may be as obvious as compensation payments or as subtle as getting more attention from a family member. In classical psychological theory, primary gain is the psychological benefit of avoiding an anxiety-producing situation through the appearance of the symptom.

27. **What is the purpose of using "pencil-and-paper" tests?**
Questionnaires can save time. They outline the patient's problem and thereby streamline the evaluation. They also help the interviewer avoid getting sidetracked by unfocused discussions with the patient, and they can act as screening tools for psychological distress. Furthermore, the results can be categorized more readily. The typical questionnaire asks the patient to outline the course of the problem, describe treatments and medications already tried, rate pain intensity, and list comorbid medical problems.

28. **What is the Multidimensional Pain Inventory? What does it measure?**
The Multidimensional Pain Inventory (MPI) is a self-report inventory designed to canvass the patient's adaptation to chronic pain and the behavioral responses displayed by both the patient and significant others. The revised edition comprises 60 items that are categorized into 12 empirically derived scales, and these 12 are grouped into three scales. Analysis of the responses provides a means to classify the patient into one of three responder groups.

29. **List the contents of the MPI scales.**
The MPI scales include the following:
- Section 1: pain severity, interference, life control, affective distress, support
- Section 2: negative responses, solicitous responses, distracting responses
- Section 3: household activities, outdoor activities, activities away from home, social activity

30. **Name the three MPI profiles and their characteristics.**
The dysfunctional group is characterized by complaints of severe pain, a diminished sense of control, impaired lifestyle and enjoyment, and a high level of emotional distress.
The interpersonally distressed group reports high levels of pain, significant emotional distress, and perceived low levels of support from significant others.
The adaptive copers group comprises patients who report lower pain intensity, are not highly distressed emotionally, and display less functional impairment despite protracted pain.

31. **What is the Pain Patient Profile?**
The Pain Patient Profile (P3) is another self-response paper-and-pencil instrument containing both validity and clinical scales. This computer-scored index provides a clinical description along with commentary regarding presumed truthfulness of the respondent and the degree of emotional distress. There is some indication that this instrument may be useful in assessing individuals feigning pain, but further research is required.

32. **Which psychological measure is most widely used to assess patients with pain?**
The Minnesota Multiphasic Personality Inventory-2 (MMPI-2) is the most broadly used and validated scale. It is a self-report instrument that asks patients to answer 567 questions as true or false and attempts to classify patients according to personality types. Analysis of response patterns yields a psychological profile.
Unfortunately, this tool was first used in psychiatric patients who did not have chronic pain. Many of the questions answered by chronic pain patients would lead to their receiving a high score on the hypochondriacal scale.

33. **What is the most appropriate application of the MMPI-2?**
    The MMPI-2 should not be employed as a means of classifying a patient as "psychosomatic." Rather, a more appropriate use is to help the clinician formulate hypotheses with regard to the presence of comorbid psychopathology and personality characteristics that have the potential to influence the patient's adaptation to the pain experience and possibly interfere with treatment efforts.

34. **How have MMPI-2 profiles been grouped to help researchers and clinicians identify relevant clinical dynamics affecting the patient?**
    Research has replicated four primary cluster profiles: within normal limits, V-type, neurotic triad, and depressed pathological.

35. **What is the neurotic triad?**
    The neurotic triad refers to scales 1, 2, and 3 of the MMPI: hypochondriasis, depression, and hysteria. However, the label "neurotic" does not mean that the pain is inorganic. Elevations on the neurotic triad were found among arthritis patients who were clinically assessed as not very distressed. The conclusion is that the presence of a physical disorder automatically elevates scores on these scales simply as an accurate reflection of the underlying disease process, rather than neurotic tendencies.

36. **How has the MMPI-2 been employed in the assessment of compensation cases?**
    Various MMPI-2 scales have been touted as predicting the probability of a patient's returning to work, recovering from surgery, and benefiting from a variety of interventions. However, the accuracy rate of these complex predictions has been unsatisfactory. Recent research has suggested that one of the validity scales, "Fake Bad Scale," distinguishes between patients who are involved in litigation and those who are not. It may be viewed as an index of symptom magnification.

37. **What is the Symptom Checklist 90, Revised (SCL-90R)?**
    The SCL-90R was designed to quantify the degree of psychological distress. It assesses nine clinical dimensions: obsessive-compulsive disorder, depression, anxiety, paranoid ideation, somatization, interpersonal sensitivity, hostility, psychoticism, and phobic anxiety. Patients are asked to rate how much they are distressed by each of 90 described situations. Ratings are quantified on a 6-point scale, ranging from zero (not at all) to 5 (extremely).

38. **What indices are commonly used for assessing depression?**
    The Beck Depression Inventory (BDI), Center for Epidemiological Studies Depression Scale (CES-D), and Hamilton Depression Scale are among the most commonly employed screening devices. The BDI is a questionnaire consisting of 21 sets of statements; each set is ranked in terms of severity and scored from 0 to 3. The statements express feelings common in depression (e.g., guilt, low self-worth, and suicidal ideation). Each set includes 10 positive and 10 negative statements, and patients sometimes find it confusing.
    The CES-D is a self-administered questionnaire consisting of 20 items to which the patient indicates the frequency of experience during the past week. Cognitive, affective, and somatic items are incorporated into this index. The Hamilton Depression Scale consists of 17 items that are rated by the observer, rather than the patient.

39. **Which rating scales are useful to measure the patient's degree of disability and responses to treatment?**
    The Roland-Morris Disability Questionnaire (RDQ), Oswestry Disability Index (ODI), and Sickness Impact Profile (SIP) are three popular instruments that have been employed both for research and clinical assessment. Collectively, these instruments assess the patient's ability to engage in everyday activities: sleep and rest, eating, work, home management, recreation and

hobbies, ambulation, mobility, body care and movement, social interaction, alertness behavior, emotional behavior, and communication. Readministration of the chosen instrument will yield change scores that can be used to measure improvement or deterioration, as well as responsiveness to treatment.

40. **What is meant by "locus of control"? How does it affect chronic pain?**
   Locus of control (LOC) refers to a patient's perception of what it is that governs experiences. There are three categories: internal (the patient feels in charge), powerful others (caregivers or family members are in charge), and chance. These last two are referred to as external locus of control, and the first is internal locus of control. Patients with an external locus of control tend to adopt passive coping mechanisms, expecting others to provide remedies for their pain and seeing these remedies as ineffective.

41. **How is the concept of LOC applied in the treatment of patients with chronic pain syndromes?**
   One of the fundamental objectives of cognitive-behavioral–based therapy is to help shift maladaptive and self-defeating thoughts to more adaptive and self-confident ones. Shifting the LOC from external sources to an internal one provides a basis for building a stronger sense of self-efficacy (i.e., patients perceive themselves as being able to manage their pain rather than being victimized by it).

42. **What are some of the medical consequences of a history of abuse?**
   A history of emotional neglect, physical abuse, or sexual abuse is commonly elicited in patients with chronic pain. Victimized patients are more likely to report chronic upper and lower abdominal pain, fatigue, headache, back pain, shortness of breath, unexplained bleeding, chest pain, more lifetime surgeries, greater use of the health care system, functional bowel disorders, drug and alcohol abuse, and attempted suicides.

43. **Is there a relationship between a history of childhood abuse and chronic pain?**
   This is one of the most discussed topics in the field of chronic pain. Numerous studies have shown a correlation between self-reports of childhood victimization and complaints of nonmalignant pain. Acts of victimization have included sexual abuse, physical abuse, and emotional neglect. Generally speaking, individuals with past histories of abuse appear to be more likely to report more sites of pain and higher pain intensities than those without histories of abuse.

44. **Are there alternate ways to interpret the data indicating a relationship between past history of abuse and benign chronic pain?**
   Critics of the proposed relationship between history of abuse and chronic pain point out that self-reported retrospective data is always subject to distortion. There may be differential recall for specific events, and a patient's current status may prompt an emotional need to supply a rationale explaining the reasons for the negative experience of chronic pain. The more chronic, widespread, and intense the pain, the greater the need to explain it or blame someone for it.

45. **Name the pain complaint most often associated with a history of abuse.**
   As cohorts, women with chronic pelvic pain, vulvar pain syndromes, and fibromyalgia tend to report high incidence of some form of abuse. However, high rates of self-reported abuse, primarily during childhood, have been reported in clinical samples of patients with a wide variety of chronic pain syndromes. The general exception is individuals with arthritis whose symptom onset occurs later in life.
   On the basis of interviews and self-report compared with either normal controls or other pain sufferers without histories of abuse, the abused group scored higher on indices of psychological distress and somatization, tended to view themselves as disabled, perceived

themselves as lacking control, experienced social and vocational impairment, amplified reports of pain, and used dissociation as a coping strategy. Those who have suffered severe abuse appear to be more vulnerable.

46. Are males also subject to the effects of victimization?
Yes. Although females have been the primary focus of research, there has been some effort to assess the impact of victimization in males. A history of trauma in a male is believed to similarly impair his ability to manage pain effectively.

47. How can prior experiences of abuse impact the current rehabilitation process?
Among the long-term sequelae of any form of abuse are depressive symptoms, low self-esteem, and a sense of powerlessness. The process of rehabilitation requires that patients be motivated to recover, assert themselves to engage in those activities that will decrease symptoms while increasing functioning, and view themselves as worthy to be helped and to recover. Abused patients may view their pain as just another way they will continue to suffer. Lacking a sense of empowerment, these patients tend to be less likely to engage in rehabilitative efforts in their own behalf.

48. What is alexithymia?
The literal meaning of alexithymia is "no words for mood." The term is applied to those individuals who have difficulty describing their emotions. This phenomenon is commonly observed among those suffering from chronic somatic problems, including chronic pain. The construct is derived from principles of Western philosophy, which places an emphasis (positive value judgment) on the verbal expression of emotions. Possessing the ability to perceive and verbally express one's emotions is regarded as a reflection of mental health and maturity. In contrast, Eastern philosophy views somatization and intellectualized description of inner experiences as normative.

49. List some of the cardinal features of the alexithymic individual.
- The patient complains about countless physical symptoms.
- The patient displays an absence of fantasy production and rarely dreams.
- Speech content lacks relevant facts and is full of repetitive details.
- Interpersonal relationships are either dependent or estranged in nature.
- Clinicians often feel bored interacting with such individuals.

50. What are some proven means of assessing alexithymia?
Two approaches to alexithymia assessment have appeared in the literature. The 20-item Toronto Alexithymia Scale (TAS-20) is an established tool used for both research and clinical assessment. A more recent tool is the Observer Alexithymia Scale, which is designed for collecting and evaluating observer data. Five factors have been identified: distant, uninsightful, somatizing, humorless, and rigid.

51. What does the term "compensation neurosis" denote?
Compensation neurosis has traditionally carried a negative connotation. The construct presumes that the patient's complaints of pain and disability are motivated by the prospect of financial rewards, are encouraged by lawyers, and have little or no organic basis and that the patient's condition would improve dramatically and quickly upon receipt of a favorable settlement.

52. Are individuals receiving compensation for pain complaints less likely than those not receiving rewards to respond positively to treatment?
This has been and remains one of the more debated topics in the field of pain management. The general clinical impression is that receipt of compensation or the prospect of a litigious

windfall acts as a disincentive to participate actively and derive maximum benefit from rehabilitative efforts. Despite this popular belief, research data have failed to substantiate it.

53. **If the patient is applying for compensation and there are no organic findings, should you conclude that the pain problem is psychogenic in origin?**
No. The neuromedical examination may be negative in a number of pain syndromes (e.g., headaches or back pain). If gross inconsistencies between pain complaints and medical findings exist, questions should be raised—but don't draw hasty conclusions.

54. **What personality characteristics make an individual more prone to claiming disability?**
Dependent individuals who have low self-esteem, poor tolerance for stress, and lack the ability to deal with stress appear more apt to become a victim of an accident. These individuals are often dissatisfied with a stressful job and may also experience family and interpersonal tensions. They typically feel unable to cope with these problems effectively. Under these circumstances, a sanctioned disability provides a face-saving way to absolve the individual of personal responsibility, place the onus for recovery on the physician, and quietly avoid the undesirable situation. When reinforced by social acceptance (because the injury or illness is not their fault), financial factors (disability payment may be equal to that received for work), attention (sympathy from family and friends along with being the focus of inquiry by health care professionals), and dysfunction can rapidly become an entrenched way of life.

55. **What single factor is most predictive for return to work in the patient with back injuries?**
Although both physicians and patients alike tend to view organic findings (e.g., herniated disc) as the critical factor in predicting a return to functioning, the literature does not support this notion. In a series of clinical studies, the patient's fear of reinjury consistently accounted for the greatest proportion of the variance for predicting successful rehabilitation.

56. **Are there specific psychological symptoms or traits associated with patients experiencing chronic headaches?**
For decades clinicians and investigators have proposed that certain personality characteristics are associated with the occurrence of chronic headaches. Migraineurs have been described as anxious, depressed, hostile, obsessive, and rigid, with a tendency toward hypochondriasis. More recent research has again pointed to a tendency of individuals with mixed headache syndromes to be at greater risk of experiencing depression and prone to suppressing their anger.

57. **Is there a strong association between migraine and depression?**
Yes. Community-based studies have pointed to a link between depression and migraine. Estimated risk for first onset of major depression among migraineurs was 3.2-fold higher than in controls. The risk for migraine was 3.1-fold higher among those with histories of depression. Findings applied equally to both males and females, although women had a higher incidence of both disorders. The study concluded that there is a bidirectional influence between the two disorders.

58. **Are migraine sufferers at greater risk for affective disorders in general?**
Yes. Epidemiologic research has pointed to a relationship between migraine and affective disorders. However, the mechanism for this relationship remains unclear. There are two perspectives: (1) Migraine either causes or is a result of affective disorders, and (2) affective disorders and migraines share some common environmental or genetic etiology.

KEY POINTS

1. The purpose of a psychological evaluation in a patient with chronic pain is to evaluate the impact of the pain on the patient's functioning and to determine the role that the patient's psychological makeup has in his or her experience of pain.

2. The psychological evaluation is not designed or intended to differentiate between organic and psychogenic pain.

3. Physical and/or other abuse is often described in patients with chronic pain. As cohorts, women with chronic pelvic pain, vulvar pain syndromes, and fibromyalgia tend to report high incidence of some form of abuse.

BIBLIOGRAPHY

1. Alexander RW, Bradley LA, Alarcon GS, et al: Sexual and physical abuse in women with fibromyalgia: association with outpatient health care utilization and pain medication usage, *Arthritis Care Res* 11(2):102-115, 1998.

2. Ambler N, Williams AC, Hill P, et al: Sexual difficulties of chronic pain patients, *Clin J Pain* 17(2):138-145, 2001.

3. Bombardier C, Hayden J, Beaton DE: Minimal clinically important difference. Low back pain: outcome measures, *J Rheumatol* 28(2):431-438, 2001.

4. Coughlin AM, Badura AS, Fleischer TD, Guck TP: Multidisciplinary treatment of chronic pain patients: its efficacy in changing patient locus of control, *Arch Phys Med Rehabil* 81(6):739-740, 2000.

5. Edwards CL, Fillingim RB, Keefe F: Race, ethnicity and pain, *Pain* 94(2):133-137, 2001.

6. Fillingim RB: Sex, gender, and pain: women and men really are different, *Curr Rev Pain* 4(1):24-30, 2000.

7. Fillingim RB, Wilkinson CS, Powell T: Self-reported abuse history and pain complaints among young adults, *Clin J Pain* 15(2):85-91, 1999.

8. French DJ, Holroyd KA, Pinell C, et al: Perceived self-efficacy and headache disability, *Headache* 40(8):647-656, 2000.

9. Haviland MG, Warren WL, Riggs ML, Gallacher M: Psychometric properties of the Observer Alexithymia Scale in a clinical sample, *J Pers Assess* 77(1):176-186, 2001.

10. Lebovits AH: The psychological assessment of patients with chronic pain, *Curr Rev Pain* 4(2):122-126, 2000.

11. Okifuji A, Turk D, Eveleigh DJ: Improving the rate of classification of patients with the Multidimensional Pain Inventory (MPI): clarifying the meaning of "significant other," *Clin J Pain* 15(4):290-296, 1999.

12. Riley III JL, Robinson ME: Validity of MMPI-2 profiles in chronic back pain patients: differences in path models of coping and somatization, *Clin J Pain* 14(4):324-335, 1998.

13. Spertus IL, Burns J, Glenn B, et al: Gender differences in associations between trauma history and adjustment among chronic pain patients, *Pain* 82(1):97-102, 1999.

14. Tsushima WT, Tsushima VG: Comparison of the Fake Bad Scale and other MMPI-2 validity scales with personal injury litigants, *Assessment* 8(2):205-212, 2001.

15. Turk DC, Okifuji A: Matching treatment to assessment in patients with chronic pain. In Turk DC, Melzack R, editors: *Handbook of pain assessment*, 2nd ed, New York, 2001, The Guilford Press, pp 400-414.

16. Venable VL, Carlson CR, Wilson J: The role of anger and depression in recurrent headache, *Headache* 41(1):21-30, 2001.

17. Vendrig AA: The Minnesota Multiphasic Personality Inventory and chronic pain: a conceptual analysis of a long-standing but complicated relationship, *Clin Psychol Rev* 20(5):533-559, 2000.

18. Weisberg JN: Personality and personality disorders in chronic pain, *Curr Rev Pain* 4(1):60-70, 2000.

19. Whyte AS, Niven CA: Psychological distress in amputees with phantom limb pain, *J Pain Symp Manage* 22 (5):938-946, 2001.

NEUROIMAGING IN THE PATIENT WITH PAIN

Howard S. Smith, MD, FACP

CHAPTER 8

1. **What is the radiographic appearance of spinal metastases?**
   One of the earliest signs of spinal metastasis that may be seen on plain radiographic films is erosion of a pedicle. Eventually, the vertebral body begins to lose height, and magnetic resonance imaging (MRI) may reveal changes in the signal intensity in the vertebral body. Progression of tumor may invade the epidural space and compress the spinal cord.

2. **What is a common difference between the MRI appearance of vertebral body destruction caused by vertebral metastases versus that caused by vertebral osteomyelitis?**
   Tumors affecting the vertebral bodies tend to spare the disc spaces. Despite the fact that two or three adjacent vertebral bodies may be destroyed by tumor, the disc spaces between them tend to be preserved. In vertebral osteomyelitis, the disc space is generally destroyed by the infection and the adjacent vertebral bodies appear to form a block of infection.

3. **What types of abnormalities are evident on MRI but not apparent on computed tomography (CT)?**
   Intrinsic spinal cord pathology such as syringomyelia and multiple sclerosis plaques are uniquely observable by MRI.

4. **How is MRI performed?**
   MRI is carried out by subjecting patients to a sequence of radiofrequency (RF) pulses while they are inside a strong, fixed magnetic field. Images are then created by using various combinations of these RF pulses known as pulse sequences to map out various differing energy-releasing characteristics of tissues.

5. **What do T1 and T2 MRI images refer to?**
   T1 and T2 refer to different relaxation constants. In general, MRI scans that emphasize T1 characteristics, known as T1-weighted images, tend to define the outline of an anatomic structure, such as the spinal cord. Alternatively, T2-weighted images tend to be better at detecting specific areas of pathology such as edema surrounding a tumor, gliosis, demyelination, or hemorrhage.

6. **When is a CT of the spine useful versus MRI?**
   In general, MRI is preferable to image the spine in most situations because the spinal cord and nerve roots can be visualized without the need for intrathecal contrast. However, CT may be useful in the postsurgical spine, where metallic internal fixation devices may degrade MRI images.
   CT is also better for bone imaging and can more reliably detect calcific lesions such as ossification of the posterior longitudinal ligament (OPLL), which may be harder to visualize on MRI images. Also, CT may be better than MRI in patients with spondylolysis.

7. **In a patient with low back pain who has been previously operated on for a herniated disc, how can clinicians use imaging to help differentiate between a new disc herniation and scar tissue?**
Distinguishing between a new disc herniation and scar tissue may be very challenging. An MRI contrast agent known as gadolinium diethylenetriamine pentaacetic acid (DTPA) may be helpful. Gadolinium is a paramagnetic rare earth metal that causes shortening of the T1 relaxing time of tissues in which it accumulates. This creates brightening or enhancement on T1-weighted images.
   Gadolinium will usually not cause enhancement of discs or noninflammatory edema but tends to cause enhancement of most spinal tumors, as well as postoperative granulation tissue and many inflammatory processes.

8. **Do "open" MRI scanners produce the same quality images as the "closed" MRI scanners?**
No. Although patients who are extremely claustrophobic may not tolerate a closed MRI while awake, the image quality of the open MRIs is poorer. The open system magnetic field strength is 10% to 20% that of a closed system. Thus, images are derived from weaker radio signals emanating from the patient, and T2-weighted images have reduced sensitivity and image quality, even after newer techniques such as constructive interference in the steady state (CISS) are utilized.
   Although the image quality of the lumbar spine may be significantly reduced with the low-field ("open") scanners, the difference in image quality between low-field ("open") scanners and high-field ("closed") scanners tends to be much less dramatic with cervical spine imaging. This is because the small diameter of the neck allows the receiving coil to be close to the cervical spine, permitting the scanner to easily detect signals arising from spinal tissues.

9. **What are some situations that may be considered contraindications to MRI?**
If the patient has any ferromagnetic aneurysm clips, certain cardiac pacemakers, metallic foreign body in the eyes, Starr Edward mechanical cardiac valve, certain stapes and cochlear prostheses, or has had coronary bypass surgery in the past 24 hours, MRI is contraindicated.

10. **A 46-year-old woman comes to the emergency department complaining of the worst headache of her life, which occurred during sexual intercourse. She has a stiff neck and is somewhat sleepy. After a complete history and physical examination, what is the most appropriate imaging technique?**
A CT scan is the most appropriate imaging technique; it shows blood in the subarachnoid space in roughly 95% of patients with subarachnoid hemorrhage.

CHAPTER 9

TENSION–TYPE HEADACHE

Richard B. Lipton, MD, and Lawrence C. Newman, MD

1. **Is there a medical term for the headaches of everyday life?**
   Yes. The most common form of primary headache is tension-type headache (TTH). Almost everyone experiences a TTH at one time or another, and about 40% of the population has had one within the past year. Although occurrence is slightly higher in females, the gender ratio is very close to 1:1. Tension-type headache affects individuals of all ages but is most common in middle life. It is seven times more common than migraine but is much less disabling. Nonetheless, because it is so common, TTH causes a societal impact equivalent to or greater than that of migraine.

2. **What is meant by "primary" and "secondary" headache?**
   In primary headaches, the headache is the problem. In secondary headaches, the headache is symptomatic of an underlying condition such as a brain tumor.

3. **What is the approach to diagnosing tension-type headache?**
   The steps in the diagnosis of TTH resemble the steps in the diagnosis of migraine. Secondary headache disorders are excluded based on a directed history and a careful general medical and neurologic examination. If red flags are present, a workup is required to diagnose or exclude secondary causes of headache. If no alarms are sounded by history or exam, the next step is to diagnose a specific primary headache disorder. If the patient fits neatly into a standard diagnostic category, a diagnosis is assigned and treatment is initiated. If the headache is atypical and does not meet criteria for a primary headache disorder, revisit the possibility of a secondary headache.

4. **How is tension-type headache defined?**
   Tension-type headaches are characterized by recurrent attacks of head pain without specific associated features. To diagnose TTH, the International Headache Society requires a history of at least 10 lifetime attacks. Early in the course of TTH, however, patients will not yet have experienced that number of attacks. To make the diagnosis, two of the following four pain features should be present:
   - Pain on both sides of the head (bilateral pain)
   - Pain that is a steady ache or a pressure pain
   - Pain that is mild or moderate in severity
   - Pain that is not exacerbated by routine physical activity

   The pain of TTH is often bifrontal, bioccipital, or nuchal. It may be described as a squeezing sensation akin to wearing a hat that is too tight, as a headband of pain, or as a pressure sensation at the vertex of the head. On occasion, the pain is associated with palpation tenderness of the pericranial muscles. Headaches typically last from 30 minutes to several days, but a duration of several hours is most common.

5. **What is the frequency of TTH?**
   TTH is the most common type of headache experienced, with a lifetime prevalence of 88% in women and 69% in men.

6. **Are there different types of tension-type headache?**
It is traditional to divide TTH into two broad groups: episodic and chronic. By definition, episodic attacks occur less than 15 days per month (or 180 days per year), and chronic headache occurs 15 or more days per month for at least 6 months (or 180 days per year). Otherwise, the clinical features of the attacks are quite similar. Chronic TTH affects about 3% of the population.

7. **Discuss chronic tension-type headache in relation to chronic migraine.**
The differential diagnosis of chronic TTH includes chronic (or transformed) migraine. Although both chronic TTH and transformed migraine are characterized by frequent attacks of mild to moderate headache, these disorders are different. As the name implies, chronic migraine evolves out of episodic migraine, as headaches increase in frequency and decrease in severity, and the specific migraine features remit. Chronic TTH may arise de novo or in individuals with episodic TTH. Those with chronic migraine may have occasional episodes of full-blown migraine.

8. **What is the differential diagnosis of tension-type headache?**
Tension-type headache must be distinguished from other primary and secondary headache disorders. Its bilateral location, mild to moderate pain intensity, and absence of autonomic features make differentiating it from cluster headache relatively easy (see Chapter 11, Cluster Headache). Its distinction from migraine is discussed in Question 9. Underlying structural or metabolic causes must be considered in patients who have headaches resembling TTH.
Unfortunately, early in their course, brain tumors and other intracranial mass lesions tend to produce bilateral, dull headaches, which may be difficult to distinguish from TTH. Headaches resulting from brain tumors tend to progress in frequency and severity, and they are often associated with focal neurologic symptoms and signs or evidence of increased intracranial pressure (see Chapter 14, Brain Tumor Headaches). When headaches of similar profile have been present for months or years and the neurologic exam is normal, secondary headaches are unlikely.

9. **How are tension-type headache and migraine differentiated?**
The diagnostic features of TTH and migraine contrast rather sharply:

Migraine Pain	TTH Pain
Unilateral	Bilateral
Throbbing or pulsatile	Steady ache or squeezing/pressure sensation
Moderate to severe	Mild or moderate
Aggravated by routine physical activity (e.g., climbing stairs)	Not aggravated

In addition, TTH is characterized by an absence of the migraine-defining associated symptoms. Specifically, episodic TTH is generally not accompanied by aura or nausea and only rarely by photophobia or phonophobia (not both).

10. **How are tension-type headache and sinus headache differentiated?**
Tension-type headache and sinus headache are often confused. This is especially likely when the headache is frontal in distribution; the location over the frontal sinuses creates diagnostic confusion. Sinus headaches are associated with sinus tenderness, fever, and purulent nasal discharge. Sinus headaches rarely cause brief, recurrent headaches.

11. **What is the pathophysiology of tension-type headache?**
The mechanism of pain in TTH remains uncertain. This disorder was once called muscle contraction headache, based on the assumption that excessive contraction of skeletal muscle produced pain. The term "tension headache" was sometimes used to suggest that stress or psychologic tension was the fundamental cause of the disorder. The term "tension-type headache" is intended to imply that we do not know what, if anything, is "tense." Although there are excess levels of muscle contraction in TTH, these levels do not exceed those found in patients with migraine. Although stress is a trigger for some people with TTH, the disorder can occur in the absence of stress, and high levels of stress can occur without TTH.

Some believe that TTH is a form of mild migraine, but response to the drug sumatriptan suggests that this is true only in some patients. According to the Spectrum Study, sumatriptan effectively treats TTH in individuals who also have migraine. In individuals without migraine, sumatriptan is ineffective (see Chapter 10, Migraine). Factors that exacerbate TTH include oromandibular dysfunction, psychosocial stress, psychiatric disorders, and drug overuse.

12. **Is tension-type headache a genetic disorder?**
There is no clear evidence that episodic TTH runs in families. Recent studies do suggest that chronic TTH, like migraine, aggregates within families.

13. **What are the approaches to treating tension-type headache?**
The treatment of TTH, like the treatment of migraine, can be divided into two major categories: nonpharmacologic and pharmacologic therapies. The pharmacologic therapies are divided into acute (abortive) and preventive (prophylactic). Note that patients with mild and infrequent TTHs may simply be looking for a diagnosis and reassurance that the headaches do not have a serious cause. These patients may not need prescription drugs.

14. **What are trigger factors?**
Trigger factors precipitate headache in a biologically vulnerable individual, but they are not the fundamental cause of headache. When devising a treatment plan, it is important to begin by identifying factors that exacerbate or trigger headaches and to distinguish trigger factors from causes. Psychologic stress, perhaps related to a job or to a family situation, may be an important trigger factor. The traditional triggers of migraine, including dietary factors, missed meals, disrupted sleep, changes in the weather, and hormonal factors, occasionally contribute to TTH.

15. **True or false: caffeine can trigger a headache.**
Partially true: caffeine withdrawal can trigger a headache. If a patient drinks several cups of caffeinated beverages or takes caffeine-containing medications on a daily basis, the absence of caffeine can trigger headache. Some patients awaken on weekend mornings with a headache because they slept through their regular cup of coffee. Caffeine withdrawal headaches are quite common even in moderate caffeine users.

16. **What are the nonpharmacologic treatment options for episodic tension-type headache?**
Resolving stressful situations sometimes improves headache control. Stress management methods, including relaxation techniques or biofeedback, often are helpful. Cognitive-behavioral therapy also can be useful (see Chapter 43, Psychological Constructs and Treatment Interventions). Some patients find that postural factors (such as working long hours with an awkward head position) contribute to headache. For these patients, ergonomic changes in the workplace or simply getting up to stretch may be helpful. Regular meals, consistent sleep patterns, and exercise can help eliminate headache.

When TTH is associated with spasm or tenderness of the pericranial or cervical musculature, physical modalities, such as local application of heat or ice packs and the use of a cervical pillow are sometimes helpful. Diathermy, massage, and trigger point injections are also employed. Transcutaneous electrical nerve stimulation has been reported to alleviate TTH.

17. **What are the acute treatment options for episodic tension-type headache?**
TTH can be treated with simple over-the-counter (OTC) analgesics such as aspirin, acetaminophen (Tylenol), ibuprofen (Advil, Nuprin), naproxen sodium (Aleve), and ketoprofen (Actron, Orudis KT). OTC combination products that contain caffeine (Excedrin, Vanquish) provide a useful alternative. Clinical trials demonstrate that the addition of caffeine to a simple analgesic significantly increases pain relief. This effect is referred to as the analgesic adjuvancy action of caffeine.
    When OTC medications do not provide adequate relief, prescription drugs can be tried. Nonsteroidal antiinflammatory agents (NSAIDs) such as naproxen sodium (Anaprox), 550 mg, or diflunisal (Dolobid), 500 mg, may succeed when OTC NSAIDs could not. Isometheptene-containing capsules (Midrin) are useful and produce few side effects. The butalbital-containing and caffeine-containing products (Fiorinal, Fioricet, Esgic) are effective. Minor opioids, including codeine combinations (acetaminophen with codeine, butalbital with codeine [e.g., Fioricet with codeine]), are also effective. Transnasal narcotics (Stadol NS) are useful for severe TTHs refractory to other treatments; one must be concerned with the potential for overuse of these types of agents. In general, acute medications should not be used more than 2 or at most 3 days per week to avoid rebound headaches.

18. **What is rebound headache?**
The medications that are used to relieve headache can become a cause of headache if overused. Virtually any medication can cause rebound headache, and therefore it is important to limit the dose of all acute medications. On average, episodic TTHs occur twice per month. In chronic TTH, with 15 or more headache days per month, the risk of rebound headache is substantial.

19. **Why is caffeine found in so many headache remedies?**
When caffeine is taken at the time of a headache, it increases the efficacy of analgesics. For this reason, patients often learn to drink a cup of coffee when they take a painkiller or use combination drugs that contain caffeine. The best advice is to limit caffeine intake on nonheadache days (to one cup of coffee or tea a day) and to save caffeine for its medicinal effects on headache days.

20. **Do preventive medications have a role in the treatment of tension-type headache?**
Preventive treatment is used for only a small minority of patients who suffer from TTH. Preventive medication should be considered in patients who have disability because of headaches 3 or more days each month. In addition, preventive medication may play a role in treatment of patients at risk for rebound headache because of a frequent need for analgesics. If acute medication is ineffective or contraindicated, preventive therapy is a treatment option. Finally, if the patient has a comorbid condition (such as depression) that requires treatment, it is appropriate to treat both the headache disorder and the comorbid condition with a single drug, when possible.

21. **What are the preventive treatments of choice for tension-type headache?**
The most widely used drugs are the antidepressants. The tricyclic antidepressants are a standard choice. We prefer nortriptyline (Pamelor) and doxepin (Sinequan) because they have fewer anticholinergic side effects than amitriptyline (Elavil). The usual regimen starts with a low bedtime dose (10 or 25 mg), and the dose is gradually increased as needed and as tolerated. The selective serotonin-reuptake inhibitors (SSRIs) are sometimes used for prevention of

TTH. Fluoxetine (Prozac) has been shown to be effective in a small controlled study of chronic daily headache. The other SSRIs have not been studied but are widely used.

If antidepressants are unsuccessful or contraindicated, many of the drugs used for the prevention of migraine may also be used for TTH. Calcium-channel blockers and divalproex sodium are generally more successful than beta-blockers. Daily administration of NSAIDs is also sometimes used for prevention.

22. **Are the management approaches for chronic TTH and episodic TTH the same or different?**
Behavioral interventions to reduce the frequency of attack are especially important for chronic TTH. Although the acute treatment options are similar, because of the frequency of attacks, patients with chronic TTH are at increased risk for rebound headache. Use of acute treatments that cause rebound headache should be avoided or severely limited. It is usually desirable to treat these patients with preventive medications.

KEY POINTS

1. Tension-type headache is the most common type of headache experienced.

2. The mechanism of TTH is uncertain.

3. Both symptomatic and prophylactic therapies are available for the treatment of TTH. Prophylactic agents should be considered for those patients with TTH who are experiencing more than 3 days of headache-related disability each month.

BIBLIOGRAPHY

1. Couch JR: Medical management of recurrent tension-type headache. In Tollison CD, Kunkel RS, editors: *Headache diagnosis and treatment*, Baltimore, 1993, Williams & Wilkins, pp 151-162.

2. Headache Classification Subcommittee of the International Headache Society: The international classification of headache disorders, 2nd ed, *Cephalgia* 24(Suppl 1):9-160, 2004.

3. Jensen R, Bendtsen L, Olesen J: Muscular factors are of importance in tension-type headache, *Headache* 38:10-17, 1998.

4. Lipton RB, Bigal ME, Steiner TJ, et al: Classification of primary headaches, *Neurology* 63(3):427-435, 2004.

5. Rasmussen BK, Jensen R, Schroll M, Olesen J: Epidemiology of headache in a general population: a prevalence study, *J Clin Epidemiol* 44:1147-1157, 1991.

6. Schwarts BS, Stewart WF, Simon D, Lipton RB: Epidemiology of tension-type headache, *JAMA* 279:381-383, 1998.

7. Selby G, Lance JW: Observation in 500 cases of migraine and allied vascular headaches, *J Neurol Neurosurg Psychiatry* 23:23-32, 1960.

8. Solomon S, Newman LC: Episodic tension-type headache. In Silberstein SD, Lipton RB, Dalessio DJ, editors: *Wolff's headache and other head pain*, 7th ed, New York, 2001, Oxford University Press, pp 238-246.

9. Warner JS: The outcome of treating patients with suspected rebound headache, *Headache* 41(7):685-692, 2001.

CHAPTER 10

MIGRAINE

Richard B. Lipton, MD, and Lawrence C. Newman, MD

1. **Is migraine an important public health problem?**

   Migraine is a major public health problem by almost any standard. It is a highly prevalent disorder that affects 11% of the U.S. population and produces enormous suffering for individuals and their families. Recent estimates indicate that 28 million Americans suffer from migraine headaches; many experience severe pain and significant levels of headache-related disability. Economic estimates show that the cost of lost labor owing to migraine in the United States is $13 billion per year; these indirect costs resulting from missed work and disability at work greatly exceed direct medical expenditures on migraine treatment. In addition, headaches are the seventh leading reason for outpatient visits in the United States and account for 2% to 4% of all emergency room visits.

2. **What are the phases of the migraine attack?**

   It is useful to divide the migraine attack into four phases: premonitory, aura, headache, and resolution. The premonitory phase typically occurs hours or days before the headache. The aura usually occurs within 1 hour of headache onset but may begin during the headache. The headache phase is characterized by pain and associated symptoms. In the resolution phase, spontaneous pain subsides, but other symptoms are present. It is important to recognize that no phase is obligatory for migraine and that most patients do not experience all four phases.

3. **Describe the premonitory phase.**

   Premonitory features include changes in mood or behavior that precede the headache by hours or days. This phase is sometimes referred to as the postdrome. Patients may feel depressed, euphoric, irritable, or restless, and occasionally report fatigue or hyperactivity. Constitutional symptoms may include changes in appetite, fluid balance, and bowel function. Some patients report food cravings; others describe a poorly characterized feeling that an attack is coming. Premonitory features vary from person to person and from attack to attack.

4. **Describe the aura.**

   The aura consists of focal neurologic symptoms that usually precede, but that may accompany, the attack. Only 20% to 30% of migraine sufferers ever experience auras, and most people who have attacks with aura also have attacks without aura. Aura symptoms typically develop slowly, over 5 to 20 minutes, and usually last 60 minutes. Auras most commonly involve changes in vision, although changes in motor and sensory function may also occur. The classic visual aura of migraine is characterized by both positive symptom features, such as flashes of light (scintillations) or zigzag lines (fortification spectra), and negative symptom features, such as visual loss (scotoma). The visual aura may begin in a small portion of the visual field and gradually expand to encompass an entire visual hemifield.

Sensory auras are also characterized by a mix of positive (tingling) and negative features (numbness), sometimes beginning on one side of the face or hand and slowly expanding to encompass an entire side of the body. Hemiparesis may occur, and if the dominant hemisphere is involved, dysphasia or aphasia may develop.

5. **How do you differentiate migraine aura from other kinds of focal episodes of neurologic dysfunction?**
Transient neurologic deficits may have several causes. These include migraine aura, epileptic seizure, stroke, metabolic derangements, and psychiatric disease. Seizure is most typically characterized by positive phenomena such as tonic or tonic/clonic movements. Stroke is most often characterized by negative phenomena, such as weakness. Both seizures and stroke tend to come on relatively suddenly. The gradual evolution of symptom features and the mix of positive and negative features, as well as the temporal association with headache help identify migraine aura. The patient's age and risk-factor profile may also point the clinician in one diagnostic direction or another.

6. **What are the characteristics of the headache phase?**
The headache phase of migraine is characterized by a combination of pain and associated symptoms. Migraine pain has four characteristic features, and most migraine sufferers experience at least two of these. Migraine pain is typically:
   - Unilateral (may be bilateral at onset or may begin on one side and then become generalized)
   - Pulsatile (85% of patients, but this description is not specific for migraine)
   - Moderate to severe in intensity
   - Aggravated by routine physical activities (e.g., climbing stairs, head movement)

By definition, the pain of migraine must be accompanied by other features. Nausea occurs in about 75% of patients and vomiting in up to one third. Many patients experience sensory sensitivity in the form of photophobia, phonophobia, and osmophobia. Other accompanying features include anorexia or food cravings, blurry vision, nasal stuffiness, abdominal cramps, polyuria, and pallor. Although impaired concentration is common, measurable memory impairment has rarely been documented.

7. **What is the resolution phase?**
The resolution phase of the migraine attack begins as the pain wanes. Following the headache, the patient may feel irritable, listless, tired, or washed-out. Many patients report residual scalp tenderness in the distribution of the remitted spontaneous pain. Some patients feel unusually refreshed or euphoric after a migraine attack.

8. **What feature or features are absolutely required to diagnose migraine?**
It is important to recognize that no single headache feature and no single associated symptom is pathognomonic for migraine. For example, 20% to 30% of migraineurs have auras; the physician who relies exclusively on aura will usually miss the diagnosis. If nausea occurs in 75% of patients, the clinician who relies exclusively on nausea will miss 25% of cases.

In 1988, the International Headache Society provided a classification system for headache disorders. That system defined seven different types of migraine. The two most important types are migraine without aura and migraine with aura (Boxes 10-1 and 10-2).

BOX 10-1. DIAGNOSTIC CRITERIA FOR MIGRAINE WITHOUT AURA

A. At least five attacks fulfilling B–D.

B. Headache attacks lasting 4–72 hours (untreated or unsuccessfully treated).

C. Headache has at least two of the following characteristics:
1. Unilateral location.
2. Pulsating quality.
3. Moderate or severe intensity (inhibits or prohibits daily activities).
4. Aggravation by walking stairs or similar routine physical activity.

D. During headache at least one of the following:
1. Nausea and/or vomiting.
2. Photophobia and phonophobia.

E. At least one of the following:
1. History, physical, and neurologic examinations do not suggest secondary headache.
2. History and/or physical and/or neurologic examinations do suggest such disorder, but it is ruled out by appropriate investigations.
3. Such disorder is present, but migraine attacks do not occur for the first time in close temporal relation to the disorder.

BOX 10-2. DIAGNOSTIC CRITERIA FOR MIGRAINE WITH AURA

A. At least two attacks fulfilling B.

B. At least three of the following four characteristics:
1. One or more fully reversible aura symptoms indicating focal cerebral cortical and/or brain stem dysfunction.
2. At least one aura symptom develops gradually over more than 4 minutes, or two or more symptoms occur in succession.
3. No aura symptom lasts more than 60 minutes. If more than one aura symptom is present, accepted duration is proportionally increased.
4. Headache follows aura with a free interval of less than 60 minutes. (It may also begin before or simultaneously with the aura.)

C. At least one of the following:
1. History, physical, and neurologic examinations do not suggest secondary headache.
2. History and/or physical and/or neurologic examinations do suggest such disorder, but it is ruled out by appropriate investigations.
3. Such disorder is present, but migraine attacks do not occur for the first time in close temporal relation to the disorder.

9. **Describe considerations for diagnostic testing.**
Diagnostic testing in migraine serves primarily to exclude secondary causes of headache. The first step is to identify red flags that suggest the possibility of secondary headache (see Chapter 14, Brain Tumor Headaches). If the patient has no history of red flags, the general medical and neurologic exams sometimes raise the possibility of secondary headache. If there is a possibility of secondary headache, an appropriate diagnostic workup is required.

In the absence of alarms, the second step is to try to diagnose a specific primary headache disorder. If the patient has typical migraine or tension-type headache (TTH), it is appropriate to proceed with treatment. If there are atypical headache features, even in the absence of red flags, consider diagnostic testing to exclude secondary causes. If treatment is initiated and the expected response to therapy is not obtained, revisit the issue of secondary headache. However, because migraine and TTH are so common, it is neither appropriate nor cost-effective to obtain neuroimaging for every patient.

10. **What diagnostic tests are required to establish the diagnosis of migraine?**
There are no diagnostic texts required to diagnose migraine.

11. **Why is migraine considered a neurologic disease?**
Migraine is viewed as a disease of the brain. Changes in the brain give rise to inflammatory changes in cranial and meningeal blood vessels, which, in turn, produce pain. The premonitory phase, with its characteristic changes in mood, behavior, and autonomic function, is best understood on the basis of central nervous system dysfunction. Neuroimaging procedures, including positron emission tomography (PET), electroencephalogram, and magnetoencephalography, demonstrate abnormalities of the brain during or between attacks in patients with migraine. Finally, the drugs used to treat migraine often act on the brain, cranial nerves, or the cranial blood vessels.

12. **Describe the mechanism of the aura.**
The phenomenon of "spreading cortical depression" may underlie the aura of migraine. Spreading depression was originally described as a wave of excitation (depolarization) followed by a wave of inhibition that spreads over the cortical surface of experimental animals after mechanical or chemical stimulation. Neuronal activity decreases during a wave of inhibition, producing decreased cerebral blood flow through the mechanism of cerebral autoregulation. As a consequence, inhibition is accompanied by a wave of spreading oligemia (decreased blood flow).
  In migraine with aura, cerebral blood flow studies demonstrate a wave of oligemia that accompanies the aura, as predicted by the model of spreading depression. This wave of oligemia progresses at a rate of 2 to 3 mm per minute, the same rate reported for spreading depression in experimental animals. In addition, the rate of spreading oligemia and spreading depression corresponds with the evolution of the scintillating scotoma that marches across the visual field of the typical migraine aura. Spreading oligemia has been demonstrated using xenon inhalation and magnetic resonance imaging (MRI).

13. **What is the substrate of migraine pain?**
The work of Michael Moskowitz and co-workers suggests that the trigeminovascular system may be a final common pathway for migraine pain. The trigeminovascular system includes the trigeminal nerve and the cranial blood vessels that it innervates. The trigeminal nerve endings contain a wide range of neurotransmitters, including substance P, calcitonin gene–related peptide, and neurokinin A. Release of these transmitters causes a sterile inflammatory response within the cranial blood vessels accompanied by extravasation of plasma proteins. The fibers of the trigeminal nerve provide an interface between the blood circulation and the brain. The pain of migraine may result from the activation of trigeminal sensory afferents and the development of a neurogenically mediated inflammatory response.

14. **What is the role of serotonin in migraine?**
Serotonin plays a prominent role in pathophysiologic models of migraine. Blood levels of serotonin decrease during a migraine attack. Urinary concentrations of serotonin's metabolites increase during a migraine attack. A serotonin-releasing factor is present in the plasma of migraine patients during attacks but not at other times. In addition, activation of the serotonergic dorsal raphe nucleus causes migrainelike headaches. Finally, evidence from PET demonstrates increased metabolism in the brainstem in the region of the serotonergic dorsal raphe nucleus during migraine attacks.

15. **Discuss the serotonin receptors. What role might they play in migraine?**
The neuropharmacology of serotonin has become increasingly complex in recent years. There are many classes of serotonin receptors in the brain and blood vessels and many subclasses as well.

The 5-HT1 receptors might play a role in acute migraine therapy on at least two levels. One subtype of the 5-HT1 receptor is found on cranial blood vessels (5-HT1b), and another is found on trigeminal nerve endings (5HT1d). Activation of 5-HT1b receptors produces a vasoconstrictor response that may also play a role in relieving the pain of migraine. Activation of the 5-HT1d receptors on the trigeminal nerve terminal blocks the release of the mediators of neurogenic inflammation. Many of the acute treatments for migraine, including ergotamine, dihydroergotamine, and the triptans, are 5-HT1 agonists. The triptans are selective agonists for the 5HT1b/1d receptors. Receptors of this class are also found within the brain. The relative importance of these receptors on blood vessels, trigeminal nerve endings, and within the brain remains uncertain.

Many of the medications used as preventive treatments for migraine act on 5-HT2 receptors. Methysergide is a 5-HT2 receptor antagonist. Tricyclic antidepressants may act by downregulating the 5-HT2 receptor.

16. **What is the role of genetics in the pathophysiology of migraine?**
We have long known that migraine is a familial disorder. Twin studies demonstrate that identical twins are more likely to be concordant for migraine than fraternal twins. More recently, specific genetic linkages have been identified for the rare subtype of migraine known as familial hemiplegic migraine (FHM). FHM is characterized by hemiplegic migraine aura and is an autosomal dominant disorder. A locus on chromosome 19 for FHM has been identified; it codes for a pq type calcium channel, which has also been implicated in cerebellar ataxia. The genetic studies suggest that migraine may be caused by abnormalities in ion channels, a "calcium channelopathy." The chromosome 19 locus plays a role in some, but not all, families with FHM. Given that FHM is genetically heterogeneous, it seems virtually certain that there are multiple genetic forms for the other types of migraine, and it is also quite likely that there are nongenetic forms of the syndrome.

17. **List the steps in managing migraine.**
The U.S. Headache Consortium Guidelines illuminate an approach to managing migraine:
    1. Make a specific diagnosis.
    2. Assess the impact of illness and comorbidities.
    3. Develop a specific treatment plan.
    4. Identify factors that trigger the patient's headache, and counsel avoidance.
    5. Introduce other behavioral interventions.
    6. Provide medications to treat acute attacks.
    7. If indicated, provide preventive medications.
    8. Follow the patient, and modify treatment as necessary.

Obtaining a thorough headache history and understanding the impact of migraine on the patient's life are critical preludes to treatment. Educate patients and their relatives about the nature of migraine and the approach to therapy.

18. **How do you help patients identify their headache triggers?**
The first step toward helping patients identify their headache triggers, is to take a history. Many dietary triggers contain biologically active chemicals that act on blood vessels or the brain to initiate an attack. Often, patients are aware that alcohol, chocolate, or certain medications trigger their headaches. Despite the long list of putative triggers (Table 10-1), it is important to recognize that triggers vary widely from one person to another. Trigger factors may be difficult to identify because they cause a headache on one day but not on another. For example, a small glass of wine may not lead to a headache, but a half bottle of wine will initiate an attack.

TABLE 10-1. SELECTED MIGRAINE TRIGGER FACTORS	
Alcohol	Hunger
Aspartame	Light (bright or flashing)
Barometric pressure changes	Medication overuse
Cheese	Menstruation
Cigarette smoke	Monosodium glutamate
Estrogens	Odors (perfume, gasoline, solvents)
Excessive or insufficient sleep	Oral contraceptives
Head trauma	Stress and worry

Chocolate may cause headache during menses or at a time of stress but not at other times of the month. Patients should understand that triggers do not necessarily initiate an attack with every exposure. In addition, vulnerability to triggers varies widely from person to person.

19. **What other nonpharmacologic options for migraine treatment are available?**
In discussing nonpharmacologic treatment with patients, it is important to distinguish exacerbating factors from the fundamental cause of migraine. Stress worsens most illnesses, including asthma, heart disease, and ulcers. Just as stress can precipitate headaches, relaxation methods, including biofeedback, can diminish their severity or frequency. Behavioral interventions are often effective treatments and help give the patient a feeling of control.
   Nonpharmacologic prevention strategies include changing the diet, learning relaxation methods, using biofeedback, and applying cognitive-behavioral therapy. Biofeedback is a relaxation method that gives patients information about a measured physiologic parameter such as muscle activity (electromyography) or skin temperature. Biofeedback training can help decrease the frequency of attacks by reducing reactivity to stress. It can also be used to treat acute attacks in patients who have learned the methods well.

20. **Is migraine associated with psychiatric disease?**
Yes. Migraine is associated with depression, anxiety disorders, and manic-depressive illness. This comorbidity does not imply that migraine has psychogenic mechanisms. Perhaps perturbations in particular brain systems, such as the serotonin system, predispose patients both to migraine and to certain forms of psychiatric illness. When comorbid psychiatric disease is present, it is important to address it in treatment.

21. **Differentiate acute and preventive pharmacotherapy for migraine.**
The drugs used to treat migraine are generally classified as acute agents and preventive agents. Acute therapy is administered at the time of the attack to relieve pain and the associated symptoms of migraine and to restore the ability to function. Preventive therapy is taken on a daily basis, whether or not headache is present, to reduce the frequency and severity of attacks. Almost everyone with migraine needs acute treatments. A minority of migraine sufferers require preventive treatments.

22. **What is an appropriate strategy for migraine pharmacotherapy?**
There are a number of acute treatment options for migraine. When migraine is mild or moderate, simple analgesics such as aspirin, acetaminophen, or nonsteroidal antiinflammatory agents (NSAIDs) may be sufficient. Caffeine enhances the effectiveness of simple analgesics and

may have special benefits in migraine (e.g., Excedrin, Anacin). The addition of a barbiturate increases treatment effects in some patients (e.g., Fiorinal, Fioricent, Esgic); however, these compounds may be associated with an increased risk of sedation, rebound headache, tolerance, or dependence, so use them cautiously. Isometheptene is a simple, safe vasoactive compound that can be used in combination with analgesics to relieve headache. When nausea or vomiting is present, adding an antiemetic/prokinetic agent, such as metoclopramide, may enhance the effectiveness of the simple analgesics.

In addition, there is a category of migraine-specific acute treatments. These include ergotamine, dihydroergotamine, and the triptans.

23. **How do the migraine-specific acute treatments work?**
Migraine-specific acute treatments are believed to act on presynaptic 5-HT1 receptors on trigeminal nerve endings, on the blood vessels, and within the brain itself. Activation of the 5-HT1 receptor blocks the release of substance P, calcitonin gene–related peptide, and neurokinin A and ameliorates the development of neurogenic inflammation. Ergotamine and dihydroergotamine activate a broad range of receptors, whereas the triptans are highly selective for the 5-HT1 class of receptors. Other 5-HT1 agonist drugs are currently in development for the acute treatment of migraine.

24. **What triptans are available?**
As of this writing there are seven triptans marketed in the United States: sumatriptan (Imitrex), zolmitriptan (Zomig), rizatriptan (Maxalt), naratriptan (Amerge), almotriptan (Axert), frovatriptan (Frova), and eletriptan (Relpax).

25. **How do the available triptans compare?**
The marketed triptans are highly effective acute treatments for migraine. They are all agonists at 5HT1b/d receptors. They differ in pharmacokinetic profiles, modes of metabolism, available routes of administration, and, to some degree, in efficacy and tolerability. Sumatriptan was the first available agent in this class and is the most extensively studied and widely used of these agents. It is marketed in three oral doses (25, 50, and 100 mg), as a nasal spray, and as a subcutaneous injection. Zolmitriptan is available as 2.5-mg and 5-mg tablets, a nasal spray, and rapidly dissolvable oral wafers (ZMT). Rizatriptan is available as 5-mg and 10-mg tablets and wafers (Maxalt-MLT); it has efficacy advantages but similar tolerability to sumatriptan. Naratriptan is available as 1-mg and 2.5-mg tablets; it is less effective than sumatriptan but has superior tolerability and a lower rate of headache recurrence. Almotriptan is available as a 12.5-mg tablet and has similar efficacy but superior tolerability to sumatriptan. Frovatriptan is available as 2.5-mg oral tablets, and eletriptan is available as 20-mg and 40-mg oral tablets.

26. **How do you choose from among the acute treatment options?**
Acute treatments should be matched to the overall severity of the patient's illness, the severity of the patient's attack, the profile of associated symptoms, and the patient's treatment preferences. This strategy of individualizing treatment from the first is termed stratified care and is recommended by the U.S. Headache Consortium. It is supported by a randomized trial.

Simple analgesics and combination analgesics may be adequate for mild to moderate migraine attacks. More severe attacks often require specific migraine therapy. In addition, when nausea or vomiting is prominent, the associated gastric paresis may limit the effectiveness of oral agents. In this context, nonoral agents such as injections, suppositories, and nasal sprays offer advantages. Patients often have strong treatment preferences for one route versus another. Some patients consider suppositories anathema, and others would prefer to avoid injections. Many patients favor nasal sprays as the nonoral route of choice.

Treatment requirements also vary with the context of an attack. If an attack begins before a major business meeting, a rapid parenteral treatment may be needed. If the attack begins on a Saturday morning, the patient may prefer to use a slower oral treatment. Optimal therapy often requires that patients receive more than one treatment. The following are some examples of how treatment is tailored to match patient needs:

- For the patient who awakens with severe, full-blown attacks with prominent nausea and vomiting, nonoral therapy may be the only effective option.
- For patients who have attacks that begin gradually or who are unsure if the attack will be mild or severe, it is best to begin with oral agents and escalate therapy if the attack increases in severity.
- For a patient with both moderate and severe attacks, treatment may begin with an NSAID (plus metoclopramide), and a triptan can be used either as an "escape medication" or for the more severe attacks.

27. **What is the role of triptans in acute migraine therapy?**
The triptans are the most effective and most specific of the available acute treatments for migraine. Response rates to the 6-mg subcutaneous injection of sumatriptan are about 70% to 90%, depending on the study. Response to 50-mg sumatriptan tablets develops more slowly, with overall response rates of about 60% at 2 hours. The choice between oral and injectable triptans should be based on the need for rapid relief and the effectiveness of the alternative routes of administration. If the headaches begin slowly and gradually progress in severity, oral triptans are appropriate and preferred by most patients. For patients who awaken with disabling headache, who require very rapid relief, or who have prominent gastrointestinal disturbances, parenteral treatment offers important advantages.
  Note that subcutaneous sumatriptan should not be given during the aura. It is best to wait until pain develops before treating.

28. **When should acute medications be given during the migraine attack?**
Acute medications work most effectively when given while pain is still mild; this has been shown in post hoc analyses for aspirin plus metoclopramide, ergotamine, and sumatriptan and in specifically designed clinical trials for sumatriptan. The benefits of early treatment need to be balanced against the risks of rebound headache caused by medication overuse. For patients who can identify headaches likely to become disabling, outcomes may improve with early treatment. Though all treatments work best if given while pain is mild, these effects appear most pronounced for triptans.

29. **What are the contraindications for the triptans?**
All of the 5-HT1 agonists are contraindicated in patients with a history of myocardial infarction, ischemic heart disease, migraine with prolonged or complicated aura, and other forms of vascular compromise. Carefully evaluate patients with risk factors for heart disease before prescribing a triptan. Serious side effects are extremely rare, but mild side effects are common. These side effects include pain at the injection site, tingling, flushing, burning, warmth, and hot sensations. In addition, noncardiac chest pressure occurs in approximately 4% of migraine sufferers; be sure to advise patients of these adverse events.

30. **How do you treat the nausea and vomiting of migraine?**
The associated symptoms of migraine, including nausea and vomiting, may be as disabling as the head pain in some patients. Gastric stasis and delayed gastric emptying can decrease the effectiveness of all medications. Most acute medications relieve the nausea and the pain together. Triptans effectively relieve both pain and nausea. Antiemetics such as metoclopramide, promethazine, or prochlorperazine may be used to treat both the nausea and the pain of migraine.

31. **What is the role of opiates in the treatment of migraine?**
Oral narcotics, usually in the form of aspirin or acetaminophen and codeine (with or without caffeine and butalbital), are widely prescribed. If these agents relieve pain and restore the ability

to function, they provide an appropriate therapeutic option. However, because of the risk of tolerance, dependence, and rebound headache, they are best reserved for compliant patients with relatively infrequent attacks.

Injectable narcotics and antiemetics are still widely used in urgent care settings. In double-blind studies, these drugs have proved to be moderately effective at relieving pain. Pain relief may be accompanied by sedation, limiting the ability of these agents to restore normal function.

32. **What is the role of transnasal butorphanol (Stadol)?**
Transnasal butorphanol (TB) is a mixed opiate agonist-antagonist available as a nasal spray and sold under the brand name Stadol. The convenient route of administration leads to rapid absorption and pain relief even in patients with prominent nausea and vomiting. This therapeutic option is especially useful in patients with nocturnal headaches or prominent gastrointestinal symptoms, as well as those with contraindications, side effects, or lack of response to the migraine-specific agents.

TB produces sedation or orthostatic hypotension in about half of patients. Use should be limited to 2 headache days per week. Patients should be instructed to lie down after administration of the drug to minimize side effects.

33. **Who should get preventive therapy?**
Acute treatment is necessary for virtually everyone with migraine, but preventive medication should be used only under special circumstances, including the following:
   - When patients have two or more attacks per month that produce disability lasting 3 or more days per month
   - If symptomatic medication is contraindicated or ineffective (Even patients with less frequent pain and disability may be good candidates for preventive treatment in this case.)
   - When abortive medication is required more than twice a week
   - When headache attacks produce profound, prolonged disruption

34. **What are the preventive treatment choices?**
The major groups of medication used for migraine prophylaxis include the beta-blockers, antidepressants, serotonin antagonists, anticonvulsants, and calcium-channel blockers. Many of these agents work either by blocking 5-HT2 receptor sites or by downregulating them.

35. **How do you choose from among the preventive treatment options?**
If preventive medication is indicated, treatments are selected primarily based on side-effect profiles (Table 10-2) and comorbid conditions. For example, in a patient with migraine and hypertension, beta-blockers or calcium-channel blockers can be used to treat both conditions simultaneously. Similarly, in a patient with migraine and depression, antidepressants may be especially useful. In the patient with migraine and epilepsy, divalproex sodium or topiramate may be appropriate for both. For a patient with migraine and manic-depressive illness, divalproex sodium provides an opportunity to treat two conditions with a single drug.

Comorbid illnesses may also impose therapeutic restrictions. For example, in the patient with migraine and low blood pressure, beta-blockers and calcium-channel blockers are difficult to use. Similarly, in the patient with migraine and epilepsy, caution is advisable because antidepressants may lower seizure threshold. The patient with migraine and asthma or Raynaud's syndrome probably should not be treated with beta-blockers. Finally, in patients concerned about sedation or increased appetite, tricyclic antidepressants are not an appropriate choice.

TABLE 10-2. PREVENTIVE AGENTS FOR MIGRAINE

Category	Drug Name	Total Daily Dose	Daily Frequency	Side Effects
Beta-Blocker	Propranolol Nadolol Atenolol Timolol	80-320 mg 40-160 mg 50-100 mg 10-60 mg	2-4 times Once Once 1-3 times	Fatigue, depression, light-headedness, impotence. Should not be used or should be used with caution if patient suffers from asthma, emphysema, heart failure, or diabetes.
Calcium-Channel Blockers	Verapamil	240-480 mg	1-4 times*	Light-headedness, constipation.
Tricyclic Antidepressants	Amitriptyline Nortriptyline Doxepin	50-150 mg 50-150 mg 50-150 mg	Divided or at bedtime	Drowsiness, dry mouth, weight gain, blurred vision, constipation, difficulty urinating. Should not be used if patient suffers from glaucoma, prostate disorders, or arrhythmias.
Other	Methysergide	4-8 mg	3-4 times with meals	Nausea, hallucinations, tingling of extremities, retroperitoneal fibrosis. Must have a 1-month drug-free period after 6 months of treatment. Use other ergot preparations with caution.
	Cyproheptadine	12-32 mg	3-4 times	Drowsiness, increased appetite, weight gain.
	Divalproex	500-2000 mg daily	2-4 times	Tremor, sedation, weight gain, hair loss, hepatic dysfunction.

*Ordinary verapamil must be administered in divided doses. There is a sustained release preparation that can be used once daily.

36. **What are the principles of using preventive drugs?**

In general, drugs should be started at a relatively low dose to avoid side effects. The dose should then be gradually increased until therapeutic effects develop, side effects develop, or the ceiling dose for the agent in question is reached. Because of the need to gradually increase the dose of most of these drugs, a therapeutic trial may take several months. Patients should be advised that treatment effects develop slowly, so that therapy is not discontinued prematurely.

If one agent fails after an adequate therapeutic trial, it is best to choose an agent from a different therapeutic category. However, in the presence of strong relative indications or contraindications, it may be appropriate to choose a second agent within the same category.

37. **What is chronic or transformed migraine?**

Chronic or transformed migraine is the single most common condition seen in headache specialty centers in the United States. The patient with chronic migraine typically begins with ordinary attacks of episodic migraine. Over time, attacks increase in frequency but may decrease in average severity. The patient is left with a condition characterized by daily or near-daily attacks that resemble tension-type headache, often with superimposed interval headaches with most or all of the features of full-blown migraine. Chronic migraine must be defined based on a longitudinal history of headache, not simply the headache features at the time of consultation.

38. **Why is chronic migraine a formidable therapeutic challenge?**

Eighty percent of patients with transformed migraine overuse analgesics, combination tablets, or ergot alkaloids. These medications sustain the cycle of ongoing daily headache through the mechanism of medication withdrawal. The key to treatment is eliminating the overused medications. Preventive therapies generally do not become fully effective until the pattern of medication overuse is broken.

39. **How is chronic migraine treated?**

The best approach to treating transformed migraine is prevention. Rebound headaches can be prevented by restricting the use of all acute medications to 2 or at most 3 days per week. Particular caution is needed with analgesics containing caffeine, narcotics, or barbiturates and ergotamine. NSAIDs can be used more frequently with minimal risk of rebound headache. Triptans have been reported to cause rebound headaches. In the outpatient setting, the treatment of rebound headache generally involves substituting a NSAID for the overused medication. Particular caution is needed to avoid barbiturate and opiate withdrawal. At times, rebound headaches may require inpatient therapy.

40. **Who needs inpatient treatment, and why?**

The overwhelming majority of migraine sufferers do not require inpatient treatment. Inpatient treatment is indicated when patients experience frequent, disabling attacks that do not respond to optimal outpatient therapy. Patients with significant medical or psychiatric comorbidities, patients who are emotionally exhausted by ongoing pain, and patients who are fearful of headache pain sometimes require inpatient therapy. For these patients, early inpatient treatment may be optimally cost-effective.

The key to inpatient treatment of transformed migraine is the use of parenteral drugs such as intravenous dihydroergotamine in combination with metoclopramide. These agents are often given every 8 hours over a period of several days to taper the pattern of medication overuse. At the same time, an effective program of migraine prevention is initiated, and various behavioral modalities of pain control are introduced.

KEY POINTS

1. Migraine is a highly prevalent health problem that affects approximately 11% of the U.S. population.

2. There are no specific tests that are required to diagnose migraine; rather, diagnostic testing is used when the clinical suspicion is high that a secondary headache disorder is present.

3. Acute migraine treatment will be necessary for virtually everyone with migraine.

4. Preventive medication should be used for patients who have two or more attacks per month that produce disability lasting 3 or more days per month, when acute migraine therapies are contraindicated or ineffective, when abortive medication is required more than twice a week, and/or when headache attacks produce profound, prolonged disruption.

BIBLIOGRAPHY

1. Goadsby PJ, Lipton RB, Ferrari MD: Migraine: current understanding and management, *New Engl J Med* 346:257-270, 2001.

2. Headache Classification Subcommittee of the International Headache Society: The international classification of headache disorders, 2nd ed, *Cephalgia* 24(Suppl 1):9-160, 2004.

3. Lipton RB, Goadsby PJ, Sawyer J, et al: Migraine: diagnosis and assessment of disability, *Rev Contemp Pharmacother* 11:63-73, 2000.

4. Silberstein SD: for the US Headache Consortium: Practice parameter: evidence-based guidelines for migraine (an evidence-based review); report of the Quality Standards Subcommittee of the American Academy of Neurology, *Neurology* 55:754-762, 2001.

5. Silberstein SD, Saper JR, Freitag FG: Migraine: diagnosis and treatment. In Silberstein SD, Lipton RB, Dalessio DJ, editors: *Wolff's headache and other head pain*, 7th ed, New York, 2001, Oxford University Press, pp 121-238.

CHAPTER 11

CLUSTER HEADACHE

Lawrence C. Newman, MD, and Richard B. Lipton, MD

1. **What is a cluster headache?**

   Like migraine, cluster is a primary headache disorder but with significantly different clinical features. Cluster headaches are characterized by attacks of excruciatingly severe, unilateral head pain. Attacks last 15 to 180 minutes and recur from once every other day up to eight times daily. These painful episodes are associated with autonomic features, including ptosis, miosis, conjunctival injection, lacrimation, and rhinorrhea, on the side of the pain.

   In episodic cluster, attacks occur in "clusters" lasting weeks to months, separated by periods of pain-free "remission" lasting months to years. Times of frequent headache are called cluster periods.

   The Second Edition of the International Classification of Headache Disorders (ICHD II) defines five clinical criteria for cluster headache (Box 11-1).

BOX 11-1. ICHD DIAGNOSTIC CRITERIA FOR CLUSTER HEADACHE

(A) At least five attacks fulfilling B-D

(B) Severe or very unilateral orbital, supraorbital, and/or temporal pain lasting 15 to 180 minutes if untreated[1]

(C) Headache is accompanied by at least one of the following signs, which have to be present on the pain side:

    (1) ipsilateral conjunctival injection and/or lacrimation

    (2) ipsilateral nasal congestion and or rhinorrhea

    (3) ipsilateral eyelid edema

    (4) ipsilateral forehead and facial sweating

    (5) ipsilateral miosis and/or ptosis

    (6) a sense of restlessness or agitation

(D) Attacks have a frequency from one every other day to 8 per day[2]

(E) Not attributed to another disorder[3]

ICHD = International Classification of Headache Disorders.

[1] During part (but less than half) of the time-course of cluster headache, attacks may be less severe and/or of shorter or longer duration.

[2] During part (but less than half) of the time-course of cluster headache, attacks may be less frequent.

[3] History and physical and neurologic examinations do not suggest any of the disorders listed in groups 5 to 12, or history and/or physical and/or neurologic examinations do suggest such disorder, but it is ruled out by appropriate investigations, or such disorder is present, but attacks do not occur for the first time in close temporal relation to the disorder.

---

2. **Are cluster headaches common? Who is affected?**

   Fortunately, cluster headache is relatively rare, affecting approximately 0.05% to 0.1% of the U.S. population. Cluster headache is one of only two headache disorders that occur more often in men. Men are affected 3.5 to 7 times more often than women. In contrast, migraine occurs in women 3 times more often than in men. Most patients begin experiencing cluster headache between the ages of 20 and 50 (mean age is 30), though the age of onset ranges from early childhood through age 80.

Women with cluster have a later average age of onset than men. Unlike migraine, there is no link between menses and cluster headaches; like migraine, clusters may disappear during pregnancy and may be triggered by the use of oral contraceptives.

3. **What are the characteristics of cluster headaches?**
The pain of cluster begins abruptly, usually without warning, and reaches maximum intensity within 1 to 15 minutes. The pain is excruciating, deep, and boring and is often described as a "red-hot poker" in or behind the affected eye. The pain is usually most severe in the orbital and retroorbital regions and may radiate into the ipsilateral temple, upper teeth and gums, and neck. Unlike migraine pain, which may alternate sides, the pain of cluster is generally unilateral; only 10% to 15% of sufferers report side-shift in subsequent bouts. Rarely, patients with typical cluster report that an aura—identical to that described in migraine—precedes an attack.

4. **When do bouts occur?**
The majority of cluster sufferers note a phenomenon called periodicity—attacks recur around the same time each day during the entire cluster cycle. Approximately 75% of attacks occur between 9 PM and 10 AM. About half of all cluster sufferers report nocturnal attacks that awaken them from sleep. Attacks typically occur within 2 hours of falling asleep and are often associated with REM sleep.

Manzoni et al studied attack characteristics in 180 cluster sufferers and noted a higher incidence of individual attacks occurring between 1 to 2 AM, 1 to 3 PM, and at 9 PM. Thus, cluster patients cycle in and out of cluster periods, but during cluster periods the individual headaches occur with regular patterns. For these reasons, cluster is considered a chronobiologic disorder.

5. **What is the explanation for periodicity of cluster headache?**
Recent evidence points to a dysfunctional hypothalamic pacemaker. The suprachiasmatic nucleus of the hypothalamus controls circadian rhythms such as the sleep-wake cycle and regulates secretion of melatonin by the pineal gland. Dysfunction of the suprachiasmatic nucleus could explain the periodicity of cluster headache. Positron emission tomography (PET) scans during acute bouts of cluster headache have revealed increased activation in the region of the hypothalamic gray matter.

6. **What is known about the pathophysiology of cluster headaches?**
Although the exact pathophysiologic mechanism is not fully understood, recent work has given us insight into the pathways and stuctures that are most likely involved. The pain of cluster is carried into the central nervous system through the nociceptive branches of the first division of the trigeminal nerve. This branch (V_1), innervates the pain-sensitive intracranial structures such as the dura and its blood vessels, and activation of the trigeminovascular pathway causes the release of substance P and calcitonin gene-related peptide (CGRP). CGRP release produces vasodilation of the dural blood vessels and induces neurogenic inflammation. Activation of this system in cluster is evidenced by the findings of increased blood levels of CGRP in the external jugular vein during an acute attack of cluster.

The autonomic features that accompany the pain suggest that there is activation of the cranial parasympathetic pathway. Fibers within this pathway originate from neurons arising within the superior salivatory nucleus. These first-order neurons travel with the seventh cranial nerve, synapsing in the pterygopalatine ganglia. The postganglionic fibers supply vasomotor and secretory innervation to the cerebral vessels, lacrimal glands, and nasal mucosal glands, which produces the clinical features seen with cluster. A marker for cranial parasympathetic activation, vasoactive intestinal peptide (VIP), is also elevated in the external jugular blood during cluster attacks. These pathways have been termed the trigeminal autonomic reflex.

The Horner's syndrome that accompanies cluster is postganglionic and likely located within the cavernous sinus because it is here that the sympathetic, parasympathetic, and trigeminal fibers meet. It is possible, therefore, that activation of both the trigeminovascular and cranial parasympathetic systems occurs in the setting of a disordered hypothalamic pacemaker that may be dysfunctional during the cluster period.

7. **Are cluster headaches triggered by the same things as migraine?**
   A very small minority of cluster sufferers report that typical migraine triggers induce their headaches. These include stress, relaxation after stress, exposure to heat or cold, and certain foods such as chocolate, dairy, or eggs. Alcohol is a common precipitant of cluster headache, affecting over half of all sufferers. Alcohol tends to trigger attacks 5 to 45 minutes after ingestion. Interestingly, this trigger is present only during the active "cluster" phase of the disorder; imbibing alcohol-containing beverages during the "remission" phase does not trigger an attack. Sublingual nitroglycerine can also induce attacks.

8. **Are there different types of cluster?**
   Yes. Typical cluster may be divided into two forms: episodic and chronic. About 90% of cluster sufferers experience the episodic form, in which discrete attacks recur in cycles, usually lasting 1 to 3 months, separated by pain-free remissions lasting from 1 month to several years. Many patients with episodic cluster headaches experience one or two bouts yearly (typically in the spring or fall).

   In chronic cluster, attacks recur on a daily or near-daily basis for more than 1 year without remission or with remissions lasting less than 1 month. Chronic cluster has two temporal profiles: (1) in some patients the chronic form begins from onset (peviously classified as primary chronic), and (2) others begin with an initially episodic form that evolves into the chronic form (previously called secondary chronic). The evolving subtype affects approximately 10% of cluster sufferers, and may occur more frequently in patients who experience a later onset of the episodic form.

   The ICHD II also considers the paroxysmal hemicranias as a form of cluster headache. (See Chapter 12, The Paroxysmal Hemicranias.)

9. **How are cluster headaches diagnosed?**
   The diagnosis of cluster headache rests primarily on the history. Despite the distinctive features of the headache, cluster sufferers consult an average of five physicians prior to receiving the correct diagnosis! Their severe headaches are often misdiagnosed as migraine. Or, if pain radiates into the upper teeth and gums, it is mistakenly related to dental pathology. Frontal pain, nasal congestion, and/or rhinorrhea may be attributed to sinus disease. Refer to Box 11-1.

10. **How is cluster headache differentiated from the paroxysmal hemicranias?**
    Features of cluster that distinguish it from the paroxysmal hemicranias include the following: an overwhelming male predominance, a lack of mechanical trigger mechanisms, a lesser number of daily attacks, a longer duration of each attack, and specific patterns of treatment response (Table 11-1).

TABLE 11-1. DIFFERENTIAL DIAGNOSIS OF CLUSTER HEADACHES

	Cluster	Hemicrania Continua	Migraine	Paroxysmal Hemicranias
Sex F:M	1:6	1.8:1	3:1	2.13:1
Age of onset	20-40	11-58	Teens-20s	6-81
Pain quality	Stabbing, boring	Baseline dull ache, superimposed throbbing/stabbing	Throbbing, pulsatile	Stabbing, pulsatile, throbbing
Site of maximal pain	Orbit/temple	Orbit/temple	Temple/forehead	Orbit/temple
Attacks per day	0-8	Varies	0-1	1-40
Duration of untreated attacks	15-180 min (average 20-45)	Minutes→days	4-72 hr	2-120 min (average 2-25)
Autonomic features	+	+ (but less pronounced than cluster)	–	+
Aura	–	–	+ in 15-20%	–
Patient's behavior during attack	Pacing/rocking	Pacing or rest	Rest/sleep	Pacing/rocking
Oxygen may abort acute attacks	+ in 80%	–	+ in 20%	–

11. **How do you determine whether a headache is cluster or migraine?**
Cluster is differentiated from migraine by a number of important features. Migraine tends to be more prevalent in females, begins at an earlier age, demonstrates side-shift from attack to attack, and is associated with nausea, vomiting, photophobia, phonophobia, and osmophobia. In migraine, attacks last longer, do not occur multiple times daily, and are usually not associated with autonomic features ipsilateral to the pain. Additionally, only rarely is there an aura in cluster (see question 3). During cluster, patients pace, sit upright in a chair, or bang their heads against a wall, whereas migraineurs lie quietly in a dark room and attempt to sleep. Of note, recumbency actually increases the pain of cluster.
    There are headaches with features of both migraine and cluster that cannot be adequately categorized in either group. These patients often have an intermediate disorder referred to as cluster-migraine variant.

12. **How is cluster headache differentiated from hemicrania continua?**
Hemicrania continua is an underrecognized, benign disorder characterized by a continuous, baseline, low-level discomfort. Sufferers report exacerbations of more severe pain, lasting from 5 minutes to a few days, superimposed on the baseline pain. These exacerbations are often associated with the ipsilateral autonomic features of cluster, although if present, they tend to be less pronounced than in cluster. The disorder is mistaken for cluster if the clinician or patient focuses on the exacerbations and misses the continuous, less severe pain. Hemicrania continua is uniquely responsive to treatment with indomethacin and fails to remit with standard anticluster therapy.

13. **Is it possible to prevent cluster attacks?**

Yes. Nearly all patients with cluster headache require preventive treatment. The short duration, high frequency, and remarkable severity of attacks make acute treatment unsatisfactory. A variety of anticluster agents can be used (Table 11-2).

Most headache specialists begin treatment with verapamil and a prednisone taper. Prednisone usually induces a rapid remission, but it has too many side effects for long-term use. Verapamil is generally safe and well tolerated, but its benefits develop over 1 to 2 weeks. Accordingly, prednisone is started at 60 to 80 mg daily for 1 week. In the second week, prednisone is tapered by 10 mg per day. Verapamil is started at a dose of 240 mg daily and often increased to 480 mg per day if tolerated. Sometimes, additional dose escalations are required. Prednisone is intended to induce a rapid remission; verapamil is intended to prevent attacks until the cluster cycle is over.

If verapamil fails, lithium carbonate may also be tried. Lithium tends to be more efficacious in the chronic form. Valproic acid has been proven useful in both forms.

TABLE 11-2. TREATMENT OF CLUSTER HEADACHES

Drug	Dose (mg/day)	Comments
Medications used preventively		
Verapamil	240-960	Useful in all forms; sometimes doses above the 480-mg maximum on the label are required
Valproic acid	500-3000	Useful in all forms
Lithium carbonate	300-1500	Best for chronic cluster
Methysergide	4-10	Best for episodic form; must discontinue every 6 months for 1 month drug-free holiday
Medications used abortively		
Oxygen	8-10 mg L/min via face mask for 10-15 min	
Sumatriptan	6 mg SQ	Maximum of two injections daily
Dihydroergotamine	0.5-1 mg SQ/IM	Maximum 2 mg/day and 6 mg/week

14. **How long should prophylactic therapy be continued?**

Patients should be maintained on preventive medications for slightly longer than their typical cycles; for example, if the cluster period usually lasts 6 weeks, keep patients on their anticluster regimen for 8 weeks and then gradually taper the preventive medications. Recurrences are treated by adjusting the dosage upward, then retapering at a later date.

15. **How are acute attacks treated?**

The two acute treatment alternatives for cluster are oxygen and sumatriptan. Oxygen is usually administered via face mask or nasal cannula for 10 to 15 minutes. Subcutaneous sumatriptan 6 mg rapidly aborts attacks of cluster in 5 to 10 minutes in most patients. Unfortunately, the drug cannot be given more than twice daily, and sufferers may have more than two attacks daily. Dihydroergotamine (DHE) administered intramuscularly or subcutaneously is also effective. Ergot suppositories at bedtime may prevent nighttime headaches in patients with nocturnal attacks.

DHE is not specifically indicated for cluster headache. Sumatriptan has received FDA approval for treatment of cluster headaches.

16. **If these medications fail to break the attacks, what else can be done?**
    Medically refractory patients can be treated in a number of ways. Hospitalization and treatment with repetitive dihydroergotamine and metoclopramide every 8 hours has been proven to break cluster cycles. Alternatively, ipsilateral occipital nerve blocks occasionally help. For patients refractory to these treatments, percutaneous glycerol injections into the trigeminal cistern, percutaneous radiofrequency trigeminal rhizotomy, or decompression of the nervus intermedius can be tried. Recently, success has been reported in a small series of patients with intractable cluster headaches treated with hypothalamic deep brain stimulation.

17. **Name a few potentially dangerous syndromes that can present with symptoms similar to cluster headache.**
    The differential diagnosis has to include any syndromes that can present with retroorbital pain and ptosis. One of the more serious syndromes is carotid artery dissection. Pain is sometimes felt behind the eye and, because the sympathetic fibers ascend with the carotid artery, there may be a Horner's syndrome. Similarly, disease in the cavernous sinus can produce periorbital pain and ptosis. However, in these patients the pupil is usually large, rather than small, because the ptosis is due to a third-nerve palsy, rather than sympathetic dysfunction.

KEY POINTS

1. Cluster headaches are characterized by attacks of excruciatingly severe, unilateral head pain; 75% of the attacks occur between 9 PM and 10 AM.

2. The pain of cluster begins abruptly, usually without warning, and reaches maximum intensity within 1 to 15 minutes. The pain is excruciating, deep, and boring and is often described as a "red-hot poker" in or behind the affected eye.

3. In contrast to migraine, men are affected more commonly than women.

4. Both acute and chronic forms of cluster headache exist.

5. The practitioner should be aware of the specific acute and prophylactic therapies that are effective for cluster headache.

BIBLIOGRAPHY

1. Bahra A, May A, Goadsby PJ: Cluster headache: a prospective clinical study with diagnostic implications, *Neurology* 58(3):354-361, 2002.
2. Ekbom K, Hardebo JE: Cluster headache: etiology, diagnosis and management, *Drugs* 62(1):61-69, 2002.
3. Headache Classification Subcommittee of the International Headache Society: The international classification of headache disorders, 2nd ed, *C. Cephalgia* 24 (Suppl 1):9-160, 2004.
4. Leone M, Bussone G: A review of hormonal findings in cluster headache: evidence for hypothalamic involvement, *Cephalgia* 13:309-317, 1993.
5. Leone M, Franzini A, Broggi G, Bussone G: Hypothalamic deep brain stimulation for intractable cluster headache: a 3 year follow-up, *Neurol Sci* 24 (Suppl 2):143-145, 2003.
6. Manzoni GC, Terzano TG, Bono G, et al: Cluster headache—clinical features in 180 patients, *Cephalgia* 3:21-30, 1983.
7. May A, Bahra A, Buchel C, et al: Hypothalamic activation in cluster headache attacks, *Lancet* 351:275-278, 1998.

8. May A, Bahra A, Buchel C, et al: PET and MRA findings in cluster headache and MRA in experimental pain, *Neurology* 55(9):1328-1335, 2000.

9. Newman LC, Goadsby P, Lipton RB: Cluster and related headaches, *Med Clin North Am* 85:997-1016, 2001.

10. Newman LC, Lipton RB, Solomon S: Hemicrania continua: ten new cases and a review of the literature, *Neurology* 44:2111-2114, 1994.

11. Swanson JW, Yanagihara T, Stang PE, et al: Incidence of cluster headaches: a population-based study in Olmstead County, Minnesota, *Neurology* 44:433-437, 1994.

12. Tahu JM, Tew JM: Long-term results of radio frequency rhizotomy in the treatment of cluster headache, *Headache* 35:193-196, 1995.

CHAPTER 12

THE PAROXYSMAL HEMICRANIAS

Lawrence C. Newman, MD, and Richard B. Lipton, MD

1. **What are the paroxysmal hemicranias?**
   The paroxysmal hemicranias are a group of rare, benign headache disorders that resemble cluster headache in most ways but do not respond to anticluster medications. The headaches are characterized by severe, excruciating, throbbing, boring, or pulsatile pain affecting the orbital, supraorbital, and temporal regions. These pains are associated with at least one of the following signs or symptoms ipsilateral to the painful side:
   - Conjunctival injection
   - Lacrimation
   - Nasal congestion
   - Rhinorrhea
   - Ptosis
   - Eyelid edema

   Attacks occur from 1 to 40 times daily, usually exceeding eight attacks in a 24-hour period. Duration is typically 2 to 30 minutes, but on rare occasions attacks last as long as 2 hours. Headaches may occur any time during the day or night, and there is often a predisposition to nocturnal attacks, in which the patient is awakened from a sound sleep by an incapacitating headache.

2. **Are there different clinical variations of the paroxysmal hemicranias?**
   Yes. Although there has been controversy regarding the nomenclature of the paroxysmal hemicranias, there appear to be three related forms:
   - Chronic paroxysmal hemicrania (CPH), in which multiple headaches occur daily for years on end without remission or with remission periods of less than 1 month
   - Episodic paroxysmal hemicrania (EPH), in which there are discrete phases characterized by frequent daily attacks separated by long-term, pain-free remissions
   - Pre-CPH, in which an initially episodic form of these headaches ultimately evolves into the chronic unremitting form

   Some authors prefer alternative nomenclature. At present, only CPH and EPH are recognized in the International Headache Society's diagnostic system as outlined in the Second Edition of the International Classification of Headache Disorders (ICHD II).

3. **What distinguishes the paroxysmal hemicranias from cluster headache?**
   The major distinguishing features of the paroxysmal hemicranias and cluster headache lie in the frequency of the attack, the duration of the attack, and the response to treatment. In addition, the paroxysmal hemicranias do not show the striking preponderance among males that characterizes cluster headache. In cluster headache, attacks are less frequent but of longer duration—one or two a day with a typical duration of 30 minutes to 2 hours. Attacks in the paroxysmal hemicranias exceed five a day and last 2 to 25 minutes each.

4. **Do the paroxysmal hemicranias differ pathophysiologically from cluster headache?**
   The paroxysmal hemicranias, like cluster headache, belong to a group of headache disorders known as the trigeminal autonomic cephalgias (TACs). The TACs are characterized by cyclical

episodes of severe headaches that are associated with cranial autonomic activation. These disorders share a common pathophysiologic mechanism, the trigeminal autonomic reflex (see Chapter 11, Cluster Headache).

Like cluster headaches, the paroxysmal hemicranias can be triggered by alcohol. Approximately 10% of patients with chronic paroxysmal hemicrania report that attacks are precipitated either by bending or by rotating the head. Headache attacks may also be triggered by exerting external pressure against the transverse process of the C4-C5, the C2 root, or the greater occipital nerve. Headaches may be precipitated within a few seconds of the trigger (range 5 to 60 seconds), sometimes in rapid succession without any refractory period.

5. **Does it matter whether we call these headaches clusters or paroxysmal hemicranias?**
Yes. The differential diagnosis is exceptionally important, as the paroxysmal hemicranias are often resistant to the medications that typically prevent cluster headaches. The paroxysmal hemicranias are uniquely responsive to treatment with indomethacin. In fact, the International Headache Society has deemed response to indomethacin therapy a sine qua non for establishing the diagnosis. Some headache specialists believe that there are patients with paroxysmal hemicrania refractory to indomethacin.

6. **Once the diagnosis of episodic or chronic paroxysmal hemicrania (EPH/CPH) is established, are any further workups necessary?**
Although the paroxysmal hemicranias are benign by definition, there have been patients with clear medical or structural etiologies of this clinical disorder. For example, to date, there have been a number of published cases of patients with CPH-like headaches associated with collagen vascular diseases, malignant brain tumors, arteriovenous malformations, and ischemic stroke. Neuroimaging is therefore recommended in all cases with the presumptive diagnosis of either CPH or EPH to exclude these or other causes of these rare headaches. Several of these patients have also responded to indomethacin.

7. **Once the diagnosis is established and neuroimaging is normal, how are these headaches treated?**
The paroxysmal hemicranias exhibit unique responsiveness to indomethacin but not to other nonsteroidal antiinflammatory agents. Initial therapy consists of 25 mg indomethacin three times a day. If there is no response or if there is a partial response after 1 week, increase the dose to 50 mg three times a day. Complete resolution of the headache is prompt, usually occurring within 1 or 2 days of initiating the effective dose. Occasionally, suppositories are better tolerated than oral indomethacin.

Advise patients of the risk of gastritis and ulcer disease, as well as the other side effects of indomethacin. In patients with CPH, consider concurrent treatment with misoprostol or histamine H-2 receptor antagonists.

Rarely, some patients require indomethacin doses as high as 300 mg/day. Recent reports suggest that a need for high indomethacin doses may be an ominous sign pointing to an underlying specific medical or structural etiology.

8. **True or false: Breakthrough headaches don't occur with indomethacin therapy.**
False. Some patients experience breakthrough headaches at the end of dosing intervals. These headaches are usually eliminated by increasing the dose or shortening the dosing interval. For patients with breakthrough headaches in the early morning hours, slow-release indomethacin at night may be helpful.

9. **If indomethacin fails to treat the headaches, what then?**
If indomethacin fails to successfully treat the headaches, reconsider the diagnosis and make sure there is no underlying cause. If upon further review the diagnosis of CPH or EPH is

still likely, partial response has been demonstrated with verapamil, acetylsalicylic acid, ibuprofen, piroxicam, naproxen, or paracetamol. These agents are not nearly as effective as indomethacin and should not be used as first-line therapy.

10. **What is SUNCT syndrome?**
SUNCT is an acronym for *s*hort-lasting, *u*nilateral, *n*euralgiform headache attacks with *c*onjunctival injection and *t*earing. It is one of the TACs (see Question 4). SUNCT is characterized by very frequent attacks of extremely short-lasting, unilateral headaches. The headaches of the SUNCT syndrome recur from 3 to 200 times per day; each attack lasts 5 to 240 seconds each. As the name suggests, individual attacks are associated with ipsilateral conjunctival injection and lacrimation.

11. **How is SUNCT treated?**
SUNCT is very refractory to treatment. Treatment with medications used for cluster and the TACs are ineffective for SUNCT. Lamotrigine has been reported to offer some benefit.

KEY POINTS

1. The paroxysmal hemicranias are a group of rare, benign headache disorders that resemble cluster headache in most ways but differ from cluster headache because they do not respond to anticluster medications and are generally more frequent and of shorter duration than cluster headache.

2. The paroxysmal hemicranias are uniquely responsive to indomethacin.

3. There are secondary causes of the paroxysmal hemicranias including collagen vascular disorders and brain tumor; therefore, for all patients who are suspected of having the diagnosis of one of the paroxysmal hemicranias, neuroimaging is recommended.

BIBLIOGRAPHY

1. Antonaci F, Sjaastad O: Chronic paroxysmal hemicrania: a review of the clinical manifestations, *Headache* 29:648-656, 1989.

2. Goadsby PJ: Trigeminal automonic cephalgias (TACs), *Acta Neurol Belg* 101(1):10-19, 2001.

3. Goadsby PJ, Lipton RB: A review of paroxysmal hemicranias, SUNCT syndrome and other short-lasting headaches with autonomic features, including new cases, *Brain* 120:193-209, 1997.

4. Haggag KJ, Russell D: Chronic paroxysmal hemicrania. In Olesen J, Tfelt-Hansen P, Welch KMA, editors: *The headaches*, New York, 1993, Raven Press, pp 601-608.

5. Kudrow L, Esperanza P, Vijayan N: Episodic paroxysmal hemicrania? *Cephalalgia* 7:197-201, 1987.

6. Medina JL: Organic headaches mimicking chronic paroxysmal hemicrania, *Headache* 32:73-74, 1992.

7. Newman LC: Effective management of ice pick pains, SUNCT, and episodic and chronic paroxysmal hemicrania, *Curr Pain Headache Rep* 5(3):292-299, 2001.

8. Newman LC, Goadsby P, Lipton RB: Cluster and related headaches, *Med Clin North Am* 85:997-1016, 2001.

9. Newman LC, Gordon ML, Lipton RB, et al: Episodic paroxysmal hemicrania: two new cases and a literature review, *Neurology* 42:964-966, 1992.

10. Newman LC, Lipton RB: Paroxysmal hemicranias. In Goadsby PJ, Silberstein SD, editors: *Headache*. Blue Books of Practical Neurology, vol. 17, Boston, 1997, Butterworth-Heinemann, pp 243-250.

11. Sjaastad O, Dale I: Evidence for a new (?), treatable headache entity, *Headache* 14:105-108, 1974.

12. Sjaastad O, Stovner LJ, Stolt-Nielson A, et al: CPH and hemicrania continua: requirements of high indomethacin dosages—an ominous sign? *Headache* 35:363-367, 1995.

CHAPTER 13

SUBARACHNOID HEMORRHAGE

Ronald Kanner, MD, FAAN, FACP

1. **What is the most common cause of spontaneous subarachnoid hemorrhage?**
   Rupture of a cerebral artery aneurysm is the most common cause of spontaneous subarachnoid hemorrhage in adults in middle life. In children and teenagers, arteriovenous malformations (AVM) are common. Small subarachnoid hemorrhages are usual after head trauma and may be the cause of early posttraumatic headache.

2. **A 40-year-old woman in the emergency department complains of the worst headache of her life that has its onset during sexual intercourse. On examination, she is slightly sleepy and has a stiff neck but no other signs. What diagnosis should be considered?**
   This is a classic story for subarachnoid hemorrhage. The sudden onset of "the worst headache of my life" is the tipoff. Most commonly, it occurs during the Valsalva maneuver—while straining at stool or during sexual intercourse. Patients commonly demonstrate stiff neck and some alteration of level of consciousness. The absence of localizing signs on neurologic exam does not contradict the diagnosis. A few specific types of subarachnoid hemorrhage will include localizing signs (see Question 3).

3. **A patient comes to the emergency department with the sudden onset of a severe headache. The patient is awake and alert, but the left eyelid is drooping, the left pupil is dilated, and the left eye is exodeviated. What is the problem?**
   The patient has a third-nerve palsy. Third-nerve palsy and headache are often thought of as signs of uncal herniation. However, the patient is awake. Furthermore, there is no hemiparesis. An isolated third-nerve paresis with severe headache is a common presentation of a ruptured aneurysm in the posterior communicating artery. The third nerve passes between the posterior communicating artery and the superior cerebellar artery. Rupture of the aneurysm may put pressure on the third nerve, causing ptosis, mydriasis, and exodeviation of the eye.

4. **What are the international headache society criteria for subarachnoid hemorrhage?**
   - Past or present bleeding demonstrated by examination of cerebrospinal fluid or by computed tomography (CT)
   - Headache of sudden onset (60 minutes) if it is an aneurysm, 12 hours if it is an AVM
   - At least one of the following:
     - Severe headache intensity
     - Bilateral headache location
     - Stiff neck
     - Increased body temperature

5. **What are the studies of choice to confirm the diagnosis of subarachnoid hemorrhage?**
   CT scan shows blood in the subarachnoid space in over 95% of patients with subarachnoid hemorrhage. In the remaining 5%, lumbar puncture may be needed to demonstrate blood.

Lumbar puncture usually shows an elevated opening pressure and an abundance of red blood cells. If the tap is done early, white blood cells and red blood cells should be in the same proportion as they are in the peripheral blood. Later, irritation of the meninges from the blood may produce a higher proportion of white blood cells. If the CT scan clearly shows a subarachnoid hemorrhage, a lumbar puncture is not necessary.

6. **What is a "thunder clap" headache?**
This term refers to a headache of very sudden onset and high severity. It is usually an indication of subarachnoid hemorrhage. However, it has also been described in unruptured aneurysms that have increased in size and produced surrounding vasospasm. In rare cases, a migraine headache can have a very sudden onset. However, this type of onset warrants neuroimaging.

7. **What is a sentinel headache?**
Sentinel headaches are brief, severe headaches that may precede a subarachnoid hemorrhage. They are presumed to be due to enlargements of the aneurysm before bleeding. However, there may be tiny hemorrhages that are not seen. If the aneurysm is in the posterior communicating artery, sentinel headaches may be accompanied by a third-nerve paresis, as described in Question 3. Sentinel headaches may occur with aneurysms in essentially any cerebral location.

8. **A patient has typical symptoms of a subarachnoid hemorrhage and severe headache. Lumbar puncture shows blood in the cerebrospinal fluid. However, angiography is negative. What are the possible causes of this syndrome?**
Subarachnoid hemorrhage with negative angiography has a number of possible causes:
- Rupture of the aneurysm, which destroys the aneurysm; therefore, the pouch itself is not seen on angiography. However, there is usually some surrounding vasospasm to point out the area of the original hemorrhage.
- Clotting of the aneurysm. An aneurysmal dome filled with clotted blood does not show up on angiography.
- Spinal subarachnoid hemorrhage (much less common).
- Severe vasospasm around the aneurysm may cause such low flow that the aneurysm cannot be visualized on angiography.

9. **What is the definitive study of choice to establish the cause of a subarachnoid hemorrhage?**
At present, selective cerebral angiography is the diagnostic tool of choice. In most cases, it shows whether or not an aneurysm or an AVM is present. As CT angiography and magnetic resonance angiography become more sophisticated, they may replace this more invasive procedure. Currently, however, most surgeons require an angiogram to define clearly the site and cause of the subarachnoid hemorrhage.

10. **A patient with a subarachnoid hemorrhage undergoes angiography, which demonstrates multiple aneurysms. What signs are helpful in determining which aneurysm caused the subarachnoid hemorrhage?**
In general, larger aneurysms (1 cm) are more likely to bleed than smaller aneurysms. If aneurysms are similar in size, a number of signs may point to the offending aneurysm. Small nipples on the aneurysm are a sign that it has ruptured and healed. A smooth-domed aneurysm is less likely to have bled than an aneurysm with small out-pouchings. Arterial spasm is more likely to be present around the site of the ruptured aneurysm. On CT scanning, a clot surrounding an aneurysm is diagnostic of the offending aneurysm. More commonly, however, there is diffuse blood throughout the subarachnoid space.

11. **A patient with severe headache from subarachnoid hemorrhage improves over a few days then experiences another severe headache. What are the possible causes?**
The most common cause is rebleeding of the aneurysm, which occurs within the first 2 weeks in up to 30% of patients who have had a subarachnoid hemorrhage. Fifty percent of

rehemorrhages are fatal. Less commonly, blood may block either the reabsorptive system or one of the foramina through which cerebrospinal fluid flows. This blockage gives rise to hydrocephalus and headache. Onset is usually much more insidious than onset of headache of repeat subarachnoid hemorrhage.

12. **What is the appropriate treatment for the headache of subarachnoid hemorrhage?**
The pain of subarachnoid hemorrhage is often severe. As such, it may require potent analgesics. Aspirin and nonsteroidal antiinflammatory drugs are to be avoided because they may increase bleeding and because they are rarely available in a parenteral form. Ketorolac is an exception because it can be administered intramuscularly. In general, however, low doses of opioids administered intravenously usually provide significant headache relief.

A balance must be struck among headache relief, obtundation, and respiratory depression. When respiratory depression occurs, it is often accompanied by an increase in cranial pressure. Doses must be titrated carefully. A 2-mg dose of morphine administered intravenously usually provides significant relief.

13. **What are the delayed complications of subarachnoid hemorrhage?**
Headache is an unusual late complication of subarachnoid hemorrhage. Most commonly, if the arachnoid granulations through which the cerebrospinal fluid is reabsorbed become blocked, a transient period of increased intracranial pressure may lead to mild headaches for weeks to months. As these subside, one theory has it that normal-pressure hydrocephalus may ensue. In such patients, dementia, gait impairment, and urinary incontinence are the classic triad. Patients also may develop seizure disorder, cognitive impairment, and focal deficits.

KEY POINTS

1. A patient's complaint of the "worst headache of my life" should prompt consideration of and evaluation for a subarachnoid hemorrhage.

2. When confirming the diagnosis of subarachnoid hemorrhage, CT scans are most often positive; however, there are times when the CT scan is negative and a lumbar puncture needs to be performed to confirm the diagnosis.

3. Rebleeding of aneurysms is not uncommon during the first 2 weeks following an aneurysmal subarachnoid hemorrhage; when it does occur, the rebleeding is frequently associated with a fatal outcome.

BIBLIOGRAPHY

1. Jamieson DG, Hargreaves R: The role of neuroimaging in headache, *J Neuroimaging* 12(1):42-51, 2002.

2. Mayer SA, Bernardini GL, Brust JCM, Solomon RA: Subarachnoid hemorrhage. In Rowland LP, editor: *Merritt's neurology*, 10th ed, Philadelphia, 2000, Lippincott Williams & Wilkins, pp 260-267.

3. Prosser RL Jr: Feedback: computed tomography for subarachnoid hemorrhage. Which review should we believe regarding the diagnostic power of computed tomography for ruling out subarachnoid hemorrhage? *Ann Emerg Med* 37(6):679-680; discussion 680-685, 2001.

4. Schwartz DT: Evidence-based emergency medicine. Feedback: Computed tomography and lumbar puncture for the diagnosis of subarachnoid hemorrhage—the importance of accurate interpretation, *Ann Emerg Med* 39(2):190-192; discussion 192-194, 2002.

CHAPTER 14

BRAIN TUMOR HEADACHES

Ronald Kanner, MD, FAAN, FACP, and Charles E. Argoff, MD

1. **What is the classic description of brain tumor headache?**
   Standard texts describe the classic brain tumor headache as a morning headache that may
   even wake the patient from sleep in the early hours. It improves as the day goes on and
   characteristically responds to aspirin and steroids. At one point, the "steroid test" was used as a
   diagnostic tool for brain tumor headaches. A dramatic response to steroid administration
   strengthened the diagnosis, on the theory that peritumor edema was resolving. Over the years,
   however, it has become increasingly clear that steroids can relieve many types of headaches—
   not just those resulting from brain tumors.

2. **What was the theoretical basis for the temporal pattern of classic brain tumor
   headache?**
   It is still believed, to some degree, that the increased intracranial pressure that may occur with
   sleep and recumbency can increase pain caused by brain tumors. Mild CO_2 retention during
   sleep leads to vasodilatation and increased pressure. Similarly, when the patient is recumbent,
   venous return from the brain decreases and intracranial pressure increases. As the patient
   awakens and ambulates, CO_2 drops and venous return increases, thus lessening the headache
   pain as the day progresses.

3. **How commonly do patients with brain tumors have the "classic history" of a
   brain tumor headache?**
   The "classic" syndrome seems to occur in only about 17% of patients with brain tumors and
   headaches. Most commonly, headaches caused by brain tumor are diffuse, nondescript,
   and tensionlike. They are usually bilateral and commonly affect the vertex.

4. **How often are brain tumor headaches unilateral?**
   Pain is unilateral in less than 50% of brain tumor headaches. However, when it is unilateral, it is
   invariably felt on the side of the tumor. A migrainous presentation is highly unusual, occurring in
   only about 9% of patients with headaches caused by metastatic brain tumors.

5. **If brain tumor headaches are most commonly tensionlike, how do you
   differentiate between a benign tension-type headache and a brain tumor
   headache?**
   There are a number of factors that differentiate a tension-type headache from a brain tumor
   headache. The most important is probably the time course. A new-onset headache that
   progresses over days to weeks is much more suspect of representing a space-occupying lesion
   than is a chronic headache that has been stable over a long period. Furthermore, abnormalities
   on the neurologic exam are virtually unheard of in benign headache syndromes (with the
   exception of Horner's sign in cluster headache) but occur in over 50% of patients with brain
   tumor headaches. Naturally, in a patient with a history of cancer and a new onset of headache,
   metastatic disease must be very high on the list.

6. **Name and describe three circumstances under which extracerebral cancer can cause headache and/or facial pain.**

Extracerebral cancer can cause headache and/or facial pain in the following circumstances: Obstruction of venous drainage of the brain produces increased intracranial pressure, with subsequent headache. Mediastinal tumors that compress the superior vena cava are a common example. Hypercoagulable states producing venous sinus thrombosis can produce severe headaches and depressed level of consciousness.

7. **Is the pathology of the brain tumor important in determining the clinical presentation?**

No. Though the pathology of the brain tumor is not important in determining the clinical presentation, the location of the tumor may be. Tumors at the base of the skull are likely to produce cranial nerve signs; tumors in the hemispheres are associated with a hemiparesis or language dysfunction; and tumors that obstruct cerebrospinal fluid (CSF) flow produce little in the way of focal neurological dysfunction.

8. **What is parinaud syndrome?**

Parinaud syndrome is characterized by difficulty with ocular convergence and upgaze. There is also light-near dissociation of pupillary reaction (pupils do not constrict well as a reaction to light, but constrict when the patient tries to look at something that is close to the nose). This constellation of signs is seen in tumors that compress the midbrain, such as pineal tumors.

9. **What is a "ball-valve" headache?**

Some tumors of the third ventricle, most commonly colloid cysts, may swing back and forth with positional changes of the head. As the patient's head swings to a new position, the cyst may shift and block off the exit foramen of the third ventricle, causing an acute increase in intracranial pressure. When the head is again shifted, the flow is released and headache decreases. The intermittent blockade by the tumor is a "ball-valve" effect. In some patients, a sharp smack on the forehead can dislodge the tumor from the foramen and produce a paradoxical cure of the headache. Do not try this unless you are very sure of what you are doing.

10. **How commonly is headache the presenting complaint in patients with metastatic brain tumors?**

About 50% of patients with metastatic brain tumors have headache as their presenting complaint. It is the single most common presenting complaint of patients with brain metastases. Of interest, headache without other focal findings is more common in patients with multiple metastases than in those with only a single metastasis.

11. **Under what circumstances do brain tumor headaches involve a sudden increase in pain rather than the usual gradual onset?**

The two most common causes for a sudden onset of headache in brain tumors are hemorrhage and obstruction of CSF flow. Certain tumors are much more likely than others to hemorrhage. Metastatic melanoma hemorrhages with great frequency. In fact, even in the absence of clinically evident hemorrhage, imaging may show blood density within the tumors. Hypernephroma and choriocarcinoma also hemorrhage with some frequency. The direction of CSF flow is from the lateral ventricles to the third ventricle (through the foramina of Monro) and from the third to the fourth (through the cerebral aqueduct). CSF leaves the fourth ventricle through the foramina of Luschka (laterally) and Magendie (medially) in the cerebellum. Tumors in these areas are particularly prone to causing obstructive hydrocephalus.

12. **Why do brain metastases cause headaches?**

Brain tissue itself is not pain-sensitive; that is, there are no nociceptors in the gray or white matter of the brain. However, the structures surrounding the brain—i.e., the meninges, tentorium cerebelli, blood vessels, and cranial nerves—are pain-sensitive. As tumors grow, they may invade or put traction on these structures. Inflammation or stretching of nociceptors in these structures causes pain.

13. **Which systemic tumors commonly metastasize to the brain?**
The most common primary sources are lung, breast, and melanoma. Small cell carcinoma of the lung and adenocarcinoma are particularly likely to metastasize. Breast cancer is a common cause of brain metastases because of its high prevalence in the population. However, given a patient with breast cancer, a patient with lung cancer, and a patient with melanoma, the patient with melanoma is most likely to suffer brain metastasis. Melanoma is also more likely than the other tumors to cause multiple metastases. With other tumors, single metastases occur with the same frequency as multiple metastases.

14. **Under what circumstances is a brain tumor likely to produce severe headaches with little or no neurologic focality?**
Tumors that involve the frontal lobes may grow to enormous sizes without producing focal neurologic deficits. Usually, however, there is some change in personality or cognition. Tumors that obstruct CSF flow may cause hydrocephalus and headache without significant neurologic focality. Finally, tumors involving the cerebellum in the midline may cause headaches without much in the way of localizing neurologic signs.

15. **Do primary brain tumors cause headaches?**
Yes. Gliomas, the most common of the primary cerebral tumors, tend to arise deep in the brain. Initially, they invaginate among brain structures and may cause little in the way of headaches. Eventually, however, they achieve sufficient size to increase intracranial pressure and cause headaches.

16. **What is the preferred treatment for brain tumor headaches?**
Because most brain tumor headaches are due to increased mass, removal of the tumor usually relieves the headaches. However, with recurrent or growing tumors, ongoing therapy is needed. Steroids reliably relieve brain tumor headaches, but complications generally preclude long-term use. Radiation therapy initially increases the headache because of increased swelling. However, as tumors resolve, the headache tends to resolve pari passu.

17. **What is pari passu?**
Pari passu is a Latin expression that means walking at the same pace. The headache that results from radiation-induced swelling tends to resolve at the same pace as the swelling resolves.

18. **How can a cerebellar metastasis cause retroorbital pain?**
The cerebellum lies just under the tentorium cerebelli. Innervation of the tentorium is through the trigeminal nerve. The trigeminal nerve also innervates the orbital structures. Referred pain is fairly common when a given nerve (or nerve roots) innervates two separate structures. As a cerebellar metastasis grows, it can stretch the tentorium cerebelli, stimulating the nociceptors that lie therein. Pain arising there is referred to the eye.

19. **What is the Foster-Kennedy syndrome?**
The Foster-Kennedy syndrome is characterized by optic atrophy in one eye and papilledema in the other eye. It is caused by large tumors of the optic nerve. As the tumor grows, it produces optic atrophy on the affected side. As it grows larger, intracranial pressure increases. Increased intracranial pressure causes papilledema. However, because the ipsilateral optic nerve is compressed, it cannot develop papilledema.

20. **A 60-year-old woman complains of progressive, unilateral headache and facial pain. On examination, she shows nystagmus, hearing loss, facial weakness, and ataxia. What is the likely diagnosis?**

This constellation of symptoms indicates dysfunction of cranial nerves V, VII, and VIII along with cerebellar dysfunction and is typical of a cerebellopontine angle tumor. Often such tumors are acoustic neuromas or meningiomas. Occasionally, however, a metastasis produces this picture.

21. **A middle-aged man has progressive headaches and is found to have a frontal glioma. His headaches become worse, and he develops diplopia that is most pronounced on distant gaze and not present on near gaze. What is a likely explanation?**

When diplopia is mainly present on distant gaze, consider a sixth-nerve palsy. The sixth nerve abducts the eye. Therefore, for reading or looking at something close, the eyes are converged and do not require sixth-nerve function. At far gaze—for example, watching television—the sixth nerve must keep the eyes focused outward. Therefore, with sixth-nerve dysfunction, diplopia is worse on far gaze. Increased intracranial pressure may lead to mild sixth-nerve dysfunction. The sixth nerve has the longest intracranial course of the cranial nerves. As pressure increases, it may be affected, even without local compression. This phenomenon is called a falsely localizing sixth nerve.

22. **A 60-year-old man with glioblastoma has undergone a full course of radiation therapy with some improvement. Six months later, he complains of increasing headache and increasing neurologic deficits referable to the area of the original tumor. What is the differential diagnosis? How would you differentiate between the two main possibilities?**

In this setting, the highest suspicion must be of recurrent tumor. However, 6 months after radiation therapy, radiation necrosis is also a possibility. The two possibilities may have relatively similar appearances on both computed tomography (CT) scan and magnetic resonance imaging (MRI). They both may appear as expanding masses. The best way to differentiate between them is with a positron emission tomography (PET) scan. However, care must be taken in the interpretation because relative activity may vary with the radionuclide used.

KEY POINTS

1. Most commonly, headaches resulting from brain tumor are diffuse, nondescript, and similar to tension headaches.

2. Gliomas, the most common type of primary cerebral tumor, tend to be associated with headache after they have grown to be sufficiently large enough to be associated with increased intracranial pressure.

3. The two most common causes for a sudden onset of headache related to brain tumors are hemorrhage and obstruction of CSF flow.

BIBLIOGRAPHY

1. Chidel MA, Suh JH, Barnett GH: Brain metastases: presentation, evaluation, and management, *Cleve Clin J Med* 67(2):120-127, 2000.

2. Forsythe PA, Posner JB: Headaches in patients with brain tumors: a study of 111 patients, *Neurology* 43: 1678-1683, 1993.

3. Jamieson DG, Hargreaves R: The role of neuroimaging in headache, *J Neuroimaging* 12(1):42-51, 2002.

4. Lovely MP: Symptom management of brain tumor patients, *Seminars in Oncology Nursing* 20(4):273-283, 2004.

5. Posner JB: Intracranial metastases. In Posner JB, editor: *Neurological complications of cancer*, Philadelphia, 1995, F.A. Davis, pp 77-110.

6. Siepmann DB, Siegel A, Lewis PJ: TI-201 SPECT and F-18 FDG PET for assessment of glioma recurrence versus radiation necrosis, *Clinical Nuclear Medicine* 30(3):199-200, 2005.

CHAPTER 15

INCREASED AND DECREASED INTRACRANIAL PRESSURE

Ronald Kanner, MD, FAAN, FACP

1. **What is the normal range for intracranial pressure?**
   Intracranial pressure is generally measured by lumbar puncture. It is presumed that, because the spinal fluid at the lumbar level is continuous with spinal fluid throughout the brain, pressures are equal. The normal pressure on lumbar puncture is 65 to 195 mm of cerebrospinal fluid (CSF) or water. This is the equivalent of about 5 to 15 mmHg.

2. **Does systemic hypertension usually cause an increased intracranial pressure headache?**
   No. Systemic hypertension is usually asymptomatic.

3. **What is the Monro-Kellie doctrine?**
   The Monro-Kellie doctrine states that an increase in the volume of any of the calvarial contents (brain tissue, blood, CSF, or brain fluids) must be accompanied by a decrease in the volume of another component, or intracranial pressure will increase markedly because the bony calvarium rigidly fixes the total cranial volume. Under normal circumstances, brief increases in intracranial pressure are associated with the Valsalva maneuver, including coughing, sneezing, or straining at stool. Some of the increased intracranial pressure is mitigated by the fact that the cerebral vessels are somewhat elastic and can be compressed. In patients who already have increased intracranial pressure or irritated meninges, transient rises may produce severe pain.

4. **Under what circumstances is the pressure measured by lumbar puncture not a true reflection of intracranial pressure?**
   If there is a block in CSF flow at a spinal level above the level of the lumbar puncture, but below the foramen magnum there may be a pressure gradient between the cerebral space and the lumbar space. Also, when the protein is extremely high, pressure may not be transmitted correctly through the thin needle.

5. **How is cerebrospinal fluid formed?**
   CSF fills the four ventricles of the brain, is distributed over the convexity, and also fills the spinal canal. It is secreted by the choroid plexus, a series of capillaries surrounded by epithelial cells. A small amount of CSF is also formed directly by brain capillaries.
   The direction of CSF flow is from the lateral ventricles (where the choroid plexuses are located) through the foramina of Monro into the third ventricle. From the third ventricle, CSF flows through the aqueduct of Sylvius to the fourth ventricle. The third and fourth ventricles are single, midline structures, whereas the lateral ventricles are bilateral. From the fourth ventricle, it exits laterally through the foramina of Luschka and medially through the foramen of Magendie. Then it goes down the spinal canal, bathing the spinal cord.

The spinal cord itself ends at about the level of the L1 or L2 vertebral body. The dural sac, however, extends to nearly the end of the spinal canal. Thus the space between L2 and the bottom of the canal is filled with some nerve roots and ample CSF. This is the area commonly used for lumbar puncture and measuring CSF pressure.

6. **What is benign intracranial hypertension?**
The clinical symptoms of benign intracranial hypertension, also known as pseudotumor cerebri, are headache and visual disturbance. No particular clinical characteristic of the headache is pathognomonic. Patients almost invariably demonstrate papilledema. Although it may occur at any age, most cases occur in the third and fourth decades. Women are much more commonly affected than men. Visual acuity is usually normal, but careful examination of the visual fields demonstrates enlarged blind spots. The neurologic examination reveals no other focal abnormalities. If focal abnormalities are present, the diagnosis of pseudotumor should not be entertained. A normal computed tomogram (CT) or magnetic resonance image (MRI) of the brain is mandatory for diagnosis. Pseudotumor cerebri is a diagnosis of exclusion; according to an old axiom, the most common cause of pseudotumor is a real tumor.
The prototype for the disease is an obese woman with chronic headaches. Papilledema is detected incidentally during routine examination. Sometimes the CT scan is rated as showing "slitlike" ventricles.

7. **Why do patients with pseudotumor cerebri have enlarged blind spots?**
On the normal visual fields, the "blind spot" is caused by the optic disk. There are no light receptors on the disk. In papilledema, the disk is swollen and enlarged, thereby causing an enlarged blind spot.

8. **What are visual obscurations?**
Visual obscurations are transient darkenings of vision that are sometimes seen in patients with increased intracranial pressure. In pseudotumor cerebri, there are two mechanisms that are theorized to cause these visual changes. The first is direct pressure on the optic nerve. This second is pressure on the posterior cerebral arteries, causing occipital blindness.

9. **What studies are important if the diagnosis of pseudotumor is entertained?**
For the diagnosis of pseudotumor to be entertained, the patient first must meet clinical criteria, including headache and papilledema with no other obvious cause. Second, an imaging procedure must rule out the presence of a structural lesion. Lumbar puncture is then performed to confirm a CSF pressure; with pseudotumor, CSF pressure is at least 200 mm (in most cases, it is well over 300 mm). Imaging studies may appear normal; that is, both the ventricles and the sulci appear quite small. An electroencephalogram (EEG) is not necessary. The vast majority of patients have normal EEGs, and even when the EEG is abnormal, it does not help with the diagnosis.

10. **Is pseudotumor cerebri exclusively a disease of women?**
Although it is much more common in women than men, there have been a number of reports of men suffering from the disease, sometimes in the setting of sleep apnea. One theory holds that the significant obesity that is often a part of sleep apnea may also play a pathogenetic role in pseudotumor cerebri. In fact, there have been therapeutic trials of relieving intraabdominal pressure as a means of decreasing intracerebral pressure.

11. **What are the most common predisposing factors in benign intracranial hypertension?**
Obesity appears to be one predisposing factor. In some cases, oral contraceptives or corticosteroid withdrawal has been implicated. The consumption of tetracyclines and large doses of vitamin A have

also been thought to be predisposing factors. Secondary causes of benign intracranial hypertension include venous hypertension, venous sinus thrombosis, and any process that impedes venous drainage from the brain.

12. **What are the main complications of untreated pseudotumor cerebri?**
Two of the most common complications are visual loss and the empty sella syndrome. Continuous pressure on the optic nerve may lead to optic atrophy. It is unclear whether surgically releasing the optic sheath eliminates this complication.

13. **Describe the treatments for pseudotumor cerebri.**
The first treatment for pseudotumor cerebri actually occurs at the time of diagnosis. When a lumbar puncture is performed, increased pressure is relieved. Relief is not due only to removal of fluid. Fluid forms so rapidly (0.4 ml/min) that the amount removed is immediately replenished. However, because lumbar puncture causes a rent in the dura, there is some leakage of fluid for a long while after the spinal tap. If a large-bore needle is used, the rent in the dura may be sufficient to serve as a shunt.
One of the most accepted medical therapies is acetazolamide, which reduces CSF production. This diuretic, a carbonic anhydrase inhibitor, presumably decreases the mechanism for production of CSF. Other diuretics also may be of value in pseudotumor cerebri.
With repeated lumbar punctures, pressure often normalizes over a few weeks. If the pressure does not normalize and cannot be restored to normal with diuretics, a shunting procedure may be necessary. The most common procedure is a lumboperitoneal shunt, which drains CSF into the peritoneal space. Glycerol, a hyperosmolar agent, is sometimes used; however, it is poorly tolerated and may cause further weight gain in already obese patients.

14. **Why does increased intracranial pressure cause headaches?**
The presumed mechanism is traction on pain-sensitive structures. However, when the pressure is diffuse, this explanation does not necessarily hold. Clearly, with brain tumors or other localized lesions, shifts of intracranial structures cause traction. With pseudotumor cerebri, however, the increase in intracranial pressure is diffuse, and it is not clear that it is associated with traction on dura or blood vessels. In healthy volunteers, infusions into the CSF, raising pressure up to 600 mm, have not produced significant headaches.

15. **What focal neurologic signs can be seen with diffuse increases in intracranial pressure?**
A mild palsy of cranial nerve VI may complicate increased intracranial pressure. The sixth cranial nerve (abducens) has a long course in the subarachnoid space, and it may be compromised by diffuse increases in pressure. When compromise occurs, the affected eye is deviated slightly medially. In contrast to tumors that directly compress the sixth nerve, diffusely increased intracranial pressure usually causes mild, rather than complete, compromise. Patients complain of diplopia on far gaze. The diplopia disappears on near gaze because the eyes tend to converge.

16. **Other than pseudotumor cerebri, what are the most common intracranial causes of increased intracranial pressure?**
In any case of increased intracranial pressure, a space-occupying lesion should be sought. Primary and metastatic brain tumors are among the most common causes.

17. **How do brain tumors cause increased intracranial pressure?**
   - Growth of the tumor may increase mass so much that intracranial pressure increases. The mass of the tumor is compounded by the surrounding edema. As in the Monro-Kellie doctrine, there is a new component of the intracranial cavity, but there has been no decrease in existing components, so the pressure goes up.

- The tumor may obstruct CSF flow. CSF flows from the lateral ventricles into the third ventricle, from the third ventricle to the fourth, and out the fourth ventricle into the subarachnoid space. A tumor obstructing the aqueduct of Sylvius (between the third and fourth ventricles) causes massive dilatation of the third and lateral ventricles, sparing the fourth. This obstructive hydrocephalus presents as rapidly increasing intracranial pressure with headache. Obstruction of CSF outflow at any point may produce hydrocephalus.

18. **What are the risks of performing lumbar puncture in patients with increased intracranial pressure?**
The risks are not as great as we were always taught. The old axiom "Pap, don't tap" does not hold. Lumbar punctures can be performed on patients with diffusely increased intracranial pressure. In fact, it may be therapeutic in these cases. The real risk occurs with a large, laterally placed mass lesion or a large mass lesion in the posterior fossa. Under these circumstances, the fear is that lumbar puncture will produce a pressure gradient between the brain and lumbar subarachnoid space, causing the brain to herniate downward. In diffusely increased intracranial pressure, as seen in pseudotumor cerebri, this risk is minimal or nonexistent.

19. **Describe the uncal herniation syndrome.**
Uncal herniation refers to a syndrome in which a large, laterally placed mass pushes the temporal lobe through the incisura. Expansion of the intracerebral mass causes contralateral hemiparesis. As the mass pushes downward, it compresses the third nerve, causing an ipsilateral third-nerve palsy (ptosis, pupillary enlargement, and exodeviation of the eye). The syndrome, therefore, is ipsilateral third-nerve palsy and contralateral hemiparesis.

20. **What historical data lead to the diagnosis of increased intracranial pressure?**
Although no symptom is pathognomonic, headaches caused by increased intracranial pressure tend to be worse in the early morning hours and improve during the day. The supine position leads to more blood pooling in the head. During sleep, mild CO_2 retention may cause vasodilatation with increased cerebral blood flow. Patients may also complain of increased headache with any Valsalva maneuver, such as coughing, sneezing, or straining at stool.

21. **What are low-pressure headaches?**
The CSF serves as a cushion for the brain, buffering its movements within the skull. When CSF pressure is markedly decreased, this cushioning ability is less effective. The clinical hallmark is a purely orthostatic headache. Patients have severe headaches when sitting or standing, but the headaches are entirely relieved by lying supine.

22. **True or false: Lesions at the base of the skull are the most common cause of low-pressure headache.**
False. CSF leaks are the most common cause. They may occur after lumbar puncture or inadvertent puncture of the dura during an attempted epidural block. Most commonly, they occur after epidural anesthesia for childbirth. The needle used for an epidural block is thicker and blunter than the one used for a usual lumbar puncture, and an inadvertent dural tear is larger than the hole caused by lumbar puncture. The results are prolonged CSF leak and postural headache. Therefore, regarding needles used for lumbar puncture, "size matters."
    Occasionally, patients develop a classic low-pressure headache without any obvious trauma. The pathophysiology is unclear. In some cases, there may have been minor trauma that went unnoticed, but was sufficient to cause a small rent in the dura. However, a search should be undertaken to look for destructive lesions at the base of the skull.

23. How can low-pressure headache be diagnosed?

Usually the history is sufficient: lumbar puncture or epidural block, followed by the classic positional headache. A CSF leak can be confirmed by injecting radionuclide into the subarachnoid space and then scanning to pick up sites of radioactivity outside the column.

24. What is the treatment of choice for low-pressure headaches?

In most patients, the causative rent in the dura heals on its own, and normal CSF production raises the pressure to baseline levels. During this process, use supportive measures. Encourage patients to increase fluid intake and use minor analgesics. If this approach fails, intravenous infusion of fluids may be helpful. Intravenous administration of 1 liter of saline with 500 mg of caffeine also has been reported to relieve low-pressure headaches. In particularly refractory cases, blood patches may be used. Autologous blood injected into the epidural space patches over the rent in the dura.

Keep in mind, however, that the vast majority of postpuncture headaches resolve within 2 weeks. If they do not, consider the possibility of a persistent fistula. In any case, the side effects of the treatment should not be worse than the effects of the headache.

KEY POINTS

1. Systemic hypertension is not likely to be the cause of a headache.

2. Pseudotumor cerebri, also known as benign intracranial hypertension, is associated with elevated cerebrospinal fluid (CSF) pressure and it is an important clinical syndrome to consider in an obese woman with chronic headache and visual complaints.

3. Low CSF pressure headaches are characterized by headaches that occur while standing or sitting and that resolve by being supine.

BIBLIOGRAPHY

1. Hagen K, Stovner, LJ, Vatten L, et al: Blood pressure and risk of headache: a prospective study of 22,685 adults in Norway, *J Neurol Neurosurg Psychiatry* 72(4):463-466, 2002.

2. Lee AG, Golnik K, Kardon R, et al: Sleep apnea and intracranial hypertension in men, *Ophthalmology*, 109(3):482-485, 2002.

3. Levine DN, Rapalino O: The pathophysiology of lumbar puncture headache, *J Neurol Sci* 192(1-2):1-8, 2001.

4. Marik P, Chen K, Varon J, et al: Management of increased intracranial pressure: a review for clinicians, *J Emerg Med* 17(4):711-719, 1999.

5. Sorensen PS, Corbett JJ: High cerebrospinal fluid pressure. In Olesen J, Tfelt-Hansen P, Welch KMA, editors: *The headaches*, 2nd ed, Philadelphia, 2000, Lippincott, Williams & Wilkins, pp 823-830.

6. Vilming ST, Campbell JK: Low cerebrospinal fluid pressure. In Olesen J, Tfelt-Hansen P, Welch KMA, editors: *The headaches*, 2nd ed, Philadelphia, 2000, Lippincott, Williams & Wilkins, pp 831-839.

CHAPTER 16

TEMPORAL GIANT CELL ARTERITIS

Robert A. Duarte, MD, and Charles E. Argoff, MD

1. **What is giant cell arteritis (GCA)?**

   Giant cell arteritis (GCA), also known as temporal arteritis (TA), is a specific form of vasculitis seen primarily in the older adult population, with a mean age of about 70 years at the time of diagnosis. However, there are documented cases of patients in their 40s with TA. It is more commonly seen in northern geographical latitudes, most commonly in people of British or Scandinavian heritage. TA is rarely seen in Asians and African-Americans. The disease is characterized pathologically by granulomatous inflammation of medium-sized arteries, resulting in the formation of multinucleated giant cells. TA can affect any artery, but it is primarily a disease of the aortic arch and its branches and not simply of the superficial temporal artery; hence the synonymous term giant cell arteritis (GCA). TA/GCA should be high on the differential diagnosis list of any person over the age of 60 presenting with new-onset headaches or any person with preexisting chronic headaches and a new headache subtype.

2. **What are the most common presenting symptoms seen in giant cell arteritis?**

   In 70% of patients headache is the most common symptom. The classic "textbook" description is of superficial scalp pain or soreness in the temporal region that is sensitive to touch. Patients will often describe a scalp or ear sensitivity, felt especially when combing there hair or wearing a hat. However, in most cases, the pain is nonspecific and not well localized. Jaw claudication (pain with chewing) is almost pathognomonic but is seen in only 40% of patients. Tongue claudication occurs in about 4% of patients. Accompanying symptoms may include generalized malaise, anorexia, and muscle pains. Occasionally, visual symptoms are the presenting complaint; this scenario is the most ominous in terms of outcome.

3. **Are there any clinical features that are most predictive of the presence or absence of TA?**

   Yes. When evaluating the patient with a complaint of headache, elevated erythrocyte sedimentation rate, advanced age, jaw claudication, and diplopia have the best positive predictive value for TA. Normal sedimentation rates markedly diminish the probability that the patient has TA.

4. **What are the common physical findings in giant cell arteritis?**

   Signs in GCA depend on the vessels involved and the end-organ damage sustained. The term *temporal arteritis* is a misnomer because this condition can involve many other arteries. The temporal artery itself is superficial and may be palpable, hard, and tender. Other signs may include fever, carotid bruits in up to 20% of affected individuals, papilledema, and extraocular muscle paresis.

5. **Are there neurological complications of giant cell arteritis?**

   Yes. The most feared complication of TA is optic neuropathy leading to blindness. Amaurosis fugax occurs in roughly 10% to 12% of patients, but there are usually no premonitory signs. Blindness occurs as a result of occlusion of the posterior ciliary arteries with anterior ischemic optic neuropathy. If left untreated, the second eye may become affected. Highest risk for visual loss is within the first 2 months. Approximately 2% of patients report having diplopia, which may fluctuate or remain static. Cerebral infarctions and transient ischemic attacks, more often affecting the vertebrobasilar circulation than the carotid circulation, have been reported frequently. Other neurological complications may include cognitive impairment, peripheral neuropathies, and, rarely, acute unilateral hearing loss.

6. **What is the most significant risk factor for visual loss in temporal arteritis?**
Significant thrombocytosis (an elevated platelet count) is a significant risk factor for permanent visual loss in temporal arteritis.

7. **List possible infectious causes for temporal arteritis.**
Possible infectious causes for TA include influenza, parvovirus B19, *Mycoplasma pneumonia, Chlamydia pneumonia,* and Borrelia burgdorferi.

8. **Which disease is frequently associated with giant cell arteritis?**
Polymyalgia rheumatica (PR) occurs in approximately 58% of patients with GCA and is the initial symptom in 25%. Conversely, GCA will develop in about 50% of patients with polymyalgia rheumatica. PR is characterized by morning stiffness and muscle aches. The proximal muscles are most affected, and patients have trouble rising from bed or from a chair. The laboratory test of choice is the erythrocyte sedimentation rate, which is markedly elevated. Treatment with 10 mg of prednisone daily usually provides dramatic relief within 4 to 5 days of starting therapy.

9. **What is the initial laboratory test that is helpful in establishing the diagnosis of giant cell arteritis?**
An erythrocyte sedimentation rate (ESR) must be done as soon as possible. The ESR is 50 mm/ hour in over 89% of cases. The ESR may be normal with TA. A C-reactive protein may also be elevated, and is more sensitive than ESR in some patients when monitoring disease activity. Other ancillary tests include a normochromic, normocytic anemia with a low reticulocyte count as well as mild elevations in serum transaminases.

10. **Are there any potential problems when obtaining a biopsy of the temporal artery?**
Yes. Involvement of the affected artery is often patchy; thus, the areas of injury are known as skip lesions. A biopsy may be directed between lesions and give a false-negative diagnosis. False positives are unusual. Nevertheless, always consider temporal artery biopsy for confirmation of GCA. Biopsy can be delayed up to 2 weeks after initiation of treatment.

11. **List other alternative investigative techniques for diagnosing TA.**
If the biopsy is negative and there remains a clinical suspicion for TA, angiography could be considered. A less invasive approach for evaluating the anatomy of medium to large vessels is magnetic resonance angiography (MRA). Because ultrasound reveals homogenous, concentric wall thickening in abnormal vessel walls, it may be a new and promising technique to assess vasculitis in TA.

12. **When should treatment be undertaken in suspected giant cell arteritis?**
As soon as the diagnosis is suspected, initiate prednisone therapy. Therapy should not be withheld pending results of a temporal artery biopsy, because the lab report may take days and may be inconclusive. Furthermore, the patient can lose vision abruptly and irreversibly if not treated in a timely fashion. Treatment consists of prednisone, 60 to 100 mg/day, for at least 1 to 2 months. If symptoms fail to improve within 1 to 3 days, consider increasing the dose of steroids until the symptoms resolve. After that, gradual tapering of less than 10% of the daily dose per week may be started. Monitor disease activity clinically and through the ESR/ C-reactive protein. After a few months, patients should be maintained on the lowest dose of prednisone that does not allow for recurrence of symptoms or elevation of the ESR/C-reactive protein. On average, duration of prednisone therapy lasts approximately 1 to 2 years.

KEY POINTS

1. Giant cell arteritis (GCA), also known as temporal arteritis (TA), is a specific form of vasculitis seen primarily in the older adult. It is characterized pathologically by granulomatous inflammation of medium-sized arteries, resulting in the formation of multinucleated giant cells.

2. When evaluating the patient with a complaint of headache, the following symptoms have the best positive predictive value for TA: elevated sedimentation rate, advanced age, jaw claudication, and diplopia. Approximately 70% of patients with TA have an elevated sedimentation rate; normal sedimentation rates markedly diminish the probability that the patient has TA.

3. The diagnosis of TA may be aided on the basis of the results of a temporal artery biopsy; however, treatment should not be delayed until after the biopsy results are known because this make take days to weeks, putting the untreated patient at risk for visual impairment.

4. Treatment consists of prednisone, 60 to 100 mg/day, for at least 1 to 2 months. After symptoms have resolved, gradual tapering of less than 10% of the daily dose per week may be started. The average duration of prednisone therapy is 1 to 2 years.

BIBLIOGRAPHY

1. Chan CC, Paine M, O'Day J: Predictors of recurrent ischemic optic neuropathy in giant cell arteritis, *Journal of Ophthamology* 25(1):14-7, 2005.

2. Foell D, Hernandez-Rodriquez J: Early recruitment of phagocytes contributes to the vascular inflammation of giant cell arteritis, *Journal of Pathology* 204(3):311-316, 2004.

3. Niederkohr RD, Levin LA: Management of the patient with suspected temporal arteritis: a decision analytical approach, *Ophthalmology* 112(5):744-756, 2005.

4. Schmidt WA, Blockmans D: Use of ultrasound and positron emission tomography in the diagnosis and assessment of large vessel vasculitis, *Current Opinion on Rheumatology* (7):9-15, 2005.

5. Smetana GW, Shmerling RH: Does this patient have temporal arteritis? *JAMA* 287(1):92-101, 2002.

6. Spiera R, Spiera H: Inflammatory disease in older adults: cranial arteritis, *Geriatrics* 59(12):25-29, 2004.

7. Weyand CM, Goronzy JJ: Giant cell arteritis and polymyalgia rheumatica, *Annals of Internal Medicine* 139 (6):505-515, 2003.

8. Younge BR, Cook BE, et al: Initiation of glucocorticoid therapy: before or after temporal artery biopsy? *Mayo Clinic Procedings* 79(4):483-491, 2004.

CHAPTER 17

HEADACHES ASSOCIATED WITH SYSTEMIC DISEASE

Robert A. Duarte, MD, and Charles E. Argoff, MD

1. **How often are headaches a manifestation of systemic disease?**
   Although headache is one of the most common pain complaints for which patients seek medical help, it is uncommonly associated with a serious systemic illness. The vast majority of headaches seen by practitioners are migraine or tension-type. A smaller number are cluster, and an even smaller number are paroxysmal hemicranias. In an emergency room setting, 10% to 15% of headaches are due to a secondary or systemic cause. Less than 1% of patients seen in a clinical practice with a complaint of headache have an underlying systemic disease that caused the headache.

2. **How do the criteria of the International Headache Society categorize headaches associated with systemic diseases?**
   The headache categorization criteria of the International Headache Society eliminate headaches caused by infection of the pericranial structures and divide headaches into those associated with noncephalic infections and those associated with metabolic disorders.

3. **What do patients believe is the most common systemic cause for episodic headaches?**
   After eliminating local complaints such as sinuses, patients most often believe that their headaches are due to a brain tumor. These suspicions can be quickly dispelled by an imaging study or by questioning the duration of the headache symptoms. Chronic headaches greater than 5 years' duration are rarely secondary to neoplastic disease. Other concerns include elevations in blood pressure. Essential hypertension is an uncommon cause for headaches. Within the range of autoregulation, elevation of blood pressure is generally asymptomatic. Clearly, in cases of hypertensive encephalopathy, with papilledema and mental status changes, headaches are a common concomitant.

4. **What is the most common systemic cause of headache?**
   Febrile illnesses are often associated with headache. Even the common cold is usually associated with a headache. However, when meningitis is superimposed, these headaches become much more severe, may be bursting in character, and rapidly increase over a period of minutes to hours. The most common cause of a sudden, severe headache in children is meningitis. In severe cases, there is stiff neck, nausea, vomiting, and photophobia. These headaches result from a direct irritation of meningeal nociceptors caused by inflammation or infection. With bacterial meningitis, signs are usually fulminant. However, with an aseptic or viral meningitis, signs may be subtle, progressive over hours to days, and the cerebrospinal fluid (CSF) commonly shows just a few cells (mainly lymphocytes) and increased protein.

5. **Describe the headache characteristics associated with Lyme disease.**
   Headache is the most common symptom of neurologic Lyme disease, but rarely is headache the presenting symptom. The headache is located bifrontally and/or in the occipital region and is intermittent. When it does occur, the headache tends to resemble migraine or tension-type headache, but is often associated with cognitive impairment or focal neurologic dysfunction.

Headaches associated with Lyme disease are usually seen as part of a meningitic process associated with early-stage dissemination, and they typically are responsive to antibiotic therapy. The CSF is usually abnormal, with pleocytosis.

Investigate for Lyme disease when a patient has new-onset headache, focal neurologic deficits, and residence in a Lyme-endemic region. In general, routine screening for Lyme disease is not recommended in patients with headache.

6. **What percentage of patients with herpes simplex encephalitis have headache?**
The incidence of headache varies with the accompanying presentation. If focal neurologic deficits are present, up to 90% of patients will also have a significant headache. If meningeal signs are present, headache is present in about 60% of cases. When there is only confusion or some obtundation, headache occurs in about 50% to 80% of patients. Overall, headache is a very common symptom in herpes encephalitis, but it is usually accompanied by focal neurologic deficits, alterations in level of consciousness, and seizures.

7. **What exogenous substances can precipitate a headache?**
The most commonly recognized exogenous substances that can precipitate a headache are the vasodilators. Amyl nitrite, a substance often used to heighten the sexual experience, is a potent vasodilator and may cause a severe, pounding headache, even in patients who do not have a headache diathesis. Similar reactions may occur in patients taking nitrates for cardiac disease. Alcoholic beverages can also cause headaches, both in the acute and the well-known hangover phase. The exact mechanism is unclear. For the acute headache, it appears to be vasodilatation. The hangover may be due to some vasoactive substances that are in the congeners in the alcoholic beverage.

Caffeine most often causes a headache as a withdrawal symptom. Cocaine, usually a vasorestrictive substance, can also cause headaches. Both of these headaches may be due to transient, severe rises in blood pressure or to a cerebral vasculitis. Monosodium glutamate (MSG) is a clear precipitant in patients who are sensitive to the substance. A generalized, throbbing headache develops within 20 to 25 minutes of eating food containing MSG.

In episodic migraine patients, certain analgesics—even those commonly used to treat headaches—can precipitate a chronic, daily headache syndrome if taken frequently. The headaches is often described as a less severe, holocephalic head pain often associated with generalized malaise and sleep disturbances. These agents include acetaminophen, aspirin, barbiturate-containing agents, ergots, and opioids. Estrogens and oral contraceptives are commonly associated with headaches.

8. **List drugs that may potentially cause headaches.**
The following drugs may potentially cause headaches:
- Cardiovascular agents
  - Nitroglycerin
- Antihypertensive agents
  - Methyldopa, reserpine
- Antiarrhythmic agents
  - Quinidine
- Central nervous system agents
- Levodopa
- Benzodiazepines
- Methylphenidate
- Analgesics
  - Nonsteroidal antiinflammatory drugs and opioids
- Gastrointestinal drugs
  - Histamine$_2$-blockers
- Respiratory agents
  - Theophylline

9. **Describe the clinical presentation of colloid cyst headache.**
Brief, short-lasting, positional headache is the most common complaint related to colloid cyst, occasionally associated with nausea and vomiting. Rarely, a patient may experience a sudden loss of consciousness at the peak of headache. The location of the headache is bifrontal, frontoparietal, or frontooccipital and is described as an intense, throbbing sensation often aggravated by exertion and relieved when lying supine. The underlying mechanism for the headache secondary to a colloid cyst is thought to be due to an intermittent obstruction of the cerebrospinal fluid flow through the foramen of Monro by a ball-valve phenomenon causing a transient and sudden increase in intracranial pressure. The physical examination is typically normal. In view of the elevated intracranial pressure, there can be signs of papilledema, nystagmus, sixth-nerve palsies, and extensor plantar responses.

10. **What systemic tumor causes headaches not secondary to metastases?**
Pheochromocytoma is the prototype of the group of systemic tumors that cause headaches not secondary to metastases. These headaches are often paroxysmal, lasting seconds to minutes, and occurring in a crescendo pattern. They are usually described as severe, bilateral, throbbing pain, sometimes associated with nausea, truncal sweating, palpitations, and tremor. The headache is usually correlated with a sudden rise in blood pressure.

11. **In what degenerative diseases of the nervous system is headache a common complaint?**
About one third of patients with Parkinson's disease report headaches. The exact mechanism is unclear, but it appears as a constant, dull pain, usually located over the cervical region. The temptation is to ascribe this to muscular stiffness secondary to the disease state, but the headaches do not necessarily correlate with the severity of the disease, nor do they usually respond to antiparkinsonian therapy.
About 10% of patients with multiple sclerosis complain of significant headaches, either secondary to the disease process or secondary to specific disease-modifying interventions. Degenerative diseases of the cervical spine often produce a headache that radiates up from the back of the head to the vertex, consistent with an occipital neuralgiform pain. This headache is usually more intense in the morning, after the patient has slept on an elevated pillow, and relieved as the day goes on. Treatment with cervical roll pillow may alleviate some of the pain. Although there are no well-controlled studies, nonsteroidal antiinflammatory drugs may provide pain relief. Less clear is the value of local nerve blocks.

12. **Describe the headache patterns that are seen in systemic lupus erythematosus (SLE).**
Prevalence of headache is as high as 70% in patients with systemic lupus erythematosus (SLE). There are three major types of headache in SLE: migraine, tension-type, or associated with lupus cerebritis. Migraine-type headaches seem most common at the onset of SLE. Later in the disease, tension-type headaches are more likely to develop. The headache of lupus cerebritis is accompanied by a clear-cut picture of cerebritis, with confusion and obtundation. Active migraines have been associated with higher disease activity, antiphospholipid antibodies, and Raynaud's phenomena.

13. **What types of headaches occur in patients with human immunodeficiency virus infection or acquired immunodeficiency syndrome?**
Recent studies indicate that about 50% of patients with HIV will experience headache at some time during the course of the disease. Most patients with HIV infection have an identifiable, organic cause for their headaches—for example, cryptococcal meningitis or central nervous system (CNS) toxoplasmosis, which usually are late complications of AIDS. Some studies indicate that cryptococcal meningitis, which features a subacute headache often without fever or significant neurologic findings, is the most common cause. CNS toxoplasmosis is also a common cause, usually with multiple toxoplasmosis lesions visible on CT or MRI. However, at the time of seroconversion, patients may develop aseptic meningitis with headache.

Note that some of the analgesics to treat these headaches may interact with the drugs to treat the HIV infection. For example, valproate increases zidovudine blood levels.

14. **Do patients with chronic obstructive pulmonary disease with hypercapnia have headaches?**
Yes. Hypercapnia from any cause, including chronic obstructive pulmonary disease (COPD), can increase cerebral blood flow, producing intracranial vasodilatation and resulting in a dull, throbbing headache. These headaches are typically worse in the morning hours upon awakening and improve as the day progresses.

15. **How frequently is headache associated with ischemic cerebrovascular disease?**
Approximately 25% of patients with carotid-middle cerebral ischemia and almost 50% of those with vertebrobasilar insufficiency describe new, recurrent, nondescript headaches. Headaches can be the presenting symptom of ischemia, can occur during the actual infarction, or can follow the event, especially if there is hemorrhagic conversion.

KEY POINTS

1. Although acute and chronic headache syndromes together represent one of the most common pain disorders experienced by patients, headaches, in fact, are uncommonly associated with a serious systemic illness.

2. Numerous febrile systemic illnesses collectively comprise the most common systemic causes of headache.

3. Ingestion of multiple exogenous substances, including prescription and nonprescription medications, may cause headaches.

BIBLIOGRAPHY

1. Appenzella S, Costallat LT: Clinical implications of migraine in systemic lupus erythematosis: relationship to cumulatuve organ damage, *Cephalgia* 24(12):1013-1015, 2004.
2. Cady RK, Schreiber CP, Farmer KU: Understanding the patient with migraine: the evolution from episodic headache to chronic neurological disease, *Headache* 44:426-435, 2004.
3. Diener HC, Dahlof CGH: Headache associated with chronic use of substances. In Olesen J, Tfelt-Hansen P, Welch KMA, editors: *The headaches*, Philadelphia, 2000, Lippincott Williams and Wilkins, pp 871-877.
4. Edmeads J: Headaches in older people, *Postgraduate Medicine* 101(5):98-100, 1997.
5. Goadsby PJ: Metabolic and endocrine disorders. In Olesen J, Tfelt-Hansen P, Welch KMA, editors: *The headaches*, Philadelphia, 2000, Lippincott Williams and Wilkins, pp 885-889.
6. Headache Classification Subcommittee of the International Headache Society: International classification of headache disorders, 2nd ed, *Cephalgia* 24:24-151, 2004.
7. Huang ST, Lee HC, et al: Acute human immunodeficiency virus, *J Microbiol Immunol Infect* 38(1):65-68, 2005.

CHAPTER 18

TRIGEMINAL NEURALGIA

Robert A. Duarte, MD, and Charles E. Argoff, MD

1. **What is the term *tic douloureux*?**

   In French, *tic* means spasm and *douloureux* means painful. Tic douloureux is synonymous with trigeminal neuralgia.

2. **What is pretrigeminal neuralgia?**

   Pretrigeminal neuralgia is a rare, prodromal pain that occurs prior to the onset of trigeminal neuralgia. Typically, the pain is described as a dull toothache. Physical examination and imaging studies are essentially unremarkable. Clinically, patients may go to the dentist and may undergo unnecessary dental procedures. Treatment often consists of trials of anticonvulsants and/or baclofen.

3. **What are the divisions of the trigeminal nerve?**

   The three main divisions of the trigeminal nerve are the ophthalmic (V1), maxillary (V2), and mandibular (V3), which supply sensation to the face.

   The ophthalmic division supplies sensation from the eyebrows to the coronal suture. However, the sensory distribution does not stop at the hairline but at the corona, which may help in differentiating anatomic lesions from factitious illness, because patients feigning sensory loss usually make the divide at the hairline.

   Innervation of the cornea is divided, being supplied by V1 in its upper half and V2 in its lower half. The cheek bones and the inside of the nares are supplied by V2.

   The mandibular branch supplies the lower jaw. However, the angle of the jaw is supplied by a cervical root rather than by the trigeminal nerve. Again, this helps in anatomic differentiation.

4. **What are the functions of the trigeminal nerve?**

   The motor functions of the trigeminal nerve include supplying the muscles of mastication. These are the temporalis, masseters, and pterygoids. The first two are involved in vertical closing of the jaw, and the third is involved in lateral motion of the jaw (grinding).

5. **Name the exit (or entry) foramina for the branches of the trigeminal nerve.**
   - Ophthalmic branch: through the superior orbital fissure, along with cranial nerves III, IV, and VI, and the ophthalmic vein
   - Maxillary branch: through the foramen rotundum in the base of the skull
   - Mandibular branch: through the foramen ovale

6. **What is the difference between primary and secondary trigeminal neuralgia?**

   Primary or idiopathic trigeminal neuralgia implies no known structural cause for the pain (even though an aberrant vessel may be found in some cases). In secondary or symptomatic trigeminal neuralgia, pain is caused by either compression or demyelination. The clinical pain syndrome is indistinguishable. However, secondary syndromes usually involve dysfunction of the trigeminal nerve between attacks. This may take the form of sensory loss in one of the distributions of the nerve or paresis of one of the muscles of mastication.

7. **What are the clinical characteristics of trigeminal neuralgia?**

   Clinically, patients with trigeminal neuralgia describe a sharp, shooting, lightninglike or electrical sensation that typically lasts seconds to minutes in the distribution of one or more branches of the trigeminal nerve. The V2 to V3 distribution is the most common location, followed by V2; the ophthalmic division is involved in only 5% of cases. Attacks of trigeminal neuralgia are severely painful, often are followed by a lucid (pain-free) interval. In the idiopathic form, the pain is unilateral, and the physical examination is unremarkable without objective sensory or motor dysfunction. In the symptomatic form, the pain can be bilateral (in up to 4% of cases), and there may be some objective sensory loss.

8. **Describe the natural history of trigeminal neuralgia.**

   In idiopathic trigeminal neuralgia, onset is most likely after the age of 50. Patients below the age of 40 with true or symptomatic trigeminal neuralgia should be investigated for an underlying demyelinating lesion. Other structural pathology may include an underlying tumor (e.g., meningioma, ependymoma). Similarly, if there is bilateral involvement, suspect multiple sclerosis.

   The disease usually follows an exacerbating but remitting course. Over 50% of individuals will have at least a 6-month remission during their lifetime. There may be months or years when the patient is pain free. Therefore, drug holidays should be attempted to see if the patient is indeed responding to the drug or simply having a remission of the disease. In some patients, the attacks become more frequent and may be nearly continuous.

9. **What is meant by "triggers" with respect to trigeminal neuralgia?**

   Triggers are a characteristic feature of trigeminal neuralgia. They include points that, when touched, bring on paroxysms of pain. These are most commonly located around the upper lip or nose. Chewing, brushing teeth, or even a breeze are other events that can trigger a painful event. Swallowing does not trigger pain in trigeminal neuralgia.

10. **How is an episode of cluster headache different from an attack of trigeminal neuralgia?**

    Although both of these pains may exhibit a V2 distribution, cluster pain rarely has the electric shock–like quality of trigeminal neuralgia. The pain in cluster headache is usually orbital or periorbital, not neuropathic (lancinating, electrical), but more of a constant, penetrating pain of 30-minute to 180-minute duration. Cluster headaches usually occur in a specific cluster period for about 3 to 6 weeks and then remit until the next attack, usually the following year. Cluster pain is often accompanied by ptosis, coryza, and lacrimation whereas trigeminal neuralgia patients do not experience these conditions.

11. **Discuss the possible pathogenesis of trigeminal neuralgia.**

    The true cause of trigeminal neuralgia is unknown. It is believed that both peripheral and central neuropathic mechanisms play a role. The central theory holds that there is a disinhibited pool of neurons in the pons, and spontaneous discharge in these neurons causes pain. The peripheral theory holds that compression of the nerve (primarily by an aberrant blood vessel) sets up an abnormal train of discharges. It is this theory that has led to treatment of trigeminal neuralgia by surgical decompression of the nerve.

12. **What imaging procedure is recommended for patients suspected of having trigeminal neuralgia?**

    The recommended imaging procedure for patients suspected of having trigeminal neuralgia is magnetic resonance imaging (MRI) of the brain with gadolinium with special attention to Meckel's cave. Meckel's cave is an indentation in the petrous bone where the gasserian ganglion (the sensory ganglion for the trigeminal nerve) is located.

13. **Is there a drug of choice for trigeminal neuralgia?**

Yes. The first-line agent for trigeminal neuralgia remains carbamazepine. The recommended starting dose to avoid adverse events is 100 mg twice a day. This can be increased by 100 mg every day or two until the patient is pain free or side effects occur. The usual maintenance dose is 600 to 1200 mg/day (serum levels of 4 to 10 mg/ml). The half-life of carbamazepine decreases with chronic dosing. Carbamazepine is effective in 80% of patients with idiopathic trigeminal neuralgia. Many clinicians report, as a general rule, if a patient responds to carbamazepine, the diagnosis of trigeminal neuralgia is confirmed. On the other hand, if patients do not respond to the drug, it does not necessarily mean they do not have trigeminal neuralgia. If individuals are pain free for 3 months, a gradual taper of this agent can be considered.

14. **What are the most common side effects of carbamazepine?**

The most feared side effect of carbamazepine is aplastic anemia. However, this is rare. There is usually a mild depression of the white blood cell count but few other side effects. The most common side effects include drowsiness, dizziness, diplopia, and dyspepsia, which are dose-related. Carbamazepine may trigger an underlying psychosis.

15. **What type of monitoring is necessary for the use of carbamazepine?**

A complete blood count and hepatic and renal profiles should be performed before starting treatment with carbamazepine. One of the pitfalls of prescribing carbamazepine is the need to obtain a weekly blood testing (white blood count with differential) for the first 2 months, then every 3 months. After the first year, blood counts should be performed every 6 to 12 months. If the white blood cell count drops below 3000, or if the absolute neutrophil count drops below 1500, discontinue carbamazepine therapy. Aplastic anemia is a very rare complication of carbamazepine therapy, but mild leukopenia and thrombocytopenia occur in about 2% of patients.

16. **List the drug interactions of carbamazepine.**

Carbamazepine induces hepatic microsomal enzymes. Therefore, it increases its own metabolism as well as the metabolism of clonazepam, ethosuximide, oral contraceptives, warfarin, and haloperidol. This increased metabolism is of particular concern with the oral contraceptives and anticoagulants, so dose adjustments will need to be made to ensure efficacy. Propoxyphene, isoniazid, and erythromycin can inhibit the metabolism of carbamazepine, causing high levels of carbamazepine. Carbamazepine may decrease the metabolism of tramadol.

17. **What are the other pharmacologic alternatives for treating trigeminal neuralgia?**

Oxcarbazepine (Trileptal) is probably as effective as carbamazepine at doses of 900 to 1200 mg/day. Its side-effect profile is better than carbamazepine. In addition, serum testing for agranulocytosis and blood levels is not necessary.

Lamotrigine at doses of 150 to 400 mg/day may be effective especially as add-on therapy. Its side-effect profile is also favorable compared to carbamazepine. However, the predominant side effect is rash, which, although uncommon, can evolve into Stevens-Johnson syndrome.

There is anecdotal evidence to support the use of gabapentin (Neurontin). Dosages range from 300 to 3600 mg/day to help control neuropathic pain.

Baclofen (Lioresal) should be considered in those patients who do not respond to, or are unable to take, carbamazepine. The starting dose is 5 mg three times/day, with an increase of 5 to 10 mg every other day, depending on the patient's response. Maintenance dose is 50 to 60 mg/day in divided doses, with a recommended maximum of 80 mg/day. Side effects include sedation and nausea. When baclofen and carbamazepine are taken together, side effects are more common.

Phenytoin (Dilantin), like carbamazepine, depresses the response of spinal trigeminal neurons to maxillary nerve stimulation in laboratory animals. Phenytoin is effective in up to 60% of patients with trigeminal neuralgia. However, it should only be considered in patients who did not respond to baclofen or carbamazepine. The initial starting dose is 200 to 300 mg/day, with a target of 300 to 500 mg/day. Dose-dependent side effects include nystagmus, ataxia, and dysarthria. Higher levels may produce ophthalmoplegia and cognitive impairment. One advantage of phenytoin over the other agents is that it can be given intravenously if a patient has severe, intractable trigeminal neuralgia.

In refractory cases, short-acting or long-acting opioids may be considered.

18. **Which surgical procedures have been used successfully for trigeminal neuralgia?**

Surgical procedures for trigeminal neuralgia are divided into two groups: decompressive and destructive. The most commonly employed decompressive technique (microvascular decompression) is based on the theory that an aberrant vessel (often one of the cerebellar arteries or veins) compresses the nerve near its entry zone. Through a small posterior fossa craniotomy, the vessel is lifted and a cushion is placed between the nerve and the vessel. Although success rates of over 90% have been reported, there have been no double-blind studies (for obvious reasons), and pain may recur, possibly from slippage of the sponge.

In a destructive technique, the offending branches of the nerve may be lesioned percutaneously, either with radiofrequency devices or alcohol injection. The latter procedure involves inserting a needle through the skin, into the foramen of the nerve where it exits the skull. Anesthesia dolorosa (pain in the denervated area) is a bothersome complication. Percutaneous injection of glycerol around the gasserian ganglion is also effective. Although these destructive lesions are less invasive than a craniectomy for decompression, they have a higher incidence of side effects and failures.

19. **What is anesthesia dolorosa?**

In surgical lesions of the trigeminal nerve, a small percentage of patients develop a secondary pain syndrome, called anesthesia dolorosa, in which pain is felt in the denervated area. The area subserved by the lesioned branch is numb, but there is spontaneous pain within that area.

KEY POINTS

1. Trigeminal neuralgia is a neuropathic pain syndrome affecting most often the V2 and V3 division of the trigeminal nerve.

2. Trigeminal neuralgia may be "idiopathic" with no known cause or "secondary" with a known cause (e.g., tumor compression or demyelinating disease).

3. Both pharmacologic and interventional treatments are available for the treatment of trigeminal neuralgia. Pharmacologic treatments include carbamazepine, oxcarbazepine, lamotrigine, baclofen, and others; interventional therapies include microvascular decompression surgery as well as percutaneous neurolytic procedures.

BIBLIOGRAPHY

1. Evans RW, Graff-Radford SB, et al: Pretrigeminal neuralgia, *Headache* 15(3):242-244, 2005.

2. Manzoni GC, Torelli CP: Epidemiology of typical and atypical craniofacial neuralgia, *Neurol Sci* 26(Suppl 2):565-567, 2005.

3. Rozen TD: Antiepileptic drugs in the management of cluster headache and trigeminal neuralgia, *Headache* 41(Suppl 1):25-33, 2001.

4. Sheehan J, Pan HC: Gamma knife surgery for trigeminal neuralgia, *J Neurosurg* 102(3):434-441, 2005.

5. Sheehan J, Steiner L: Trigeminal neuralgia, *J Neurosurg* 102(6):1173-1179, 2005.

6. Sindrup SH, Jensen TS: Pharmacotherapy of trigeminal neuralgia, *Clin J Pain* 18(1):22-27, 2002.

7. Watson CP: Management issues of neuropathic trigeminal pain from a medical perspective, *J Orofacial* 18(4):366-373, 2004.

CHAPTER 19

GLOSSOPHARYNGEAL AND OTHER FACIAL NEURALGIAS

Robert A. Duarte, MD, and Charles E. Argoff, MD

1. **What is the clinical presentation of glossopharyngeal neuralgia?**
   The pain of glossopharyngeal neuralgia is similar in many ways to that seen in trigeminal neuralgia, but it has a different distribution. It presents with paroxysms of lancinating pain that involve the glossopharyngeal and vagus nerves. Pain is felt around the jaw, throat, ears, larynx, and/or base of the tongue. The pain is typically unilateral and lasts for about 1 minute. Multiple attacks can occur throughout a day and may even awaken the patient out of a sound sleep. The usual triggers are talking and chewing. Odynophagia is a specific trigger in glossopharyngeal neuralgia that is rarely, if ever, seen in trigeminal neuralgia. When glossopharyngeal neuralgia is not caused by an underlying tumor, spontaneous remissions often occur.

2. **Define odynophagia.**
   Odynophagia is pain upon swallowing.

3. **How common is glossopharyngeal neuralgia?**
   Glossopharyngeal neuralgia is an uncommon disorder with a prevalence of only about 1/100 that of trigeminal neuralgia. Symptoms of the primary disorder usually begin when the patient is in his or her 60s.

4. **A patient experiences neck pain upon swallowing and a sudden loss of consciousness. What is a likely explanation?**
   Swallow syncope is a syndrome of unclear mechanism that occurs in patients with glossopharyngeal neuralgia. It is thought that a barrage of impulses from the glossopharyngeal nerve, through the tractus solitarius, to the dorsal motor nucleus of the vagus nerve produces bradycardia or brief asystole. It is most commonly seen in patients with tumors of the neck and, in previously operated-on patients, usually represents tumor recurrence.

5. **What is the difference between idiopathic glossopharyngeal neuralgia and secondary glossopharyngeal neuralgia?**
   The difference between idiopathic and secondary glossopharyngeal neuralgia is a clearly identified underlying cause. Clinically, idiopathic glossopharyngeal neuralgia rarely, if ever, shows objective sensory impairment on physical examination. If there is sensory loss, a causative lesion (oropharyngeal tumor, peritonsillar infection, or vascular compression) must be sought. Tumors at the base of the skull, particularly around the jugular foramen, may also cause pain radiating to the throat, so careful imaging of the oropharynx and the base of the skull must be undertaken.

6. **What are the recommended treatments for idiopathic glossopharyngeal neuralgia?**
   Anticonvulsant or Baclofen therapy is the recommended treatment for idiopathic glossopharyngeal neuralgia, and agents such as carbamazepine, gabapentin, and phenytoin are preferred. In refractory cases, intracranial sectioning of the glossopharyngeal nerve and the upper rootlets of the vagus nerve and microvascular decompression of the glossopharyngeal nerve have been performed with some success.

7. **A patient has severe ear pain followed by ipsilateral facial weakness. What extremely important objective sign should be investigated?**
In any case of facial palsy, the search for a causative lesion is imperative. When there is severe ear and face pain, the lesion to be sought is a herpetic eruption. The vesicles most commonly affect the external auditory canal and ear but may be seen on the ear, palate, or pharynx. The syndrome of facial nerve palsy with a herpetic eruption is called Ramsay Hunt syndrome, a particularly painful neuralgia caused by zoster in the geniculate ganglion.

8. **What is the most common presentation of acute herpes zoster in the face?**
Ophthalmic zoster (a V1 distribution of the trigeminal nerve) is the most common and most troublesome. The forehead and upper lid are involved with a vesicular eruption. Pain may precede the eruption for as long as 3 to 4 days. Viral vesicles may involve the eye itself. Aside from the general symptomatic treatment for zoster, the eye must be protected from secondary infection. The complication of postherpetic neuralgia is far more common in the older person than in the young and seems to be more common when the zoster rash affects the V1 distribution.

9. **Describe the clinical features of occipital neuralgia.**
In occipital neuralgia, a sharp pain originates at the base of the skull and shoots up the back of the head. It may go as far forward as the coronal suture. It is generally unilateral and stabbing in nature. In idiopathic cases, there is no sensory loss, and some of the triggering mechanisms may be the same as those in other cranial neuralgias. However, occipital neuralgia may be a harbinger of more serious disease. Metastases to the occipital condyle can reproduce this syndrome, as can lesions at the C2 to C3 level of the spine. In these cases, local pressure will reproduce the pain, and there may be some accompanying sensory loss. Computerized tomography with overlapping cuts and bone windows can usually demonstrate the lesion. Occasionally, lesions around the foramen magnum can also produce this type of syndrome. Trauma is also a common cause; infection and chronic compression are less frequent causes.

10. **What is superior laryngeal neuralgia?**
The superior laryngeal nerve, a branch of the vagus nerve, innervates the cricothyroid muscle of the larynx. This muscle stretches, tenses, and adducts the vocal cord. Superior laryngeal neuralgia usually appears as a postsurgical complication. There are paroxysms of unilateral submandibular pain, sometimes radiating to the eye, ear, or shoulder. This pain may be indistinguishable from glossopharyngeal neuralgia. It lasts from seconds to minutes and is usually provoked by swallowing, straining the voice, turning the head, coughing, sneezing, yawning, or blowing the nose.

11. **What are the typical characteristics of Villaret's syndrome?**
Villaret's syndrome is characterized by unilateral paralysis of the ninth, tenth, eleventh, and twelfth cranial nerves, sometimes accompanied by a Horner's syndrome on the same side. The syndrome may include glossopharyngeal neuralgia and is associated with lesions in the posterior retroparotid space.

12. **What is Eagle's syndrome?**
Eagle's syndrome involves elongation of the styloid process of the temporal bone, which may cause impingement on the glossopharyngeal nerve and is thought to be one of the causes of secondary glossopharyngeal neuralgia.

13. **Define sphenopalatine neuralgia.**
Sphenopalatine neuralgia has been given a number of names, including lower half headache, greater superficial neuralgia, Sluder's neuralgia, and atypical facial pain. It is an uncommon form of facial neuralgia. The key clinical features include unilateral pain in the face (usually around the nasal region) lasting for days and associated with nasal congestion, otalgia, and tinnitus.

Unlike trigeminal and glossopharyngeal neuralgia, sphenopalatine neuralgia is usually not associated with a trigger zone. Some authors believe that this is not a separate syndrome and may simply be a variation of cluster headache. Sphenopalatine ganglion blocks have been tried with minimal success, but this treatment remains controversial.

KEY POINTS

1. The typical triggers of glossopharyngeal neuralgia are talking and chewing.

2. Because idiopathic glossopharyngeal neuralgia rarely if ever is associated with objective sensory loss, when such sensory loss is present glossopharyngeal neuralgia secondary to a structural abnormality (vascular anomaly or tumor) or infection should be considered and evaluated for.

3. Occipital neuralgia, a sharp paroxysmal that originates at the base of the skull and shoots up the head as far as the coronal suture, is a common source of chronic neck and head pain.

BIBLIOGRAPHY

1. Rozen TD: Trigeminal neuralgia and glossopharyngeal neuralgia, *Neurol Clin* 22(1):185-206, 2004.

2. Sampson JH, Grossi PM, et al: Microvascular decompression for glossopharyngeal neuralgia: long-term effectiveness and complication avoidance, *Neurosurgery* 54(4):884-890, 2004.

3. Elias J, Kuniyoshi R, et al: Glossopharyngeal neuralgia associated with cardiac syncope, *Arq Bras Cardiol* 78(5):510-519, 2002.

4. Mortellaro C, Biancucci P, et al: Eagle's syndrome: importance of a correct diagnosis and adequate surgical treatment, *J Craniofac Surg* 13(6):755-758, 2002.

5. Ashkenasi A, Levin M: Three common neuralgias: how to manage trigeminal, occipital and postherpetic pain, *Postgrad Med* 116(3):16-18, 21-24, 31-32, 2004.

CHAPTER 20

LOW BACK PAIN

Ronald Kanner, MD, FAAN, FACP

1. **What are the most common causes of acute back pain?**
   In most cases of acute back pain, no clear pathophysiologic mechanism is defined, and patients are diagnosed as having "back strain." Episodes are usually preceded by minor trauma, heavy lifting, or a "near fall." Direct trauma is rarely a cause. A small minority of patients have acute medical illnesses that cause back pain.

   The first urgent crossroad in the diagnosis of low back pain is to decide whether the patient has a medically emergent condition (tumor, infection, or trauma) or not. The signs and symptoms that should alert the clinician to impending disaster are focal spine tenderness, fever, weight loss, or bowel or bladder dysfunction. More than 90% of cases of so-called benign acute low back pain resolve spontaneously.

2. **Why does the back hurt?**
   Erect posture forces the spine into a position in which it is constantly exposed to minor trauma and to stress on pain-sensitive structures. These pain-sensitive structures are the supporting bones, articulations, meninges, nerves, muscles, and aponeuroses. The vertebral body, despite being short, is actually a long bone with endplates of hard bone and a center of cancellous bone. It is innervated by the dorsal roots. In general, the periosteum, including the periosteum associated with the spine, is markedly pain-sensitive. (This is why, for example, banging the shin is so painful: the periosteum is unprotected.) The articulations (facet joints) are true diarthrodial joints and have a capsule and meniscus. The capsule and bones are richly innervated with nociceptors and are subjected to stress every time the spine turns or bends.

3. **Why do some patients with absolutely no evidence of spine injury complain of chronic, disabling back pain?**
   The answer here is the same as the answer in any other significant chronic pain syndrome: the absence of a demonstrable lesion does not confirm the diagnosis of psychogenic pain, and the presence of psychopathology does not mean that the patient is not suffering. Although our intellectual grasp of nociceptive systems is good, these systems are not sufficient to explain all types of pain. Chronic pain must be viewed as a biopsychosocial phenomenon.

4. **Some patients who had clearly defined causes for back pain continue to suffer from the same pain, even after the causative agent is eliminated. Why?**
   There is evidence to suggest that chronic, ongoing pain can actually restructure signaling within the central nervous system. There are synaptic changes and there may be neuronal hyperactivity, expression of new genes, and other central phenomena that perpetuate the perception of pain.

5. **What characteristics of pain help to define its origin?**
   The type of pain suffered varies with the structure involved. Pain originating in a vertebral body (from osteoporosis, tumor, or infection) tends to be local and aching. It is somatic, nociceptive pain, made worse by standing or sitting and relieved by lying supine. Even though it

is usually local, it may refer to other sites. Characteristically, the L1 vertebral body refers pain to the iliac crests and hips. When facet joints are involved, pain is most pronounced when the back is extended. Limitation of active range of motion is a hallmark of facet pain.

6. How do the intervertebral discs ("slipped discs") contribute to back pain?
The intervertebral disc is composed of a firm anulus fibrosus, with a spongier nucleus pulposus inside. The fibrous ring is innervated by nociceptors, but the nucleus pulposus is not. When strong vertical stress is applied to the spine, the nucleus pulposus bulges outward through the anulus fibrosus. Stretching of the fibrous ring is painful; in general, it produces localized low back pain. Once the anulus breaks, disc material may extrude and press against a nerve. Pressure on the nerve root is felt as radicular pain ("sciatica"). Of interest, as the anulus bursts, the intense low back pain tends to subside and is replaced by radicular pain.

A bulging disc in itself is usually not painful. Anything that increases pressure on the spine increases pain from a disc. Thus, pain is exacerbated by standing, sitting, and the Valsalva maneuver.

7. What is the usual outcome of a patient with acute low back pain?
The vast majority of the general population will have acute back pain at some point in their lives. Over 90% of cases resolve, without specific therapy, in less than 2 weeks. As mentioned earlier, in most cases no specific diagnosis is made.

8. How helpful are radiographs in determining the etiology of acute low back pain?
Most patients with acute low back pain require no imaging procedures. It may not be easy to convince a patient who is writhing in pain that no radiographs are needed. However, plain radiographic findings of degenerative disease are as common in asymptomatic patients as in patients with acute back pain. Furthermore, magnetic resonance imaging (MRI) is far too sensitive and nonspecific to be used as a screening procedure. More than one half of adults with no history of back pain may show asymptomatic bulging of discs at one or more lumbar levels, and fully one fourth show disc protrusion.

Reserve imaging procedures for patients with acute low back pain when the diagnosis is in question. Specifically, if fever or point tenderness on the spine raises the suspicion of infection or tumor, an imaging procedure is imperative.

9. A patient complaining of left lower back pain stands with his buttocks protruding and with his shoulders tilted to the left. What does this stance indicate?
The spine has a number of normal curvatures. With the patient standing erect, the normal position of the spine shows cervical lordosis, thoracic kyphosis, and lumbar lordosis. In low back pain with muscle spasm, the lumbar lordosis may be lost or hyperaccentuated. If the patient tilts toward one side, there may be muscle spasm or foraminal encroachment. With lateral tilt, the ipsilateral intervertebral foramen narrows. Therefore, if there is nerve root compression in the foramen, pain increases. Conversely, when the patient tilts away from an affected side, the foramen on that side opens, lessening neural pain but possibly accentuating pain from muscle spasm. In lateral disc herniations, patients tend to lean away from the side of the herniation.

10. What is the normal range of motion of the spine?
The lumbar spine should be able to flex forward 40 to 60 degrees from the vertical. As the patient extends backward, range is somewhat reduced (to about 20 to 35 degrees). Severe pain on extension of the spine may indicate pathology in the articular facets.

11. **Describe the significance of the straight-leg raising maneuver.**

Straight-leg raising is used to diagnose nerve root compression from disc disease. It is most commonly used to look for lower lumbar root pathology. The patient lies supine, and the leg is elevated from the ankle, with the knee remaining straight. Normally, patients can elevate the leg 60 to 90 degrees without pain. In disc herniations, elevations of 30 to 40 degrees produce pain.

Ipsilateral straight-leg raising is more sensitive, but less specific, than contralateral straight-leg raising. That is, nearly all patients with herniated discs have pain on straight-leg raising on the affected side, but straight-leg raising elicits pain in many other conditions (e.g., severe hip arthritis). However, contralateral straight-leg raising does not produce pain on the affected side unless the pain is due to root disease.

Use Patrick's maneuver to differentiate between hip and lumbar root pathology. The thigh is flexed on the abdomen and the knee is externally rotated, putting stress on the hip joint but not on the nerve root. The patient with hip pathology experiences pain, but the patient with root pathology does not.

12. **What is the significance of pain on percussion of the spine?**

Benign disease (disc protrusion and muscle spasm) rarely, if ever, produces pain on percussion of the spine. This sign usually indicates bone disease, most often metastases or infection; it requires immediate investigation with imaging procedures.

13. **What historical data raise suspicion of infection or tumor, rather than benign disease?**

Most patients with herniated discs or other benign mechanical causes of back pain state that the pain improves with bed rest. When they are no longer weight bearing, pain is relieved. Patients with tumor or infection often say that their worst pain is at night when they are in bed. Nocturnal exacerbation is a clear danger signal.

14. **Describe the most common scenario for a herniated intervertebral disc.**

In the most common scenario for a herniated intervertebral disc, patients report severe back pain after lifting something heavy, and a few days later pain radiates down the leg. This sequence of events is due to the pathologic process underlying a herniated disc. With the initial exertion, the nucleus pulposus pushes against the anulus fibrosus, causing it to distend. This distention causes local back pain. As the anulus ruptures, the back pain is relieved, but the nucleus then presses against a nerve root, causing radiated pain down the leg.

15. **What is the most common symptom for vertebral metastases?**

Patients with vertebral metastases almost invariably experience localized back pain. More than 95% of patients with malignant epidural spinal cord compression have pain as their first complaint. Pain is usually described as deep, localized, and aching. As neural structures become involved, the pain radiates in the distribution of the affected nerves. The thoracic spine is the site most commonly affected; thus, pain radiates in a band around the chest. Over time, further neurologic problems ensue. If epidural spinal cord compression progresses, patients have paraparesis, sensory loss, and bowel and bladder involvement. Epidural spinal cord compression from tumor is a medical emergency.

Pain usually resolves fairly quickly with the administration of high doses of dexamethasone. Definitive treatment with radiation therapy or surgery is then undertaken.

16. **Describe the radiographic appearance of spinal metastases.**

On plain films, one of the earliest signs of spinal metastasis is erosion of a pedicle. Over time, the vertebral body begins to lose height. MRI reveals a change in signal intensity in the vertebral body. As the tumor progresses, it may be seen invading the epidural space and compressing the spinal cord.

17. **Both vertebral metastases and vertebral osteomyelitis can cause destruction of vertebral bodies and changes on MRI signal. How can they be differentiated?**
When tumors affect the vertebral bodies, they tend to spare the disc spaces. Even though two or three adjacent vertebral bodies may be destroyed by tumor, the disc spaces between them are generally preserved. In the case of vertebral osteomyelitis, the disc space typically is destroyed by the infection, and the adjacent vertebral bodies appear to form a block of infection.

18. **What is the difference between an osteoporotic vertebral collapse and vertebral collapse caused by tumor involvement?**
Clinically, the pain from an osteoporotic collapse is almost invariably relieved by a brief period of bed rest. Tumor-related pain is often unrelieved by bed rest.
   Pathologically, an osteoporotic collapse is essentially an accordion of the vertebral body. A hollow body collapses on itself. With tumor involvement, collapse of the vertebral body causes extrusion of tumor material.
   Tumor extrusion may compress the spinal cord. Compression from osteoporosis is exceedingly rare.

19. **What treatment should be used for the pain from metastatic destruction of a vertebral body?**
Pain from vertebral metastases is due to destruction of bone trabeculae, expansion of the periosteum, and stretching of the dura. This is a classic somatic nociceptive pain syndrome. As such, it is well treated by a combination of either nonsteroidal antiinflammatory drugs (NSAIDs) or steroids and an opioid. As bone metastases grow, they elaborate prostaglandin E_2, which continues destruction of bone trabeculae. The administration of an NSAID or steroids decreases production of prostaglandin E_2 and slows destruction.

20. **Why is osteoporosis painful?**
In general, osteoporosis is not painful in the absence of fractures. In weight-bearing bones, microfractures can occur with minor trauma. Unfortunately, the patient with this type of pain generally stays in bed, and the absence of weight bearing leads to further demineralization of the bone and additional fractures upon weight bearing. In such patients, progressive exercise is of paramount importance. Weight bearing leads to greater bone density and fewer fractures. Of interest, when a vertebral body collapses completely, it is painful at first, but the pain subsides once the fracture is complete.

21. **How should pain from an osteoporotic vertebral collapse be treated?**
First, be sure that the pain is due to benign osteoporotic collapse. Although postmenopausal women and patients treated with corticosteroids are at high risk, do not assume that the osteoporosis is idiopathic. Evaluate serum protein electrophoresis, sedimentation rate, alkaline phosphatase, phosphorus, serum calcium, and plain films to rule out a secondary cause for the osteoporosis. Once a secondary cause has been ruled out, treat the patient with therapy directed at reversing the osteoporosis and with analgesics and exercise. Vertebroplasty and kyphoplasty are radiologic procedures for the treatment of the intense pain caused by vertebral compression fracture when the pain has been inadequately controlled with more conservative means. Each procedure involves the intraosseous injection of acrylic cement under local anesthesia and fluoroscopic guidance to control the pain of vertebral fractures associated with osteoporosis.

22. **What is the most common symptom of vertebral osteomyelitis?**
A patient with vertebral osteomyelitis usually has subacute back pain that increases over days to weeks. Progressive pain is felt in the low back and, if untreated, focal weakness and bowel and bladder problems ensue. Focal tenderness is present, and usually another source of

infection is found. Although previously the most common incidence was in the lumbar spine in men over age 50, the AIDS epidemic has changed the epidemiology somewhat. Younger men are affected, and the cervical spine is becoming a more common site of vertebral osteomyelitis.

23. **What is the most common cause of vertebral osteomyelitis?**
In immunocompetent hosts, *Staphylococcus aureus* infection is the most common causative agent. Infection involves the vertebral bodies, endplates, and disc spaces, but generally spares the posterior elements. In the rare cases of actinomycosis or coccidioidomycosis, the posterior elements may be involved, and the spine becomes unstable.

24. **What is sciatica?**
The term *sciatica* has come into rather broad usage and usually refers to any sharp pain that radiates down the posterior aspect of the leg. Its initial formulation was for pain in a sciatic nerve distribution. However, it is used to describe pain of L5 root compromise, S1 root compromise, and true sciatic neuropathy.

25. **What is piriformis syndrome?**
The sciatic nerve passes through the piriformis muscle as it exits the pelvis. Occasionally, the muscle has a fibrous band or area of contraction. Pain is felt in the distribution of the sciatic nerve, but there is no back pain. Pain radiates from the buttocks down the posterior aspect of the thigh. Deep palpation of the piriformis muscle, either through the buttocks or through a rectal examination, exacerbates the pain and reproduces the patient's clinical syndrome. Therapy involves repeated stretching of the piriformis muscle or, in extreme cases, injection of lidocaine and steroids into the piriformis.

26. **What are the common areas of pain radiation in lumbar and sacral radiculopathies?**
- L1 Iliac crest and inguinal canal
- L2 Inguinal canal
- L3 Anterior thigh
- L4 Anterior thigh and medial calf
- L5 Buttocks and the lateral aspect of the shin
- S1 Buttocks to the posterior thigh

27. **If a patient has severe back pain radiating into the anterior thigh accompanied by weakness of the leg, how can you differentiate between an L4 radiculopathy and a femoral nerve lesion?**
The L2, L3, and L4 roots split into anterior and posterior divisions. The anterior divisions come together to form the obturator nerve, and the posterior divisions come together to form the femoral nerve. The quadriceps muscle is innervated by the femoral nerve, and the adductors of the thigh are innervated by the obturator nerve. In an L4 radiculopathy, both the quadriceps and the adductors are affected. In a femoral nerve lesion, the quadriceps are affected, but the adductors are spared.

28. **Which nerve roots subserve the knee jerk reflex?**
The L2, L3, and L4 roots, through the femoral nerve, form the afferent and efferent arc of the knee jerk. When the patellar tendon is tapped, the quadriceps contracts.

29. **Which nerve root subserves the Achilles reflex?**
The Achilles reflex is mediated through the S1 nerve root. Tapping of the Achilles tendon produces contraction of the gastrocnemius muscle.

30. **What is the role of MRI in the diagnosis of herniated discs?**

The MRI scan is highly sensitive for disc pathology. Even slight bulges in the disc can be picked up with an appropriate MRI; however, it may be overly sensitive. The fact that a disc is seen to be bulging or herniated on MRI does not mean that it causes the pain syndrome. Nearly one half of a sample of asymptomatic patients was shown to have disc bulges on MRI. The advantage of MRI over computed tomography (CT) scan is that the nerve root can be seen.

31. **In a patient with low back pain and a previously operated-on herniated disc, how can you differentiate between a new disc herniation and scar tissue?**

Differentiating between a new disc herniation and scar tissue can be a particularly vexing clinical problem. On MRI scan, discs do not enhance with gadolinium, but inflammatory tissue may.

32. **If a patient has acute low back pain and there are no findings on clinical examination, how much bed rest is required?**

No evidence indicates that bed rest influences the ultimate outcome of low back pain. In general, patients with acute pain feel more comfortable with a day or two in bed. However, more prolonged bed rest leads to deconditioning and may prolong recovery time (see Questions 20 and 49).

33. **What weight of traction should be used for low back pain?**

The theoretical benefit of traction is to lower intradiscal pressure. Simply lying supine reduces pressure, and no evidence indicates that traction significantly alters the outcome of low back pain. Traction from 5 pounds to total body inversion has been used without clear demonstration of lowering pressure beyond the levels achieved by recumbency.

34. **Describe the role of myelography in low back pain.**

Myelography has been almost completely supplanted by MRI scanning in low back pain. However, in cases in which the exact location or morphology of a disc herniation is in doubt, myelography can be combined with CT scanning to provide exquisite anatomic images.

35. **What is meant by a facet syndrome?**

The articular facets are the means by which the vertebral bodies articulate with each other. When these joints become inflamed or arthritic, range of motion is diminished. Maximal stress is put on these joints when the spine is hyperextended. Thus, when the patient reports no pain on anterior flexion, but severe pain on extension, a facet syndrome is believed to be present. The diagnosis is confirmed by CT scanning of the affected area with demonstration of marked arthritic changes of the specific facet. In some patients, direct instillation of a steroid solution and lidocaine into the affected facet produces dramatic relief.

36. **What is meant by degenerative disease of the spine?**

The term degenerative joint disease (DJD) is probably overused. Most joints, after age 40, show osteophytes or other signs of deterioration. In the spine, these signs are particularly common and may not correlate with pain states.

37. **What is spondylolisthesis?**

Spondylolisthesis refers to slippage of one vertebral body on the adjacent one. It is fairly common in the older person (10% to 15% of even asymptomatic patients over the age of 70). Most cases are caused by lysis of the posterior elements, which may be due to advanced age or trauma. When pain is markedly exacerbated by movement, imaging should be performed with flexion and extension views, which show whether there is any increase in movement at the abnormal joint.

38. **What is meant by a lateral recess syndrome?**
The lumbar spine contains a triangular space (the lateral recess) bordered by the pedicle, vertebral body, and superior articular facet. Facet hypertrophy or a disc fragment may encroach upon this triangular space and compress a nerve root on its way to exit at the next lower level. Pain is often neuropathic and is characterized by lancinating jabs or by a burning, dysesthetic pain in the distribution of the affected nerve root.

39. **Define lumbar arachnoiditis.**
Lumbar arachnoiditis refers to thickening of the arachnoid lining around the nerve roots. It is most commonly iatrogenic, produced by repeated myelography or by surgery. Nerve roots may become matted in an inflamed arachnoid or by scar tissue. On MRI, the nerve roots appear matted together. They may form a clump in the center of the canal or be matted to the sides of the canal.

40. **What is spinal stenosis?**
Spinal stenosis is a narrowing of the spinal canal. Facet hypertrophy, ligamentous hardening, and spondylolisthesis can narrow the diameter of the lumbar canal as a result of normal aging. In some cases, this may lead to a syndrome called neurogenic claudication, in which patients are pain-free at rest, but develop pain upon walking. The pain is felt as an ache in both legs. Patients characteristically say that they get relief after stopping for a few minutes and leaning forward at the waist. According to one theory, compromise of the radicular arteries gives rise to the claudication.

41. **What is the role of epidural steroid injections in low back pain?**
There are not enough well-controlled clinical trials in select patient populations to define accurately the indications for epidural steroid injection. However, clinical experience shows that many patients have dramatic responses. A small amount of a corticosteroid is mixed with a small amount of lidocaine, and the mixture is instilled into the epidural space. Patients report early pain relief from the lidocaine, exacerbation of pain in the evening, and then gradual diminution of pain as the steroids take effect. In good hands, epidural steroid injections are a relatively low-risk procedure. In any case, no more than three injections should be performed in any 6-month period, because epidural steroid injections may lead to ligamentous laxity.

42. **What are the indications for laminectomy and discectomy?**
The indications are open to great dispute. Some surgeons believe that the only cure for lumbar radiculopathy is surgical removal of the causative disc. However, in many cases of low back pain, the herniated disc may not be the causative factor. A conservative approach dictates that progressive pain with neurologic impairment is an indication for surgical intervention.

43. **Is the timing of surgery important?**
There is evidence to suggest that the long-term outcome is better when patients undergo surgery before the pain has become chronic.

44. **Why is there no definitive answer about the benefit of surgical procedures that have been performed for decades?**
The problem lies in a number of areas. An appropriate study of laminectomy and discectomy would have to control for the cause of back pain, anatomical location, surgical procedure performed, neurologic and psychological status of the patient, skill of the surgeon, intensity of pain, compounding social factors, duration of pain, and specific criteria for outcome. This study would have to be prospective, involve a large number of patients, and have a sham surgery control. Such a study would be prohibitively expensive and have a number of ethical issues.

45. **Is transcutaneous electrical nerve stimulation (TENS) effective in low back pain?**
Here again, studies have yielded conflicting results. In a large metaanalysis, a definitive statement could not be made. When TENS is compared with inactive placebo, it appears to have an effect. However, an appropriate control would have to deliver some type of stimulus. Much the same can be said for acupuncture.

46. **What are the recent surgical innovations in the treatment of lumbar disc disease?**
Surgical interventions are becoming "less invasive." Some of the newer techniques include intradiscal electrothermal therapy (IDET), radiofrequency ablation (RFA), percutaneous endoscopic laser discectomy (PELD), and cryoablation. These are all aimed at removing or repairing disc material, without the need for extensive laminectomies.

47. **What is the role of acupuncture in low back pain?**
A systematic review of the literature recently updated a prior study. Because acute low back pain tends to be self-limited, firm conclusions could not be drawn regarding the efficacy of acupuncture in that setting. For chronic low back pain, it did seem to show some advantages for pain relief and functional improvement in the short term. In the current context, given the lack of well-controlled studies, acupuncture should probably be viewed as a useful adjunct to other therapies in chronic low back pain.

48. **What is the role of exercise in low back pain?**
Individually tailored exercise programs, aimed at stretching, strengthening, and general conditioning, may improve pain and function in chronic low back pain, when the exercises are supervised by a trained individual. The exact characteristics of the exercise pattern that best treats low back pain have not been elucidated.

49. **What is the role of prolonged bed rest in low back pain?**
There is no evidence to suggest that bed rest of more than 2 days is beneficial. In fact, for people with acute low back pain, bed rest may be less effective than staying active. There is little or no difference in outcome in patients with sciatica.

50. **What is the best method for treating acute and chronic low back pain?**
Systematic reviews have covered areas as diverse as psychological interventions and extensive surgical exploration with instrumentation. Almost invariably, these studies end with the phrase "further studies with adequate controls are required for definitive statement."

51. **What phrase most clearly demonstrates that we do not fully understand the relative indications of specific treatments for low back pain?**
"Further studies with adequate controls are required for definitive statement."

KEY POINTS

1. Most cases of acute low back pain are not associated with a clearly defined pathophysiologic mechanism, and most resolve spontaneously. In most cases imaging is not required for patients with acute low back pain.

2. Chronic low back pain is associated with many known causes, including degenerative disc and joint disease, neoplasm, osteoporosis, and infections, but frequently a known cause cannot be determined.

3. Numerous treatments are available and should be considered for patients with chronic low back pain. Treatment should be individualized to the patient's needs and specific circumstances.

BIBLIOGRAPHY

1. Armon C, Argoff CA, Samuels J, Backonja MM: Therapeutics and Technology Assessment Subcommittee of the American Academy of Neurology. Assessment: use of epidural steroid injections to treat radicular lumbosacal pain: report of the Therapeutics and Technology Assessment Subcommittee of the American Academy of Neurology, *Neurology* 68(10):723-729, 2007.
2. BenDebba M, Torgerson WS, Boyd RJ, et al: Persistent low back pain and sciatica in the United States: treatment outcomes, *J Spinal Disord Tech* 15(1):2-15, 2002.
3. Boos N, Semmer N, Elfering A, et al: Natural history of individuals with asymptomatic disc abnormalities in magnetic resonance imaging: predictors of low back pain-related medical consultation and work incapacity, *Spine* 25(12):1484-1492, 2000.
4. Brosseau L, Milne S, Robinson V, et al: Efficacy of the transcutaneous electrical nerve stimulation for the treatment of low back pain: a meta-analysis, *Spine* 27(6):596-603, 2002.
5. Deyo RA, Weinstein JN: Low back pain, *N Engl J Med* 344(5):363-370, 2001.
6. Furlan AD, Clarke J, Esmail R, et al: A critical review of reviews on the treatment of chronic low back pain, *Spine* 26(7):E155-162, 2001.
7. Furlan AD, van Tulder M, Cherkin D, Tsukayama H, Lao L, Koes B, Berman B: Acupuncture and dry-needling for low back pain: an updated systematic review with in the framework of the Cochrane collaboration, *Spine* 30(8):944-963, 2005.
8. Hagen KB, Hilde G, Jamtvedt G, Winnem MF: The Cochrane review of bed rest for acute low back pain and sciatica, *Spine* 25(22):2932-2939, 2000.
9. Hagen KB, Jamtvedt G, Hilde G, Winnem MF: The updated Cochrane review of bed rest for low back pain and sciatica, *Spine* 30(5):542-546, 2005.
10. Hayden JA, van Tulder MW, Tominson G: Systematic review: strategies for using exercise therapy to improve outcomes in chronic low back pain, *Annals of Internal Medicine* 142(9):776-785, 2005.
11. Jensen ME, Dion JE: Percutaneous vertebroplasty in the treatment of osteoporotic compression fractures, *Neuroimaging Clin N Am* 10(3):547-568, 2000.
12. Kanner RM: Low back pain. In Portenoy RK, Kanner RM, editors: Pain Management: theory and practice, Philadelphia, 1996, F.A. Davis, pp 126-144.
13. Onesti ST: Failed back syndrome, *Neurologist* 10(5):259-264, 2004.
14. Portenoy R, Lipton R, Foley K: Back pain in the cancer patient: an algorithm for evaluation and management, *Neurology* 37:134-138, 1987.
15. Singh K, Ledet E, Carl A: Intradiscal therapy: a review of current treatment modalities, *Spine* 30(Suppl 17): 20-29, 2005.
16. Truchon M: Determinants of chronic disability related to low back pain: towards an integrity of biopsychosocial model, *Disabil Rehabil* 23(17):758-767, 2001.
17. Van Tulder MW, Ostelo R, Vlaeyen JW, et al: Behavioral treatment for chronic low back pain: a systematic review within the framework of the Cochrane Back Review Group, *Spine* 26(3):270-281, 2001.

CHAPTER 21

NECK AND ARM PAIN

Ronald Kanner, MD, FAAN, FACP, and Gary McCleane, MD

1. **What factors predispose a person to the development of neck pain on the job?**

   In the work setting, high quantitative job demands and low co-worker support appear to be independent risk factors for neck pain. In the general population, women are more likely than men to develop neck pain. A history of previous neck injury is a risk factor for subsequent chronic pain. A past history of low back pain also may predict the appearance of neck pain. Psychosocial factors may be as important as physical abnormalities in the development of chronic neck pain, paralleling the prevalent issues in low back pain.

2. **What precautions can reliably diminish the risk of neck pain?**

   Although many occupational standards have been established to reduce neck pain, the literature supports only exercise as a clear preventive agent. There are relatively few controlled studies that have yielded a positive outcome for ergonomic reconfiguring, avoidance of repetitive stress injury, and lumbar supports. These interventions may have some role, but their benefit has not been demonstrated adequately in controlled trials.

3. **Who had the first case of neck pain?**

   In his book on neck and arm pain, Dr. Rene Cailliet cites writings in the *Papyrus*, over 4600 years ago, describing cervical vertebral dislocation and sprains. He goes on to say that Tutankhamen described what may have been the first cervical laminectomy. At any rate, it appears that cervical pain has been present since humans walked erect.

4. **Why does the neck hurt?**

   As in the lumbar spine, there are a number of pain-sensitive structures in the cervical spine. These include the vertebral bodies, laminae, dura, and surrounding muscles. Inflammation or destruction of any one of these structures produces pain.

5. **What is the normal configuration of the cervical spine?**

   In the pain-free, normal cervical spine, there is a gentle lordosis from C1 to T1. As the head flexes forward, this lordosis normally disappears. Anterior flexion should be pain free, even with the chin touching the chest. On lateral flexion, the ears should come within a few centimeters of the shoulder. Flexion and extension have a combined excursion of about 70 degrees. Rotations about the vertical axis (left and right) are approximately 90 degrees in each direction. Lateral flexion should be about 45 degrees in each direction.

   When testing range of motion (ROM) of the cervical spine, always have the patient try active ROM before passive ROM. If there are structural abnormalities, the patient will guard the area.

6. **What is an early sign of neck pain?**

   One of the earliest signs is straightening of the cervical lordosis. Normally, the cervical spine demonstrates a gentle curve with the convex to the posterior. As the patient tries to guard the neck from movement, the lordosis disappears.

7. **What is the prevalence of neck pain?**
Neck pain appears to be less common than low back pain in the general population. There are very few demographic studies of neck pain in the literature. The vast majority of pain prevalence studies have been done on low back pain. Acute attacks of stiff neck appear to be relatively common, occurring in 25% to 50% of workers. Chronic neck pain, however, is less prevalent.

8. **How many cervical vertebrae and roots are there?**
There are seven cervical vertebrae and eight cervical spinal nerves. C1, however, has no sensory root and innervates the muscles that support the head.

9. **How do the exiting characteristics of the nerves in the cervical spine differ from those in the rest of the spine?**
In the thoracic and lumbar spines, the spinal nerves exit through the intervertebral foramen subjacent to the vertebral body numbered for that root. Therefore, the L1 root exits between the L1 and L2 vertebral bodies, L2 between L2 and L3, and so on. The root is numbered for the body under which it exits. In the cervical spine, however, the numbering is somewhat different. Except for the C8 nerve root, the cervical roots exist above its corresponding vertebrae. The C8 root exits between the seventh cervical and the first thoracic vertebrae. C7 exits between C6 and C7, and so on in a cephalad direction.

10. **What is whiplash injury?**
Whiplash refers to acceleration/deceleration of the head, whipping the neck. It most commonly occurs in motor vehicle accidents, usually when a car is struck from behind. Patients complain of soreness and tenderness in the neck, usually occurring a day or two after the initial injury. In most cases, pain resolves spontaneously. In some, it can go on for many months or years. On examination, there is tenderness of the neck muscles and limitation of ROM. Focal neurologic dysfunction is uncommon.

11. **What is the presumed mechanism of whiplash injury?**
Whiplash is a widely disputed entity. The mechanistic theory holds that a rear impact causes the sixth cervical vertebrae to be rotated back into extension before movement of the upper cervical vertebrae. This produces an "S-shaped" deformity in the cervical spine. The neck mobility is reduced immediately after trauma, but may be normal when measured more than 3 months later. Whiplash, much like chronic low back pain, should probably be viewed as a biopsychosocial phenomenon.

12. **Which articulations in the neck are critical to anteroposterior flexion?**
Fifty percent of the AP flexion of the neck is centered on the atlantooccipital joint, and 50% is divided relatively evenly among the other cervical vertebral articulations. Therefore, even with relatively severe cervical spondylosis, some degree of nodding ability is maintained.

13. **How does movement of the head affect the intervertebral foramina through which cervical roots exit?**
Anterior flexion of the head opens the neuroforamina. As the head turns from side to side or tilts from side to side, the ipsilateral intervertebral foramen closes. If there is nerve root compromise, tilting or turning the head toward that side increases radicular pain.

14. **What is the most benign cause of cervical pain?**
Stress, with accompanying muscle tension, can produce neck pain and tenderness. With tension and anxiety, the shoulders are held shrugged and muscle pain ensues. The ideal treatment for this would be removal of the stress, though this is rarely possible. More practically, local applications of heat or cold or relaxation techniques may be useful.

15. **What is meant by spondylosis?**

Spondylosis refers to pathologic changes in the spinal column. It is also called degenerative disc disease and osteoarthritis of the spine. Radiographically, there is hypertrophy of the facet joints, narrowing of disc spaces, and osteophyte formation. All of these changes narrow the spinal canal and compromise nerve roots as they exit through the intervertebral foramina. Neurologic compromise may be at the root or cord level.

16. **What is a central cord injury?**

In severe trauma to the neck there may be hemorrhage into the central canal of the spinal cord. With time, this can progress to form a true syrinx. Patients initially complain of burning in the hands. With time, atrophy of the hand muscles and a "suspended sensory loss" may develop. This suspended sensory loss, or "cape distribution" of loss of pinprick and temperature sense, is due to the anatomy of the crossing, second-order, nociceptive fibers. The second-order neurons that are going to form the lateral spinothalamic tracts cross anterior to the central canal in the spinal cord (see Chapter 3, Basic Mechanisms). An injury at that level produces suspended sensory loss, without sensory loss below or above the point of injury.

17. **List the signs and symptoms of cervical epidural spinal cord compression.**

- Pain: the first symptom; usually local, with some radicular radiation depending on the level at which the compression occurs
- Myelopathy: characterized by sensory loss below the level of compression and paraparesis
- Hyperreflexia
- Babinski signs
- Bowel and bladder involvement

18. **What are the common causes of cervical cord compression?**

The most common causes are trauma, infection, and tumor. Cervical spondylosis can produce spinal cord compression, but it is usually insidious and progresses over many years.

Prognosis in spondylitic cord compression is poorest in the older person and in patients with sphincter disturbances.

19. **What roots form the brachial plexus?**

Cervical roots 4, 5, and 6 form the upper trunk of the brachial plexus; C7 forms the middle trunk; and C8 and T1 form the lower trunk.

20. **What is the sensory distribution of the cervical nerve roots?**

- C1 has no sensory representation.
- C2 covers the occiput.
- C3 and 4 cover part of the neck and trapezius.
- C5 goes over the cap of the shoulder and part of the lateral arm.
- C6 produces sensory symptoms over the lateral forearm, lateral hand, and first and second digits.
- C7 mainly affects the third and fourth digits.
- C8 covers the medial part of the forearm and the fifth finger.

21. **What reflex changes are commonly seen with cervical nerve root compression?**

C5 lesions commonly lead to diminished biceps and brachioradialis reflexes, whereas C7 affects the triceps. There is some C6 contribution to the biceps and brachioradialis, but isolated C6 lesions are unusual, and they tend not to affect the reflexes because C5 is the main innervation.

22. **Which muscles are innervated by the C5 root?**

The main muscles that are innervated by the C5 root are supraspinatus, infraspinatus, deltoid, biceps, and brachioradialis.

23. **Describe thoracic outlet syndrome.**
Thoracic outlet syndrome refers to compression of the neurovascular bundle as it crosses the first rib and enters the arm. It may be compressed by a cervical rib, by the scalenus muscle, or by fibrous bands. Pain is usually felt in the forearm and is exacerbated by movement and by elevation and abduction of the arm.

24. **What is Adson's sign?**
Adson's sign refers to disappearance of the radial pulse when the arm is abducted and the head is turned contralaterally. It is thought to be a sign of vascular compression at the thoracic outlet.

25. **What is the Phalen test?**
The Phalen test is a test for median nerve compression at the wrist. The wrists are held fully flexed (usually one against the other) for 1 minute. If the test reproduces the patient's symptoms in the distribution of the median nerve, it is considered positive.

26. **What is Tinel's sign? How does it apply to the carpal tunnel syndrome?**
Following nerve injury, a neuroma sometimes forms. Neuromata are more sensitive to percussion than are uninjured nerves. Tinel's sign is considered to be present if percussion over a specific point produces discomfort in the distal distribution of the injured nerve. If there is median nerve entrapment and injury under the carpal tunnel, tapping the wrist over the median canal may produce a jolt of sensation over the thumb and index finger.

27. **A 19-year-old man has severe pain in his shoulder and upper arm. The pain resolves over a few days, but is replaced by weakness in the deltoids, biceps, brachioradialis, and triceps. What is the most likely diagnosis?**
Brachial plexitis is a relatively common syndrome in young men. Inflammation of the brachial plexus produces severe pain that gradually subsides and is replaced by weakness that depends on the distribution of the plexus inflammation. Commonly, only the upper plexus is involved, affecting the deltoids, biceps, and brachioradialis. Occasionally, inflammation is more widespread.

28. **What is Pancoast syndrome?**
Tumors affecting the superior pulmonary sulcus can grow upward into the brachial plexus. This causes severe pain in the arm, with weakness of the muscles subserved by the lower trunk of the brachial plexus—primarily the intrinsic muscles of the hand; this condition is known as Pancoast syndrome. Early in the disease, pain may be the only symptom. As the disease progresses, the full syndrome is characterized by an ipsilateral Horner's syndrome (ptosis, myosis, and anhydrosis), atrophy of the muscles of the hand, decreased reflexes, and sensory loss in a C8 to T1 distribution. If the tumor progresses further, it can involve the entire brachial plexus and spread medially to invade the epidural space. In very advanced cases, epidural spinal cord compression occurs. On average, pain is present for 7 to 12 months before an accurate diagnosis is made.

29. **What is tennis elbow?**
Lateral epicondylitis, or tennis elbow, is a very common clinical condition that produces pain on the extensor surface of the lateral forearm. The cause is thought to be an inflammatory lesion at the insertion of the extensor tendons, mainly of the extensor carpi radialis brevis.

30. **What is carpal tunnel syndrome (CTS)?**
Carpal tunnel syndrome (CTS) is characterized by numbness and tingling over the thumb, index, and middle fingers. It is most pronounced upon awakening. Patients state that they have to "shake the hand to wake it up." Sensory loss maps out to the distribution of the median nerve,

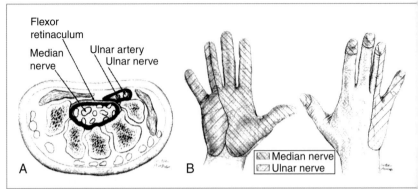

Figure 21-1. *A,* Wrist anatomy showing the median nerve through the carpal tunnel in close proximity to Guyon's canal, where the ulnar nerve passes. *B,* Median and ulnar sensory distributions. (From West SG: *Rheumatology secrets,* Philadelphia, 1997, Elsevier.)

affecting the thumb, index finger, and radial side of the ring finger. CTS is due to entrapment of the median nerve as it passes under the ligamentous canal in the wrist (Fig. 21-1). Weakness, when it occurs, is in the muscles innervated by the median nerve: the opponens and the abductor pollicis brevis.

Initial treatment is with nighttime splints. If treatment fails and weakness progresses, surgical decompression of the nerve at the wrist may be necessary.

31. **What is the value of electrodiagnostic studies in the evaluation of radicular pain in the neck and arm?**
Electromyography (EMG) and nerve conduction velocities (NCVs) help in localizing lesions and quantifying their severity. They can be used to determine which level is involved and at what point that nerve or root is injured. In lesions proximal to the dorsal root ganglion, sensory nerve action potentials (SNAPs) are preserved. Signs of denervation in a group of muscles innervated by a single root and their absence in other muscles are indicative of compression of that root. However, it takes up to 3 weeks after nerve injury for those signs to appear.

32. **What are some of the EMG signs of denervation?**
Normal muscles show electrical silence at rest. After denervation, there is increased insertional activity (spontaneous electrical discharges after an EMG needle is inserted into the muscle). Fibrillations and sharp waves may also be seen.

33. **Clinically, how can a root lesion be differentiated from injury to a peripheral nerve?**
A number of muscles may be innervated by the same root, but through different nerves. For example, the biceps, brachioradialis, and deltoids are all innervated by the C5 nerve root, but also by the musculocutaneous, radial, and axillary nerves, respectively. A root injury at the C5 level produces changes in all three muscles, while injury to one of the peripheral nerves produces weakness only in the muscle supplied by that nerve.

34. **What is the value of NCVs in carpal tunnel syndrome?**
With median nerve compression at the wrist (as in carpal tunnel syndrome), nerve conduction is locally slowed. The velocities are normal in the upper part of the extremity and then show a major drop-off over the wrist. In most laboratories, a median nerve delay of more than 4 to 4.5 milliseconds at the wrist is considered indicative of carpal tunnel syndrome.

KEY POINTS

1. There are multiple causes of acute and chronic neck pain. History and physical examination are necessary to help identify the cause. Diagnostic studies may be necessary as well.

2. Cervical spinal cord compression also has multiple causes and is characterized by pain and signs of myelopathy including bowel and bladder dysfunction, sensory changes below the level of the lesion, hyperreflexia, and the presence of Babinski responses.

3. Electrophysiologic studies (EMG/NCV) to help differentiate nerve root (radicular) abnormalities from peripheral nerve dysfunction. This may be especially valuable in distinguishing between cervical radiculopathy and carpal tunnel syndrome for example.

BIBLIOGRAPHY

1. Ariens GA, Bongers PM, Hoogendoorn WE, et al: High quantitative job demands and low coworker support as risk factors for neck pain: results of a prospective of cohort study, *Spine* 26(17):1896-1901, 2001.

2. Brazis PW: The localization of spinal and nerve root lesions. In Brazis PW, Masdeu JC, Biller J, editors: *Localization in clinical neurology*, Boston, 1990, Little, Brown.

3. Cailliet R: *Neck and arm pain*, Philadelphia, 1991, F.A. Davis Company.

4. Cote P, Cassidy JD, Carroll L, et al: A systematic review of the prognosis of acute whiplash and a new conceptual framework to synthesize the literature, *Spine* 26(19):E445-458, 2001.

5. Croft PR, Lewis M, Papageorgiou AC, et al: Risk factors for neck pain: a longitudinal study in the general population, *Pain* 93(3):317-325, 2001.

6. Eck JC, Hodges SD, Humphreys SC: Whiplash: a review of a commonly misunderstood injury, *Am J Med* 110(8):651-656, 2001.

7. Kasch H, Stengaard-Pedersen K, Arendt-Nielsen L, Staehelin Jensen T: Headache, and neck pain, and neck mobility after acute whiplash injury: a prospective study, *Spine* 26(11):1246-1251, 2001.

8. Linton SJ, van Tulder ME: Preventive interventions for back and neck pain problems: what is the evidence? *Spine* 26(7):778-787, 2001.

9. Persson LC, Lilja A: Pain, coping, emotional state and physical function in patients with chronic radicular neck pain. A comparison between patients treated with surgery, physiotherapy or neck collar—a blinded, prospective, randomized study, *Disabil Rehabil* 23(8):325-335, 2001.

10. Strausbaugh LJ: Vertebral osteomyelitis: how to differentiate it from other causes of back and neck pain, *Postgrad Med* 97(6):147-154, 1995.

CHAPTER 22

ABDOMINAL PAIN

Ronald Greenberg, MD, and Charles E. Argoff, MD

1. **What are the three afferent relays that mediate perception of abdominal pain?**
   - Visceral, or splanchnic, pathway
   - Somatic, or parietal, pathway
   - Referral pathway

   Visceral abdominal pain is produced by stimulation of nociceptors located in the walls of the abdominal viscera. Somatic abdominal pain is produced by stimulation of nociceptors located in the parietal peritoneum and intraabdominal supporting structures. Referral pain occurs when strong visceral impulses enter the spinal cord at the same level as afferents from other areas; this is mistakenly "read" as pain arising from the second area (e.g., shoulder pain in gallbladder disease).

2. **Can abdominal pain have any other causes?**
   As well as arising from abdominal structures, pain can be felt in the abdomen and yet be generated by distant structures. In the same way as abdominal pathology can cause a pain to be referred elsewhere in the body, irritation of distant structures can cause a pain to be referred to the abdomen. For example, pathology of the thoracic vertebra can be referred to the abdomen, giving the mistaken impression that intraabdominal problems exist. If the causal lesion is midline, then the referred pain can be to both sides of the abdomen. Similarly, irritation of thoracic nerves can cause radiation of neuropathic pain to the abdomen. For example, intercostal neuralgia will produce pain in a dermatomal distribution of the involved nerve, which, if arising from a lower intercostal nerve, will then be felt in the abdomen. Because allodynia is one of the features of neuropathic pain, care must be taken to ensure that intense pain on palpation of the abdomen is not in fact allodynia.

3. **How can visceral, somatic, and referred abdominal pain be clinically distinguished?**
   Visceral pain tends to be poorly localized and felt in the midline, and it is often experienced as a dull soreness that fluctuates in severity. Visceral pain can be very difficult for patients to describe and may be referred to as an aching, gnawing, burning, or cramping discomfort or as pain commonly attended by restlessness and associated symptoms of autonomic disturbance (i.e., nausea, vomiting, diaphoresis, and pallor).

   In contrast, somatic pain is typically more acute, intense, sharp, localized, and aggravated by movement.

   Referred pain combines features of both visceral and somatic pain and is well localized in areas distant from the precipitating stimulus.

4. **Can the location of abdominal pain be useful in determining the origin of the problem?**
   Information on the location, depth, and radiation of pain can provide helpful clues, but can also be misleading. Pain mediated along visceral afferent pathways tends to be poorly localized

and referred to the midline, regardless of the lateral location of the pathologic process. However, the level of midline pain can provide helpful clues. Pain from gastroduodenal and hepatobiliary structures is usually perceived in the epigastrium; pain from the small bowel is usually periumbilical; and pain from the colon tends to be perceived in the lower abdomen.

5. **What four classes of stimuli generate abdominal pain?**
The abdominal visceral organs are insensitive to many stimuli that would ordinarily provoke cutaneous pain such as burning, pinching, stabbing, and cutting. The abdominal visceral organs generate pain in response to the following four general classes of stimuli:
- Distention and contraction
- Traction
- Compression and torsion
- Stretch

6. **The paucity of visceral afferent nerves and the bilateral symmetric innervation of most abdominal organs results in abdominal pain that is poorly localized and midline. What is the significance of abdominal pain that is clearly lateralized?**
Clearly lateralized abdominal pain may arise either from one of the few intraabdominal organs with predominant one-sided innervation (e.g., kidney, ovary, ureter) or from structures with somatic rather than visceral innervation.

7. **What determines where in the abdomen pain is experienced?**
Afferent nerves from the abdominal viscera enter the spinal cord at different levels, and the level of entry governs where within the abdomen pain is experienced. Foregut structures, including the distal esophagus, stomach, duodenum, pancreas, liver, and biliary tree, are innervated by spinal segments T5–T6 to T8–T9 and manifest pain between the xiphoid process and umbilicus. Midgut structures, including the small bowel, appendix, and colon up to the distal transverse part, are innervated by spinal segments T8–T11 and L1 and manifest pain in the periumbilical region. Hindgut structures, including the distal colon and rectum, are innervated by spinal segments T11–L1 and result in pain between the umbilicus and pubic symphysis.

8. **What historical attributes must always be enquired of when obtaining the history from a patient with abdominal pain?**
The mnemonic PQRST provides a framework that ensures a full exploration of a given patient's abdominal pain:
P: Factors that either *p*alliate or *p*rovoke abdominal pain. For example, pain relieved by defecation suggests a colonic origin.
Q: *Q*ualities of the pain (i.e., burning, sharp, crampy).
R: *R*adiation of pain. For example, biliary tract pain radiates to the right periscapular region; pancreatic pain radiates to the back; and subdiaphragmatic pain may be referred to the shoulder tips.
S: *S*everity of the pain.
T: *T*emporal events associated with the pain (i.e., duration of pain, constant or intermittent, association with eating or defecation).
In addition, any relationship to other associated gastrointestinal symptoms (e.g., vomiting, diarrhea) or dysfunction of other contiguous organ systems (e.g., genitourinary or thoracic) must be sought.

9. **Is chronic abdominal pain purely a disease of adults?**
No. More than one third of children complain of abdominal pain lasting 2 weeks or longer. Commonly, simple issues such as constipation are the cause. In general, the response to an empirical course of medical management may give a higher yield than an exhaustive diagnostic workup. Employ behavioral, psychological, and nutritional strategies.

10. **What historical symptoms suggest the presence of an uncomplicated peptic ulcer?**
   Peptic ulcer pain is commonly described as a burning or gnawing pain in the midepigastric or subxiphoid region. Occasionally patients with peptic ulcer deny any pain and complain of discomfort and distress with a "hunger" or "empty stomach feeling" in the epigastrium. Peptic ulcer pain may vary from patient to patient, but is commonly classic for a given patient and occurs in an episodic and rhythmic fashion. Episodic pattern refers to the way in which ulcer pain recurs over a long period of weeks, months, and years. Rhythm refers to the pattern in which pain recurs during a 24-hour period, typically adhering to the sequence of pain-food-relief. Ulcer pain typically occurs when the stomach is empty and is relieved by eating or drinking, especially for ulcers located at or near the pyloroduodenal junction. Pain from more proximal ulcers may be exacerbated by eating.

11. **A 39-year-old man with a history of duodenal ulcer experiences sudden, severe pain throughout his abdomen. What may have happened?**
   Any alteration in the previous pattern of pain in a patient with a peptic ulcer should raise the suspicion of perforation (see Question 12). Acute free perforation (see Question 12) occurs suddenly and with almost immediate peak intensity. Severe pain may be felt throughout the abdomen and may be referred to the shoulders or flanks and lower abdomen. Physical examination demonstrates abdominal wall rigidity and involuntary guarding related to peritoneal irritation. In extreme cases of peritonitis, the abdominal rigidity is boardlike.
   Note that palpation for muscular rigidity and guarding must be gentle. Do not attempt to elicit "rebound tenderness," because it can be misleading, may cause the patient significant discomfort, and provides no more information than can be obtained using gentle palpation for underlying muscular rigidity.

12. **What clinical features suggest the complication of ulcer penetration?**
   Ulcer penetration signifies the presence of a confined perforation where the ulcer crater has extended beyond the stomach or duodenum but is walled off by an adjacent structure (as opposed to acute free perforation). For example, a posterior wall duodenal ulcer may penetrate into the head of the pancreas. The presence of a penetrating ulcer must be considered when a patient's previous typical pattern of pain-food-relief is disrupted, giving way to more constant and unrelenting pain. In addition, pain that is not relieved by previously effective measures (e.g., antisecretory drugs); pain that radiates to the upper lumbar back; occurrence of night pain; and change in the location, radiation, and intensity of anterior epigastric discomfort should also raise the suspicion of ulcer penetration.

13. **A 68-year-old woman with a long history of duodenal ulcer has recently been experiencing her typical intermittent discomfort of epigastric burning and gnawing pain, relieved by food, but recurring 2 hours later. However, for the last week she notes an upper abdominal cramping spasm, early satiety, and postprandial vomiting. What complication of ulcer disease may have ensued?**
   Peptic ulcer disease, especially at or near the pyloroduodenal junction, may be complicated by gastric outlet obstruction. Symptoms of gastric stasis include upper abdominal distention, crampy spasm, early satiety, loss of the usual rhythm of ulcer pain, and postprandial vomiting.

14. **What are some of the characteristics of small bowel pain?**
   Pathologic processes of the small bowel typically give rise to pain felt in the periumbilical and midabdominal regions. The pain is poorly localized and varies in quality depending on the underlying pathologic process. Small bowel obstruction resulting in spasm of small intestinal smooth muscle provokes cramping pain. Mucosal inflammatory or ulcerative processes result in a vague soreness and ache. An inflammatory or neoplastic process that extends through to the

serosa and adjacent parietal peritoneum will stimulate somatic pain pathways and become manifest as more sharply localized pain at the site of the lesion (i.e., characteristic parietal pain).

Small bowel pain, as opposed to peptic ulcer pain, is typically precipitated by eating and palliated by fasting. Progressive vomiting and obstipation occur with small bowel obstruction. In severe cases, vomitus may be feculent.

15. **What are the most common causes of small bowel obstruction?**
    - Adhesions
    - External hernias
    - Internal hernias
    - Crohn's disease
    - Primary or metastatic carcinoma

16. **You are called to examine an 88-year-old woman with a history of atrial fibrillation, peripheral vascular disease, and diabetes who now complains of severe, diffuse, constant abdominal pain. She is quite distressed. Examination reveals the abdomen to be soft and nontender without guarding or peritoneal signs. What is the likely diagnosis?**
The likely diagnosis is acute mesenteric ischemia (AMI) secondary to an embolism to the superior mesenteric artery. AMI typically manifests as severe, acute abdominal pain out of proportion to physical findings. The absence of peritoneal signs must not deter this diagnosis from being considered, because potentially reversible vasospasm precedes bowel infarction and necrosis. AMI may result from embolization, thrombosis, or a low flow to the superior mesenteric artery. Thrombosis of the superior mesenteric vein produces a similar syndrome.

Colonic ischemia caused by atherosclerotic disease of the inferior mesenteric artery results in crampy lower abdominal pain and bloody diarrhea.

17. **What is abdominal angina?**
The syndrome of chronic, postprandial, periumbilical crampy pain and weight loss due to anorexia and aversion to eating is sometimes referred to as abdominal angina.

18. **What is the pelvic floor tension syndrome?**
The pelvic floor tension syndrome is a syndrome of chronic pelvic pain that occurs predominantly in women. It presents as chronic, unremitting lower abdominal pain aggravated by standing or walking. It is commonly associated with dysmenorrhea, dyspareunia, and depression.

19. **A 22-year-old woman with recent onset of polyuria and polydipsia presents with lethargy, vomiting, and severe abdominal pain with associated rigidity and tenderness. A high anion gap metabolic acidosis is noted. What is the likely diagnosis?**
This patient has diabetic ketoacidosis; her clinical signs and symptoms simulate the acute abdomen. Additional systemic or metabolic disorders that can simulate an acute abdomen include acute porphyria, lead poisoning, hemolytic crisis, periarteritis nodosa, familial Mediterranean fever, black widow spider bite, and Addisonian crisis.

20. **A 72-year-old man with severe tricuspid valve regurgitation complains of a chronic right upper quadrant (ruq) pain felt as a constant, nonradiating, dull ache. Physical examination reveals tender hepatomegaly with a soft, blunted, pulsatile liver edge. What is the likely diagnosis?**
This case illustrates the type of pain that originates from the liver. The hepatic parenchyma is insensitive to pain. However, Glisson's capsule (around the liver) is rich in nociceptors and readily gives rise to pain in response to penetration, stretching, or distention. The pain is felt in

the subcostal area, but especially in the right hypochondrium because of the larger size of the right hepatic lobe. The severity and intensity of hepatic pain depends on the rapidity with which the liver capsule is stretched. Abrupt distention can cause sudden, sharp pain that may mimic gallstone disease, whereas more gradual distention typically causes a dull ache.

21. **Why is the commonly used term *biliary colic* a misnomer?**
Biliary tract pain is not colicky but is typically a sustained pain that steadily rises to a peak that may be sustained for several hours and then subsides (crescendo/decrescendo). Although biliary tract pain may fluctuate in intensity and severity, it does not remit and recur as would the colic of small bowel obstruction.

22. **A 42-year-old woman with abdominal pain reports a history of chronic, intermittent, recurrent attacks of severe dull epigastric pain that typically occur during the night, radiate to the right periscapular region, and last 4 to 6 hours. She has had four such episodes several months apart; she was asymptomatic during intervening periods. She now complains of severe ruq pain, nausea, and nonbloody emesis, and she is noted to have ruq abdominal tenderness that is accentuated on inspiration. What is the likely diagnosis?**
This patient is suffering from symptomatic gallstones. Her previous episodes typify biliary colic where a gallstone is transiently impacted in the cystic duct or bile duct, stimulating nociceptors served by visceral afferent pathways. As is typical of visceral pain, this is poorly localized to the epigastrium. Her current episode is notable for more localized RUQ pain with marked tenderness and a positive Murphy's sign compatible with a diagnosis of acute cholecystitis. Continued obstruction of the cystic duct provokes an inflammatory process in the gallbladder wall, which may progress to involve the serosal surface of the gallbladder and parietal peritoneum, resulting in a more intense, localized, somatic type of pain.

23. **How might a patient with chronic pancreatic disease describe his or her pain?**
Chronic pancreatic pain results from stimulation of visceral afferent pathways and is a midline, midepigastric, deep, dull ache, which may spread to the right or left hypochondrium. It characteristically penetrates to the back. Patients with chronic pancreatic pain report that lying in the fetal position or sitting up and leaning forward decreases the severity of the pain, and hyperextension of the back typically exacerbates it. Chronic pancreatic pain from either carcinoma or chronic pancreatitis is provoked by eating and is often associated with significant weight loss, diarrhea, steatorrhea, and diabetes.

24. **What is dyspepsia?**
Dyspepsia has been defined as the presence of persistent or recurrent pain or discomfort that is centered in the upper abdomen or epigastrium. Dyspepsia suggests that the symptoms are arising from a disorder of the upper gastrointestinal tract. Additional symptoms may include bloating, early satiety, nausea, anorexia, and postprandial fullness.

25. **Which diagnostic technique can help distinguish chronic abdominal pain caused by disease of the abdominal wall from that of intraabdominal origin?**
Carnett's test can help make this distinction. The site of maximum tenderness is identified, and the patient is asked to assume a partial sitting position with arms crossed, which causes the abdominal wall muscles to generate increased tension. Carnett's test is positive if increased tenderness on repeat palpation is noted. The differential diagnosis of chronic abdominal wall pain includes rectus sheath hematoma, rib tip syndrome, abdominal wall hernia, myofascial pain syndrome, and cutaneous nerve entrapment syndromes.

26. **A 33-year-old woman has made multiple visits to the emergency department with complaints of abdominal pain and tingling in her feet. She has also exhibited bizarre behavior. She was sent home with some medications for sleep, but came in with a severe exacerbation of her abdominal pain and sensory complaints. What uncommon disease should be considered?**

    Acute intermittent porphyria is characterized by intermittent abdominal pain, peripheral neuropathy, and psychiatric symptoms. Barbiturates can precipitate an acute attack.

27. **What is the significance of differing pain patterns in patients with chronic abdominal pain?**

    Two distinct pain patterns should be recognized, because they have implications with regard to the differential diagnosis and response to therapy:

    - Abdominal pain that occurs in intermittent, discrete attacks with intervening asymptomatic periods can usually be explained by specific pathophysiologic disorders (e.g., symptomatic cholelithiasis).
    - Chronic abdominal pain lasting days to weeks may have no clear pathophysiologic explanation and may be deemed functional in origin. Examples include nonulcer dyspepsia, which presents with chronic epigastric ulcerlike pain but without any ulcer; and irritable bowel syndrome, which presents with lower abdominal cramping pain, bloating, and disordered bowel function (most notably alternating diarrhea and constipation). Chronic abdominal pain that lasts longer than 6 months, remains undiagnosed, and lacks features of nonulcer dyspepsia and irritable bowel syndrome is termed chronic intractable abdominal pain.

    In all of these patients, a detailed psychosocial history is crucial. Recognition of depression or anxiety may be key.

28. **Patients with chronic abdominal pain commonly exhibit many of the same psychologic responses that other chronic pain patients exhibit. What are they?**

    Many patients with chronic abdominal pain also suffer from depression, insomnia, loss of libido, fatigue, withdrawal, and anxiety. The predisposition to these responses is in part mediated by social and family circumstances, culture, and the patient's psychologic state. Many patients with chronic intractable abdominal pain, the majority of whom are women, report a history of childhood physical or sexual abuse.

29. **What clinical features suggest the presence of chronic idiopathic abdominal pain?**

    Patients with chronic idiopathic abdominal pain commonly have nearly constant discomfort and pain that is relatively unchanging in location, character, and intensity. The pain follows no consistent pattern and cannot be explained by known pathophysiologic mechanisms. Patients rarely show weight loss or fever; commonly have a history of other chronic pain; and may show associated psychopathology.

30. **List some of the well-recognized disorders of organs in the thorax that can present as abdominal pain.**

    Abdominal pain can occur in patients with disorders at extraabdominal sites. Thoracic pathologic processes that can cause abdominal pain include pneumonia, myocardial infarction, pulmonary embolism, pneumothorax, esophagitis, emphysema, and myocarditis.

31. **Patients who are immunocompromised by virtue of disease or immunosuppressive therapy may present with abdominal pain. What are some diagnostic considerations?**

    The immunocompromised host with acute intraabdominal pathology may have few abdominal signs and symptoms, blunted systemic manifestations, and minimal change in biochemical and hematologic parameters. The differential diagnosis includes any of the diseases that can occur in the general population independent of immune function as well as problems unique to the immunocompromised host. Specific considerations include neutropenic enterocolitis, graft versus host disease, opportunistic infections (e.g., cytomegalovirus infection, atypical mycobacterial infection, fungal infection), and tumors arising from immune deficiency (e.g., lymphoma, Kaposi's sarcoma).

32. **What are some of the caveats about atypical presentations of abdominal pain?**
In certain circumstances, such as in older or immunosuppressed patients or in those receiving corticosteroids, common abdominal disorders may present in an atypical fashion. Fever may be absent or low grade; signs of peritoneal irritation may be blunted; and an altered mental status (e.g., dementia) may modify the history and physical examination.

33. **True or false: All abdominal pain is caused by gastrointestinal pathologic processes.**
False. In particular, and especially in women, disorders of the pelvic organs must always be considered in the differential diagnosis of either chronic or acute lower abdominal pain.

34. **What are some diagnostic considerations in women with abdominal pain?**
A full history and physical is required of all women with lower abdominal pain, including a detailed sexual and menstrual history, pelvic examination, and pregnancy test (for women of childbearing age). Diagnostic considerations include pelvic inflammatory disease, endometriosis, ectopic pregnancy, uterine obstruction, ovarian cyst torsion, ovulatory pain (mittelschmerz), ruptured ovarian cyst, and dysfunction of pelvic floor muscles. Pain occurring at monthly intervals suggests endometriosis or ovulatory pain.

35. **What are some of the theories regarding the pathophysiology of the irritable bowel syndrome (IBS)?**
IBS is a functional disease of the gastrointestinal tract defined as chronic abdominal pain and/or discomfort in association with altered bowel habits (i.e., diarrhea, constipation, or a combination of both). A specific pathophysiologic mechanism remains to be established, but postulated mechanisms include abnormal gastrointestinal motor function, abnormal visceral perception, psychosocial factors (e.g., somatization, phobia, anxiety), and postinfectious gastroenteritis.

36. **What pharmacological options exist for the treatment of irritable bowel syndrome?**
Antispasmodics, such as hyoscine and mebeverine, have formed the mainstay of IBS treatment. More recently the 5-HT3 antagonist alosetron has been shown to help in the treatment of IBS pain but only in females with diarrhea-predominant IBS.

37. **Is irritable bowel syndrome associated with any other conditions?**
IBS is associated with the fibromyalgia syndrome and interstitial cystitis.

38. **What general considerations should be made when assessing a patient with abdominal pain?**
As with any medical condition, diagnosis is based on the following progression: history, examination, differential diagnosis, investigation, and tentative diagnosis.
   Specifically in relation to abdominal pain, a differentiation between abdominal and nonabdominal causes of pain must be considered. In the case of pain definitely arising from the abdomen, a decision as to whether the pain is arising from within the abdomen or from the abdominal wall must be considered.

KEY POINTS

1. Abdominal pain is either visceral, somatic, or referred in nature.

2. Abdominal pain is not always caused by abdominal pathology: it may be caused by problems at a distant site and referred to the abdomen.

3. Pain arising from small bowel is often felt in the periumbilical region.

4. Irritable bowel syndrome is often associated with interstitial cystitis and fibromyalgia.

BIBLIOGRAPHY

1. Beard RW, Reginald PW, Wadsworth J: Clinical features of women with chronic lower abdominal pain and pelvic congestion, *Br J Obstet Gynaecol* 95:153-161, 1988.

2. Camilleri M, Chey WY, Mayer EA, et al: A randomized controlled clinical trial of the serotonin type 3 receptor antagonist alosetron in women with diarrhea-predominant irritable bowel syndrome, *Arch Intern Med* 161:1733-1740, 2001.

3. Camilleri M, Choi MG: Review article: irritable bowel syndrome, *Aliment Pharmacol Ther* 11:3-15, 1997.

4. Chui DW, Owen DL: AIDS and the gut, *J Gastroenterol Hepatol* 9(3):291-303, 1994.

5. DeBanto JR, Varilek GW, Haas L: What could be causing chronic abdominal pain? Anything from common peptic ulcers to uncommon pancreatic trauma, *Postgrad Med* 106(3):141-146, 1999.

6. Gallegos NC, Hobsley M: Abdominal wall pain: an alternative diagnosis, *Br J Surg* 77(10):1167-1170, 1990.

7. Haubrich WS: Abdominal pain. In Berk JE, Haubrich WS, editors: *Gastrointestinal symptoms: clinical interpretation*, Philadelphia, 1991, BC Decker, pp 23-58.

8. Klein KB: Approach to the patient with abdominal pain. In Yamada T, editor: *Textbook of gastroenterology*, 2nd ed, Philadelphia, 1995, JB Lippincott, pp 750-771.

9. Lake AM: Chronic abdominal pain in childhood: diagnosis and management, *Am Fam Physician* 59(7): 1823-1830, 1999.

10. Silen W: Diseases that may simulate the acute abdomen. In *Cope's early diagnosis of the acute abdomen*, 20th ed, New York, 2000, Oxford University Press, pp 269-280.

11. Thompson WG, Creed F, Drossman DA, et al: Functional bowel disease and functional abdominal pain, *Gastroenterol Int* 5:75-91, 1992.

12. Talley NJ, Colin-Jones D, Koch K, et al: Functional dyspepsia: a classification with guidelines for management, *Gastroenterol Int* 4:145-160, 1991.

CHAPTER 23

CHRONIC PELVIC PAIN

Helen Greco, MD, and Charles E. Argoff, MD

1. **What is chronic pelvic pain?**
   Chronic pelvic pain is pain that is recurrent or persistent for 6 months or longer. There may or may not be an identifiable causative lesion. (The time frame is a measurement used to categorize most types of chronic pain, not just chronic pelvic pain.)

2. **What are some other hallmarks of chronic pelvic pain?**
   With chronic pelvic pain, pain and disability appear out of proportion to physical abnormalities, and are unrelieved by usual medical or surgical therapies. There may be signs of depression, such as loss of appetite, weight change, and sleep disturbance. Pain interferes with daily lifestyle, causing inability to perform normal household or job-related tasks, exercise, or sexual intercourse. A history of physical or sexual abuse may be elicited.

3. **Describe the impact of chronic pelvic pain on family interaction.**
   Pain may become an interpersonal device through which family members communicate. Caregivers may infantilize the patient, and the patient may use the pain to manipulate the family. Although the process is difficult, patient and family education is needed to interrupt this cycle.

4. **Is chronic pelvic pain purely a disease of women?**
   No. Men may have a syndrome that mimics prostatitis but does not include acute infection or inflammation. Objective findings may be absent. These patients are similar in many ways to women with interstitial cystitis.

5. **Identify important information that can be obtained from the history.**
   Findings from the history should include the following: What aggravates or alleviates the pain? Is it related to the menstrual cycle or stress? Is it continuous, or intermittent? Characteristics such as quality, severity, and location of the pain are all important factors to elicit.

   Age, parity, and use of contraception are important in respect to the ovulatory cycle, as well as the possibility of prolapse of the uterus.

   Menstrual history may give insight as to duration of discomfort and at which point of the menstrual cycle the pain occurs.

   A history of endometriosis may be significant, because this may cause scarring and adhesions that give rise to pain.

   Sexual history may reveal introital pain, dyspareunia, or sexual abuse. Vaginal spasm may be due to an inflammatory reaction or scarring or may have a psychologic origin. A history of sexually transmitted infection or pelvic inflammatory disease is relevant because these can lead to adhesion formation.

   Any associated pain in other areas of the body, including the lower back, gastrointestinal tract, and the urinary tract should be discussed. Radiation of pain is important in ruling out other etiologies of pain, including a neuropathy or radiculopathy.

   Previous operative procedures may be significant for adhesion formation and scarring in the area.

6. **How can the physical examination contribute to the diagnosis?**
   A vaginal, rectal, and rectovaginal examination with direct visualization, where possible, should be performed in an attempt to reproduce the pain. A Pap smear and cervical cultures for *Chlamydia trachomatis* and *Neisseria gonorrhoeae* should be done, as well as a pregnancy test, if warranted. During bimanual and rectovaginal examination, evaluate areas of tenderness by assessing the uterosacral ligaments, which are commonly thick and tender in endometriosis. Also, assess adnexal or uterine tenderness, and mobility. Infection and scarring from endometriosis can affect normal mobility, as well as thicken and damage tissue.

7. **From what pelvic structures can chronic pelvis pain arise?**
   - Vulva (e.g., vulvodynia)
   - Vagina (e.g., atrophy, chronic infection)
   - Cervix (e.g., tumor, cervical stenosis)
   - Uterus (e.g., dysmenorrhea)
   - Fallopian tube (e.g., chronic infection)
   - Ovary (e.g., cyst, tumor, adhesions, torsion)
   - Uterine ligaments (e.g., endometriosis)
   - Bowel (e.g., IBS, constipation, diverticulitis, obstruction)
   - Bladder (e.g., interstitial cystitis)
   - Perineum (e.g., perinea neuralgia)

   Nonpelvic structures (e.g., nerve, joint, and ligament) can give rise to radiated and referred pain to the pelvic area.

8. **Is a retroflexed uterus a cause for pain?**
   Approximately 20% of normal women have a uterus in the retroflexed position. A retroflexed uterus may be due to adhesions from a postoperative or postinflammatory process or to endometriotic lesions. Pain in these patients is not due to the position of the uterus but rather to the primary disease. On occasion, anterior displacement of the uterus alleviates the pain. In this case, a pessary or uterine suspension may be considered.

9. **What are the common signs and symptoms of endometriosis?**
   Pain tends to follow the menstrual cycle. Pain on defecation and intercourse may occur because the disease affects the cul-de-sac and/or uterosacral ligament. In severe cases, the bowel wall may be involved, causing cramping or even obstruction.

10. **What is the pelvic congestion syndrome?**
    This syndrome is due to pelvic vascular engorgement, which presents as heaviness and pain. Symptoms start after arising in the morning and worsen as the day continues. The diagnosis is made by laparoscopy: the uterus looks dusky and mottled, and the broad ligament veins demonstrate varicosities.

11. **What is the relationship among bowel habits, menstrual cycle, and lower abdominal pain?**
    Lower abdominal cramping pain that is intermittent in nature may be due to constipation or irritable bowel syndrome (IBS). IBS is characterized by bouts of abdominal cramping and frequent bowel movements. Pain caused by IBS may be aggravated in the luteal phase of the menstrual cycle. Progesterone has a slowing effect on visceral contractions and may relieve IBS, but exacerbate constipation.

12. **Which medications may contribute to lower abdominal pain?**
    - Anticholinergic drugs
    - Opioids
    - Antipsychotic agents
    - Antihypertensives
    - Cold relief preparations
    - Over-the-counter diuretics

13. **When is evaluation of the urinary tract necessary?**
    Urinary tract evaluation is necessary when symptoms such as dysuria, urgency, incontinence, discomfort in the suprapubic area, colicky flank pain, or hematuria are present.

14. **Give nine gynecologic causes of chronic pelvic pain.**
    1. Mittelschmerz describes midcycle pain caused by peritoneal irritation from follicular fluid or blood that has been released from the ovary at the time of ovulation.
    2. Pain can result from any inflammatory process that irritates the peritoneal lining, e.g., endometriosis or acute chronic salpingitis.
    3. Adenomyosis can create cramping with a mildly boggy, enlarged, tender uterus, especially during menses.
    4. Myomata can create pressure and degeneration, thereby causing inflammation.
       ○ Uterine anomalies and cervical stenosis can create an obstruction of menstrual outflow.
    5. Prolapse of reproductive organs can cause significant lower abdominal pressure.
    6. Primary dysmenorrhea is usually due to prostaglandin-induced uterine contractions with ischemia.
    7. Secondary dysmenorrhea is due to an organic pathology.
    8. A fallopian tube prolapsed through the vaginal cuff after a hysterectomy, residual ovarian syndrome with one or both ovaries adherent to the vaginal apex, or a chronically infected vaginal cuff with granulation tissue can cause deep dyspareunia.
    9. Pelvic malignancy may compress or invade various organs as well as cause severe adhesions.

15. **What are the common extragenital causes of chronic pelvic pain?**
    - Gastrointestinal causes: colitis, diverticulitis, appendicitis, pancreatitis, perihepatitis, obstruction, and irritable bowel syndrome
    - Urinary tract dysfunction: infectious process, obstruction, calculus, tumor, adhesions
    - Orthopedic conditions: facet joint arthritis may give referred pain while neural compression by disc, osteophyte or spinal stenosis, for example, may give radiated pain to the pelvic area.

16. **What is interstitial cystitis?**
    Interstitial cystitis is a painful syndrome characterized clinically by excessive urinary urgency and frequency of urination, suprapubic pain, dyspareunia, and chronic pelvic pain, in the presence of repeatedly negative urine cultures. Women account for 95% of cases. Pathological examination of the bladder may reveal glomerulations and Hunner's ulcers.

17. **What are Hunner's ulcers?**
    Hunner's ulcers are small, denuded areas seen on the mucosal surface of the urinary bladder in some patients with long-standing interstitial cystitis.

18. **What associated symptoms may suggest a gynecologic etiology of pain?**
Dyspareunia, menorrhagia, amenorrhea, any other type of menstrual disturbance, as well as vaginal/cervical discharge or pain related to ovulation suggest a gynecologic etiology. If pain occurs when changing from a combination oral contraceptive to one that does not suppress ovulation, the pain is likely to be of gynecologic origin.

19. **What are the most common causes of pelvic pain in a woman who is of postreproductive age?**
Gastrointestinal problems can create lower abdominal pain. Bladder dysfunction, pelvic relaxation, and genital atrophy are other potential etiologies. Muscular spasm, pressure pain, and easily inflamed tissue further complicate the problem.

20. **How does knowledge of a woman's parity contribute to the assessment of pelvic pain?**
Patients who are parous are more likely to have pelvic relaxation with symptomatic cystocele, rectocele, or enterocele than are nulliparous women.

21. **Why would a patient who is anovulatory or oligoovulatory experience pelvic pain?**
Patients who are anovulatory or oligoovulatory may develop enlarged ovaries from multiple cysts. There may be chronic pain caused by enlargement or adhesions or acute pain caused by rupture.

22. **Which laboratory tests may aid in making a diagnosis?**
An elevated white blood count and erythrocyte sedimentation rate may reveal an inflammatory process. An abnormal urinalysis or positive urine culture may point to a kidney stone, urinary tract infection, or other urologic etiology. Stool positive for blood may reveal an inflammatory or infectious process of the bowel. An elevated serum amylase may indicate pancreatitis. Hormone analysis (luteinizing hormone [LH], follicle stimulating hormone [FSH], estrogen, prolactin) should be undertaken to exclude a hormonal factor in the pain.

23. **What special diagnostic procedures, where appropriate, can help in diagnosing the etiology of pain?**
Gynecological examination by an experienced gynecologist should have been undertaken before a diagnosis of "chronic pelvic pain" is made. Further, ultrasound assessment (transabdominal and/or vaginal) of the pelvis should be undertaken. Hysteroscopy, cystoscopy, and laparoscopy may enable direct vision of pelvic organs to be obtained so that the presence or absence of macroscopic pathology may be ascertained.

24. **If no apparent organic cause can be demonstrated, what other possibility could there be for chronic pelvic pain?**
Levator ani muscle spasm or spasm of other local pelvic muscle groups may cause chronic pelvic pain. Digital palpation must reproduce the pain and local anesthetics may relieve it before the diagnosis can be made with assurance. Interstitial cystitis is another possibility.

25. **How do you approach the patient with chronic idiopathic pelvic pain?**
Psychological and pharmacologic approaches can be used. Carefully question the patient to identify underlying depression, anxiety, or somatoform disorder. Cognitive-behavioral techniques may be helpful. In addition, antidepressant medications can be employed but in lower doses than used for chronic depression. The long-term use of opioids is not effective nor is it appropriate for this condition.

26. **Does a response to nonsteroidal antiinflammatory drugs (NSAIDs) mean there is no structural cause for dysmenorrhea?**

    No. Endometriosis may respond to NSAIDs because the dysmenorrhea experienced with endometriosis is in part caused by prostaglandin release by the ectopic endometrium and the intrauterine endometrium. Therefore, do not immediately assume that endometriosis is not present just because there is a response to NSAIDs.

27. **How do fibroids cause chronic pelvic pain?**

    In general, fibroids do not cause chronic pelvic pain. However, when they are large, they may create pressure on other organs or tissues or outgrow their blood supply and degenerate. If they compress the anterior vaginal mucosa, they can cause dyspareunia. Partial bladder obstruction may cause incomplete emptying of the bladder, leading to recurrent urinary tract infections. Direct bladder pressure may cause urgency.

28. **How can the diagnosis of adenomyosis be made?**

    Patients with adenomyosis usually develop dysmenorrhea in their 30s, and it tends to be unresponsive to NSAIDs or ovulation-suppression agents. Sonography can demonstrate a globular, boggy type of uterus, which may also be felt on pelvic examination. Definitive diagnosis can only be made histologically.

29. **What other medical approach can be used for adenomyosis?**

    Combination estrogen-progestin oral contraceptives may be effective in suppressing ovulation and decreasing the amount of menstrual blood flow, thereby decreasing the amount of prostaglandins released. Sometimes the use of continuous oral contraceptives without withdrawal bleeding may alleviate the pain. NSAIDs are usually ineffective.

30. **If no organic condition is found despite extensive evaluation, can a hysterectomy help?**

    The patient often insists on having a hysterectomy out of desperation to feel better. However, the physician must keep in mind that hysterectomy often does not relieve the pain and, in fact, may aggravate it because of the formation of new scar tissue from a laparotomy. Chronic pain of unknown etiology should rarely, if ever, be addressed surgically.

31. **Is laparoscopy only a diagnostic tool?**

    No. Laparoscopy can be used as a therapeutic measure whereby adhesions may be lysed, endometriosis ablated with laser or electrocautery, and other pathology handled in an appropriate manner.

32. **If chronic pelvic pain caused by endometriosis continues, despite treatment with both medical and conservative surgical intervention, what is the next step?**

    A hysterectomy with removal of both fallopian tubes and ovaries is usually the next step. However, there is no guarantee of reduced pain because adhesions may contribute to this disease process. Furthermore, extragenital deposits of endometriosis (on the bowel or peritoneum) can be an ongoing source of pain.

33. **What types of treatment can be helpful in a patient with chronic pelvic pain?**

    The type of treatments used should depend on which anatomical structures are considered to be the origin of the pain. For example:
    - Endometriosis: hormonal treatment, surgical treatment (cautery, laser removal)
    - Vulvodynia: topical NSAIDs, topical tricyclic antidepressants (which can have a local analgesic effect), topical nitrates (reduce inflammation and pain), antiepileptic and antidepressant medications
    - Cervical stenosis: dilatation, NSAIDs
    - Adhesions: surgical division (but likely to reoccur)

KEY POINTS

1. Chronic pelvic pain may result from a variety of etiologies, including intrapelvic sources and pain that is referred from nonpelvic sources.

2. Numerous medications may contribute to chronic lower abdominal pain; thus, this needs to be considered when evaluating a patient with chronic pelvic pain.

3. Chronic pelvic pain does not only occur in women.

BIBLIOGRAPHY

1. American College of Obstetrics and Gynecologists Technical Bulletin: *Chronic Pelvic Pain*, No. 223, May 1996.

2. Bjerklund Johansen TE, Weidner W: Understanding chronic pelvic pain syndrome, *Curr Opin Urol* 12(1):63-67, 2002.

3. Herbst AL, et al: *Comprehensive gynecology*, 3rd ed, St. Louis, 1997, Mosby, pp 156-159.

4. Moldwin RM, Sant GR: Interstitial cystitis: a pathophysiology and treatment update, *Clin Obstet Gynecol* 45(1):259-272, 2002.

CHAPTER 24

FIBROMYALGIA AND MYOFASCIAL PAIN

Mark A. Thomas, MD, and Ronald Kanner, MD, FAAN, FACP

1. **What are the chronic pain syndromes that involve muscle and fascia?**
   Myofascial pain syndrome and fibromyalgia are chronic pain syndromes that involve the muscle and soft tissues. Myofascial pain syndrome is regional in distribution whereas fibromyalgia involves the entire body. These diagnoses may represent two points in a spectrum of disease, as subgroups of fibromyalgia have been identified on the basis of differing clinical findings and prognoses.

2. **Describe the myofascial pain syndrome.**
   The myofascial pain syndrome is a chronic, regional pain syndrome that involves muscle and soft tissues. It is characterized by trigger points and taut bands (see Questions 7 and 8). Originally described by Travell and later elaborated on by Travell and Simons, myofascial pain syndrome occurs in most body areas, most commonly in the cervical and lumbar regions.

3. **What is fibromyalgia?**
   Fibromyalgia is a clinical syndrome characterized by chronic, diffuse pain and multiple tender points at defined points in muscle and other soft tissues. Periosteal tender points are frequently present. Widespread pain can be felt both above and below the waist and bilaterally. Other characteristic features of the syndrome include fatigue, sleep disturbance, irritable bowel syndrome, interstitial cystitis, stiffness, paresthesias, headaches, depression, anxiety, and decreased memory and vocabulary.

4. **What are the American College of Rheumatology 1990 criteria for the classification of fibromyalgia?**
   - History of widespread pain
   - Pain in 11 of 18 tender point sites

   Pain is widespread when it is present both in the left and right sides of the body, and both above and below the waist. In addition, axial skeletal pain (cervical spine, anterior chest, thoracic spine, or low back) must be present. Low back pain is considered lower segment pain.
   Pain must be present in at least 11 of the following 18 trigger point sites (9 pairs) on digital palpation:
   Occiput—bilateral, at suboccipital muscle insertions
   Low cervical—bilateral, at anterior intertransverse spaces C5–C7
   Trapezius—bilateral, at midpoint of upper border of muscle
   Supraspinatus—bilateral, above scapular spine near medial border
   Second rib—bilateral, at second osteochondral junctions
   Lateral epicondyle—bilateral, 2 cm distal to epicondyles
   Gluteal—bilateral, in upper outer quadrants of buttocks
   Greater trochanter—bilateral, posterior to trochanteric prominence
   Knee—bilateral, at medial fat pad proximal to joint line
   Digital palpation should be performed with an approximate force of 4 kg/1 cm^2. For a trigger point to be considered "positive," the subject must state that the palpation is painful. "Tender" is not to be equated with "painful."

5. **Do all fibromyalgia patients have the same symptoms?**
   No. There is a high degree of variability in the presentation of fibromyalgia. Subgroups of the syndrome have been identified based on the number of active tender points, sleep quality, and cold pain threshold. These subgroups have different prognoses. Patients may also be grouped according to related disease. Of patients with irritable bowel syndrome (IBS), 20% demonstrate findings consistent with fibromyalgia. Fibromyalgia is more common in diabetics than in the general population, and the severity of pain correlates with the duration of diabetes. These may constitute additional subgroups of fibromyalgia.

6. **Name syndromes that are associated with fibromyalgia.**
   - Chronic fatigue syndrome
   - Irritable bowel syndrome
   - Restless leg syndrome
   - Interstitial cystitis
   - Temporomandibular joint dysfunction
   - Sicca syndrome
   - Raynaud's phenomenon
   - Autonomic dysregulation with orthostatic hypotension
   - Mood disorder

7. **What are trigger points?**
   Trigger points are sites in muscle or tendon that, when palpated, produce pain at a distant site. These occur in consistent locations with predictable patterns of pain referral. Trigger points are often associated with prior trauma, "near falls," or degenerative osteoarthritis.

8. **What are "taut bands"? How are they associated with trigger points?**
   In patients with myofascial pain, deep palpation of muscle may reveal areas that feel tight and bandlike. Stretching this band of muscle produces pain. This is a taut band. Trigger points are characteristically found within taut bands of muscle. Despite the muscle tension, taut bands are electrophysiologically silent (i.e., the electromyogram [EMG] is normal). Rolling the taut band under the fingertip at the trigger point (snapping palpation), may produce a local "twitch" response. This shortening of the band of muscle is one of the cardinal signs of fibromyalgia.

9. **What are some of the most common sites of tender points in fibromyalgia?**
   - Midtrapezius
   - Lower part of sternocleidomastoid muscle
   - Lateral part of pectoralis major muscle
   - Midsupraspinatus muscle
   - Upper outer quadrant of gluteal region
   - Trochanteric region
   - Medial fat pad of knee

10. **Describe the prevalence and typical demographics of the fibromyalgia patient.**
    In most reported series, 80% to 90% of patients with fibromyalgia are female, with a peak incidence in middle-age and a prevalence of 0.5% to 5% of the general population.

11. **What laboratory investigations are useful in fibromyalgia?**
    All laboratory values in fibromyalgia are used for exclusionary purposes. There are no characteristic chemical, electrical, or radiographic laboratory abnormalities. However, several consistent investigational serum markers of the disease have been reported in the literature. An increase in cytokines, with a direct relationship between pain intensity and interleukin-8, has been reported. Other investigational findings include a decrease in circulating cortisol (this may play a role in decreased exercise tolerance), a decrease in branched-chain amino acids (perhaps correlating with muscle fatigue), and decreased lymphocyte Gi protein and cAMP

concentrations. At present, these findings are not clinically useful for the diagnosis, prognosis, or monitoring of the treatment response of fibromyalgia patients. Sleep studies are often abnormal ("alpha-delta," nonrestorative sleep), but the abnormalities are also seen in other chronic painful conditions.

12. **What treatments are commonly used for fibromyalgia and for myofascial pain?**
A combination of physical, anesthesiologic, and pharmacologic techniques are employed. Some of the most common treatments involve lidocaine injection or dry-needling of trigger points. These approaches are based on the concept that trigger points represent areas of local muscle spasm. However, the efficacy of trigger point injections has never been fully substantiated, although they do offer transient relief to some patients. Physical techniques, such as stretching, spray and stretch (see Question 19), massage, and heat and cold application have all been advocated, but none are fully validated by well-controlled studies.

13. **Describe the role of physical therapy modalities in the treatment of myofascial pain.**
Most studies documenting the efficacy of physical therapy modalities are anecdotal and include relatively small subject numbers. They suggest the efficacy of transcutaneous electrical nerve stimulation (TENS), balneotherapy, ice, massage, ischemic compression (acupressure), and biofeedback in the treatment of myofascial pain. Low-power laser has been studied for its effect on myofascial pain associated with fibromyalgia. This modality seems to significantly reduce pain, muscle spasm, stiffness, and number of tender points.

14. **Which medications are commonly used in the treatment of fibromyalgia and myofascial pain syndrome?**
Tricyclic antidepressants are widely used drugs for these disorders. They are used because they have the potential to regularize sleep patterns, decrease pain and muscle spasm, and because of their mood-enhancing properties. Selective serotonin-reuptake inhibitors (SSRIs) are used to elevate mood, but have little analgesic effect. Serotonin-norepinephrine reuptake inhibitors (SNRIs), such as duloxetine, have recently been shown to have pain-reducing properties in patients with fibromyalgia and can also improve mood. The use of antidepressants as analgesics in these conditions is not a recognized indication for these drugs, although their use is widespread in practice. Pregabalin and duloxetine have recently received an indication for the treatment of fibromyalgia in the United States. Nonsteroidal antiinflammatory drugs (NSAIDs), opioids, and nonnarcotic analgesics are also frequently used, but their role is also unclear and not evidence based. Many medications, such as cyclobenzaprine, baclofen, tizanidine, and chlorzoxazone, have been used to achieve symptom relief. However, a treatment effect has not been consistently supported. Medications that target associated symptoms are often employed. Among the most common of these are sleep medications such as zolpidem, and fludrocortisone to treat postural hypotension and adynamia.

15. **What are some other interventions that have been studied for the treatment of fibromyalgia?**
There is a large series investigating the role of diet in treating fibromyalgia. Some studies promote a raw vegetarian diet; others tout *Chlorella pyrenoides* (algae) as a dietary supplement. Monosodium glutamate and aspartame have both been implicated in producing symptoms common to fibromyalgia and may play a role in pathogenesis for certain fibromyalgia subgroups.
Botulinum toxin injection and acupuncture have also been studied. They appear to be helpful in certain instances, but consistent efficacy has not been proven.

16. **Is exercise useful in the treatment of fibromyalgia and myofascial pain syndrome?**
Yes! The most consistent improvement in fibromyalgia and myofascial pain syndrome occurs with exercise. The exercise hormonal response is abnormal in patients with fibromyalgia

(increase in growth hormone concentration, the opposite of normal response), so the frequency and intensity of exercise needs to be carefully adjusted to the patient's tolerance. Although strengthening (progressive resistive or isokinetic) exercise can be helpful, the best outcome appears to result from conditioning, or aerobic, exercise.

17. **What are the proposed pathophysiologic mechanisms for fibromyalgia?**
Fibromyalgia is associated with an augmentation of sensation. Pathophysiologic explanations for fibromyalgia have ranged from primarily central, to a combination of central and peripheral, to primarily peripheral. Examples:
   - Fibromyalgia is a variation of an affective disorder. This idea was based on its common association with depression, IBS, and chronic fatigue syndrome.
   - A sleep abnormality is the main disturbance, leading to altered pain perception.
   - Peripheral factors, especially musculoskeletal derangements, are most important, along with the depression resulting from chronic pain.
   - Travell and Simons believed that the muscle problem was primary.

It remains unclear whether there is one pathological mechanism for fibromyalgia or a variety of etiologic factors. Nevertheless, current hypotheses under investigation hold some promise that the pathogenesis and pathophysiology of fibromyalgia may soon be clarified:
   - The cause is neuroendocrine in origin. This concept is largely based on the observation of decreased circulating cortisol levels and abnormal 5-HT metabolism.
   - Peripheral C-fiber and central nociceptive sensitization occurs following a painful stimulus.
   - High levels of circulating immunoglobulin M (IgM) in response to an enteroviral infection have been demonstrated in some fibromyalgia patients.
   - A Chiari I malformation, with brainstem compression, leads to an altered autonomic response, orthostasis, and fibromyalgia syndrome.

18. **How is sleep disturbance related to fibromyalgia?**
Sleep disturbance is one of the most common complaints of patients with fibromyalgia. It was initially described as "nonrestorative sleep." Some patients were shown to have an intrusion of alpha rhythms into their stage-IV sleep ("alpha-delta" sleep). However, the same electroencephalographic pattern is often seen in other chronically painful conditions. Moreover, other disorders frequently found in association with fibromyalgia, such as the restless leg syndrome, can contribute to a sleep disorder. The incidence of sleep disturbance seems more related to the duration of chronic pain than to the specific diagnosis of fibromyalgia.

19. **What is the "spray and stretch" technique?**
The spray and stretch technique is based on the theory that trigger points located in taut muscle bands are the principle cause of pain in fibromyalgia and in myofascial pain syndrome. A taut band in the muscle is identified, and then a vapo-coolant spray (ethylchloride or fluoromethane) is applied directly along the muscle band. Once cooled, the muscle is stretched along its long axis. This helps to relax muscle tension (via muscle spindle and Golgi tendon organ stimulation), improve local circulation, decrease the number of active trigger points, and reduce the amount of pain.

20. **True or false: There are a number of controlled studies that demonstrate the efficacy of the various treatments used for fibromyalgia.**
False. There is a paucity of controlled studies with adequate outcome measures. Most studies have small cohorts and are largely anecdotal. Studies have been performed using tricyclic antidepressants, EMG biofeedback, education, physical training, hypnotherapy, a variety of drug combinations, and many other treatment strategies. In 145 reports of outcome measures, only 55 were able to differentiate the active treatment from placebo.

The treatment of fibromyalgia and myofascial pain syndrome remains a significant challenge to the practice of evidence-based medicine.

21. **Are there any factors that can precipitate the onset of fibromyalgia?**
Fibromyalgia can occur without any identifiable precipitating factors. However, it seems that it can also be initiated by trauma (e.g., surgery, childbirth, accident, severe infection, severe emotional strain) and can then be classified as "posttraumatic fibromyalgia."

22. **What drugs have recently been added to the list of medications used in the symptomatic treatment of fibromyalgia?**
Although only Pregabalin and duloxetine have received a specific indication for use in the treatment of fibromyalgia, a number of others have recently been used in increasing volumes. These include SRNIs such as the muscle relaxant/analgesic tizanidine and the 5-HT3 antagonists such as ondansetron, granisetron, and tropisetron.

23. **Are there any alternative therapeutic options for the treatment of myofascial syndrome?**
Pregabalin and duloxetine are examples of oral drugs, indicated for other disease states, which can be used with benefit in the treatment of myofascial syndrome. A number of topical options also exist. These include topical capsaicin, glyceryl trinitrate (which has a localized antiinflammatory effect), lidocaine (Lidoderm patch), and doxepin (a tricyclic antidepressant with localized analgesic effects). Injection of local anesthetic into tender points can be used, as well as injection with corticosteroid. Corticosteroids stabilize nerve membranes, reduce ectopic neural discharge, and have a specific effect on dorsal horn cells as well as their well known antiinflammatory effects.

24. **Are there any acute treatments that can be used to lessen the pain of fibromyalgia during a flare-up of this condition?**
It has recently been shown that parenteral injection of the 5-HT3 antagonist tropisetron can reduce the pain of fibromyalgia.

KEY POINTS

1. Myofascial pain syndrome is regional in distribution whereas fibromyalgia is bodywide.

2. Fibromyalgia is more common in females.

3. Laboratory investigations cannot be used to diagnose fibromyalgia but can be used to exclude other conditions.

4. The cause of fibromyalgia is not known.

BIBLIOGRAPHY

1. Arnold LM, Rosen A, Pritchett YL, et al: A randomized, double-blind, placebo-controlled trial of duloxetine in the treatment of women with fibromyalgia with or without major depressive disorder, *Pain* 119:5-15, 2005.

2. Bergman S, Herrstrom P, Jacobsson LTH, Peterson IF: Chronic widespread pain: a three-year follow-up of pain distribution and risk factors, *J Rheumatol* 29:818-825, 2002.

3. Bohr WT: Fibromyalgia syndrome and myofascial pain syndrome. Do they exist? *Neurol Clin* 13(2):365-384, 1995.

4. Clark SR, Jones KD, et al: Exercise for patients with fibromyalgia: risks versus benefits, *Curr Rheumatol Rep* 3(2):135-146, 2001.

5. Criscuolo CM: Interventional approaches to the management of myofascial pain syndrome, *Curr Pain Headache Rep* 5(5):407-411, 2001.

6. Garland EM, Robertson D: Chiari I malformation as a cause of orthostatic intolerance symptoms: a media myth? *Am J Med* 111(7):546-552, 2001.

7. Gowans SE, deHueck A, Voss S, et al: Effect of a randomized, controlled trial of exercise on mood and physical function in individuals with fibromyalgia, *Arthritis Rheum* 45(6):519-529, 2001.

8. Gur A, Karakoc M, et al: Cytokines and depression in cases with fibromyalgia, *J Rheumatol* 29(2):358-361, 2002.

9. Hurtig IM, Raak RI, Kendall SA, et al: Quantitative sensory testing in fibromyalgia patients and in healthy subjects: identification of subgroups, *Clin J Pain* 17(4):316-322, 2001.

10. Moldofsky H: Fibromyalgia, sleep disorder and chronic fatigue syndrome. In Bock C, Whelan J, editors: *Chronic fatigue syndrome*, CIBA Foundation Symposium 173, 262-271, Chichester, UK, 1993, Wiley.

11. Muller W, Stratz T: Results of the intravenous administration of tropisetron in fibromyalgia patients, *Scand J Rheumatol* 113 (Suppl):59-62, 2000.

12. Offenbacher M, Stucki G: Physical therapy in the treatment of fibromyalgia, *Scand J Rheumatol* 113 (Suppl): 78-85, 2000.

13. Park DC, Glass JM, Minear M, Crofford LJ: Cognitive function in fibromyalgia patients, *Arthritis Rheum* 44(9):2125-2133, 2001.

14. Parker AJ, Wessely S, Cleare AJ: The neuroendocrinology of chronic fatigue syndrome and fibromyalgia, *Psychol Med* 31(8):1331-1345, 2001.

15. Simons DG, Travell JG, Simons LS: *Myofascial pain and dysfunction: the trigger point manual*, 2nd ed, Baltimore, 1999, Williams & Wilkins.

16. vanWest D, Maes M: Neuroendocrine and immune aspects of fibromyalgia, *BioDrugs* 15(8):521-531, 2001.

17. West SG: *Rheumatology secrets*, 1997, Philadelphia, Hanley & Belfus.

18. White KP, Harth M: An analytical review of 24 controlled clinical trials for fibromyalgia syndrome, *Pain* 64:211-219, 1996.

19. White KP, Harth M: Classification, epidemiology, and natural history of fibromyalgia, *Curr Pain Headache Rep* 5(4):320-329, 2001.

CHAPTER 25

POSTOPERATIVE PAIN MANAGEMENT

Michael M. Hanania, MD, and Charles E. Argoff, MD

1. **What is the pathophysiology of acute postoperative pain?**
   Postoperative pain is mainly nociceptive (see Chapter 2, Classification of Pain), but central sensitization also occurs. At the periphery, inflammatory mediators (prostaglandins, histamine, serotonin, bradykinin, and substance P) increase the sensitivity of nociceptors. Central sensitization is a result of functional reorganization in the dorsal horn of the spinal cord. Both of these processes result in an exaggerated response to noxious stimuli, spread of hyperresponsiveness to noninjured tissue, and a reduced threshold for producing pain.

2. **Describe the deleterious physiologic effects of postoperative pain.**
   Muscle splinting secondary to pain in the abdomen or chest results in a decreased vital capacity and, ultimately, decreased alveolar ventilation. Atelectasis is therefore a common postoperative complication. If coughing is very painful and performed with minimal effort or infrequently, retention of secretions and subsequent pneumonia may result. Release of stress hormones and catecholamines secondary to pain may cause persistent tachycardia and hypertension, resulting in increased cardiac work and myocardial oxygen consumption. Increased sympathetic activity decreases intestinal motility and prolongs recovery.

3. **What are the principles of postoperative pain management?**
   Pain is a normal accompaniment of surgical intervention. The severity and duration of postoperative pain can be predicted from a knowledge of the surgical procedure involved. Therefore provision of analgesia for the postoperative period should be planned and should reflect the expected severity and duration of pain. Timed administration of analgesia should be the norm, rather than reliance on an "as required" basis. Logical combinations of analgesics should be used (e.g., opioid and acetaminophen; opioid and nonsteroidal antiinflammatory drugs [NSAIDs]; opioid, acetaminophen and NSAIDs) and side effects predicted (e.g., nausea, vomiting, constipation) with prophylactic measures instituted (e.g., antiemetics, laxatives).

4. **What is preemptive analgesia?**
   Preemptive analgesia provides pain relief prior to surgery and throughout the perioperative period. Acute postoperative pain is associated with alterations in synaptic function and nociceptive processing within the spinal cord dorsal horn, neuroendocrine responses, and sympathoadrenal activation. Theoretically, preemptive analgesia minimizes these responses and prevents the spinal cord "wind-up phenomenon" (central sensitization), which is more resistant to treatment and is associated with chronic pain conditions. Although the concept of preemptive analgesia is well proven in animal pain models, human studies have as yet failed to provide conclusive evidence that analgesia provided before the nociceptive stimulus is inflicted alters the extent or duration of subsequent pain.

5. **What evidence is available that preemptive analgesia may work?**
   According to a study by Brodner and colleagues, patients having more intense pain preoperatively used more patient-controlled analgesia (morphine) following surgery. Patients who received epidural bupivacaine and fentanyl (local anesthetic and opioid) before the surgical

incision for a prostatectomy had less pain and were more active postoperatively while hospitalized and 9 weeks later. Preemptive thoracic epidural infusion of an opioid and local anesthetic in patients undergoing abdominothoracic esophagectomy resulted in faster extubation and a shorter intensive care unit (ICU) stay.

6. **What is intravenous patient-controlled analgesia (PCA)?**
   Intravenous patient-controlled analgesia (PCA) is a system of opioid delivery that consists of an infusion pump interfaced with a timing device. It allows the patient to titrate the analgesic dose required for optimal control of pain. The patient presses a button, and a preset dose of analgesic is delivered. A programmed "lockout" period (usually 6 to 15 minutes) prevents inadvertent overdoses and excessive sedation. This system may be used on top of a baseline continuous infusion. The parameters that can be set therefore include the presence, or absence, of a background continuous infusion, the bolus dose of opioid administered, and the "lockout" period (during which further opioid cannot be delivered).

7. **What are the advantages of a PCA system over nurse-administered intramuscular (IM) opioids?**
   There are a number of problems with the traditional nurse-administered intramuscular (IM) opioids, including the following:
   - Lack of knowledge regarding analgesic pharmacodynamics and overconcern about respiratory depression and addiction liability
   - A long lag period between the onset of pain and the administration of opioid, because of the process involved in calling for a nurse, obtaining and recording narcotics, and administration of the drug. This lag period is extended by the time required for absorption of an IM dose and further complicated by the pain of IM administration. Intravenous PCA eliminates these factors.

   The dose of opioid is titrated with PCA use (the patient will continue to seek a dose until pain relief is achieved). With nurse-administered opioid, a fixed dose is given, and because it is given IM, the lag time to effect is long.

8. **Is a continuous background infusion necessary with intravenous PCA?**
   A continuous background infusion does not improve pain scores and is even associated with more side effects, such as sedation and respiratory depression, when used after less-painful abdominal surgeries such as cesarean section. A continuous background infusion is usually not necessary with other abdominal procedures, but probably serves a useful role in extensive abdominal and thoracic operations; definitive data are not available. Certainly, if a patient has been taking opioids preoperatively, the daily equivalent dose should be administered as a continuous infusion in addition to the PCA bolus.

9. **Which opioids are commonly used for intravenous PCA?**
   Morphine is most commonly used because it is relatively inexpensive and has an intermediate duration of action. The typical adult bolus dose is 1 mg with a 5- to 10-minute lockout (see Question 6). Other opioids used include meperidine (10-mg bolus dose), hydromorphone, and fentanyl. Ultralong-acting opioids, such as methadone, require very long lockout intervals; ultrashort-acting opioids, such as alfentanil, require a very short lockout with a basal infusion, making them suboptimal choices for PCA. An agonist-antagonist such as butorphanol may be used when pain is not severe, because a ceiling effect for analgesia is characteristic of this drug. However, mixed agonist-antagonists cannot be used with pure agonists.

10. **What is the youngest age for which PCA is appropriate?**
    Seven-year-olds do very well with PCA, but those ages 5 to 6 have variable success. Patients age 4 and under do not use PCA successfully. Preoperatively, each patient has to be evaluated individually, but PCA appears to be inappropriate for those 5 years of age and younger.

11. **What types of PCA devices are available?**
   PCA devices are generally of two types: (1) programmable pumps where background infusion rate, bolus dose, and lockout can be varied, or (2) disposable devices where lockout and bolus doses are fixed.

12. **What is spinal or neuraxial opioid analgesia?**
   Spinal or neuraxial opioid analgesia is a technique of managing postoperative pain by epidural or intrathecal delivery of opioids. Epidural opioids can be delivered through an indwelling epidural catheter by intermittent injections or continuous infusion or both (i.e., epidural PCA). Intrathecal or subarachnoid opioid delivery is usually a single bolus injection via a spinal needle, but it can be given through a catheter placed in the subarachnoid space. These techniques have become widely accepted for the management of moderate to severe postoperative pain, because of their ability to provide prolonged and profound analgesia.

13. **What is the mechanism of action of spinal opioids?**
   Epidural or intrathecal administration of opioids provides analgesia at least in part through opioid receptor binding in the dorsal horn of the spinal cord. Binding to opioid receptors occurs in Rexed's laminae II and III (substantia gelatinosa). Some analgesia is a result of systemic absorption and rostral flow of drug acting at the level of the brain. In the case of epidural opioid administration, the molecular size of the opioid determines its analgesic efficacy, because it has to pass through the dura (a connective tissue membrane) prior to contact with the spinal cord. With intrathecal opioid use, efficacy is dependent on the lipophilicity of the opioid in question.

14. **List some of the commonly used epidural opioids in order of most hydrophilic to most lipophilic.**

Drug	Lipid Solubility*
Morphine	1
Hydromorphone	6
Meperidine	30
Methadone	100
Fentanyl	800
Sufentanil	1500
* Partition coefficient relative to morphine	

15. **What are the advantages of delivering opioids using a thoracic versus lumbar epidural catheter?**
   When lipophilic opioids are used for pain in the abdominal area, it is advantageous to place the catheter at the level of the nerve roots involved in the afferent transmission of pain. For example, a thoracic epidural catheter for fentanyl infusion provides excellent analgesia for abdominal surgical pain. Adding a dilute concentration of local anesthetic may reduce opioid requirement and improve analgesia. If a hydrophilic opioid such as morphine is used, it is less important where the catheter is located because the drug will spread. Good analgesia is obtained with a lumbar catheter for abdominal pain. Hydrophilic opioids such as morphine and hydromorphone must be used cautiously at the thoracic level, because respiratory depression as a result of cephalad spread is a possibility.

16. **What are the advantages of combining regional anesthetic techniques with postoperative spinal analgesia for lower extremity orthopedic and vascular surgery?**
    There is a decreased incidence of thromboembolic events after lower extremity orthopedic surgery and a decreased incidence of graft thrombosis after vascular procedures when regional anesthesia is used. Postoperative pain management is then usually provided by epidural opioid and local anesthetic. In the case of amputations, phantom limb pain is less likely to develop if preemptive spinal analgesia is provided and a regional technique is used for the procedure.

17. **What are the side effects of spinal opioids?**
    The most common side effects of spinal opioids are urinary retention, pruritus, nausea, and vomiting. Less frequent side effects are hypotension, oversedation, and respiratory depression. Even after injection of a single bolus dose of opioid, occasionally respiratory depression can occur many hours after injection. In a study of more than 1100 patients, Ready et al. found an incidence of 0.2% for respiratory depression in those given epidural morphine postoperatively. A Swedish study by Rawal documented a respiratory depression incidence of 0.09% following epidural morphine and 0.36% following intrathecal morphine. A recent study by Liu and colleagues of 1030 patients on PCA epidural reported 13% incidence of nausea and 0.3% incidence of respiratory depression.

18. **How should respiratory depression be monitored on a surgical ward?**
    Hourly or 2-hour respiratory rate checks are ordered for the first 24 hours after a bolus of epidural or intrathecal morphine. The level of sedation should also be assessed, although less frequently. In severely sick and debilitated patients or those who had extensive surgery of the upper abdomen or thorax, monitoring may be done in the ICU with pulse oximetry and respiratory rate monitors.

19. **Explain the early and late respiratory depression associated with spinal opioids.**
    The early respiratory depression associated with spinal opioids is a reflection of vascular absorption and is typically seen 1 to 2 hours after injection of morphine. The late respiratory depression is thought to be due to rostral migration of the drug in the cerebrospinal fluid (CSF) affecting the respiratory centers in the brain. These phenomena are more common with large doses of opioid, advanced age, and the Trendelenburg position.

20. **How does analgesia differ between epidural and intrathecal opioid administration?**
    Intrathecal opioid administration results in much higher CSF concentrations of opioid and potent analgesia, so that a reduced dose is required (one-tenth the dose of epidural morphine). Onset of analgesia is also faster with intrathecal administration.

21. **List the contraindications to epidural or intrathecal injection.**
    Absolute contraindications include significant coagulopathy, septicemia, local skin infection at the insertion site, and the patient's refusal to have the procedure. Relative contraindications include presence of dural puncture (because of the risk of inadvertent spread to CSF after epidural injection), central sleep apnea (because of increased risk of respiratory depression), and history of latent herpes simplex labialis (reactivation in obstetric population).

22. **How is the side effect of pruritus treated?**
    The typical axial pruritus seen with spinal opioids involves mainly the face and torso. An antihistamine such as diphenhydramine may be administered, or a low-dose intravenous infusion of naloxone may be started (1 to 3 mg/kg/hr). The analgesia of spinal opioids

(especially morphine) is usually not lost with such a low-dose infusion of naloxone. Oral naltrexone and propofol also have been reported to relieve pruritus.

23. **How is the side effect of nausea and vomiting treated?**
Metoclopramide, droperidol, prochlorperazine, and ondansetron are commonly used to treat nausea and vomiting associated with opioids. Transdermal scopolamine has also been shown to be effective after epidural morphine. Nausea is also somewhat related to position, so the patient can reduce nausea by remaining still.

24. **How is the side effect of respiratory depression treated?**
Naloxone should be kept at the bedside and may be administered intravenously as 0.4-mg bolus for severe respiratory depression and in increments of 0.04 mg for mild to moderate depression. An infusion of naloxone may be required with long-acting opioids, because naloxone has a relatively short half-life. If the patient has had significant exposure to opioids, naloxone may precipitate withdrawal. Some other form of analgesia will be needed because naloxone reverses the opioids. Remember that the duration of action of the opioid may be longer than the duration of the effect of naloxone. Therefore further doses of naloxone may need to be administered.

25. **Why are local anesthetics used in spinal analgesia?**
Bupivacaine and levobupivacaine are long-acting local anesthetics that provide greater sensory than motor blockade and are often used in conjunction with an opioid in epidural analgesia. When infused with an opioid at the level of the nerve roots involved in pain transmission, a synergism results in improved pain relief associated with decreased opioid requirement and (sometimes) decreased side effects. Therefore, the local anesthetic is used at a concentration which if used on its own would have an inadequate analgesic effect, along with an opioid, again at a dose that would be insufficient if administered alone but when used in combination can provide good quality pain relief. However, the disadvantages of potential motor and sympathetic blockade with local anesthetic use must be realized—ambulation must be restricted, and precautions against hypotension must be implemented.

26. **How are epidural opioids cleared from the CSF?**
Opioid that has gained access to the CSF may remain there or bind to opioid receptors in the substantia gelatinosa. Removal of opioid from the dorsal horn primarily occurs through local spinal cord blood flow, including uptake into epidural veins in close proximity to the arachnoid granulations. Highly lipid-soluble agents are rapidly absorbed into blood vessels and epidural fat from receptor sites, and analgesic duration is short. Hydrophilic opioids preferentially remain in CSF and diffuse more slowly into blood vessels; thus, analgesia is prolonged.

27. **Where is the site of action for local anesthetics when used epidurally for management of postoperative pain?**
Local anesthetics, when injected epidurally, pass through arachnoid granulations of the dural cuff region to enter the CSF and nerve roots. Local anesthetics block the sodium channels of nerve axons and therefore block nerve conduction. Small-diameter nerve fibers are more susceptible than larger ones. Therefore, sympathetic blockade occurs at low concentrations and is followed by sensory and eventually motor blockade.

28. **How else can local anesthetics be used in postoperative pain management?**
It should be normal practice for the surgeon to infiltrate the operative area with local anesthetic such as levobupivacaine or bupivacaine at the end of the surgical procedure, particularly when no other nerve block or spinal use of local anesthetic has been used. When the

wound is being infiltrated with local anesthetic, thought must be given to the safe dose of that local anesthetic, which is a compromise between the concentration of the local anesthetic and the volume used.

29. **What are other modalities of postoperative pain management?**
Regional nerve blocks such as intercostal nerve blocks may be used for one-sided abdominal or thoracic postoperative pain. Upper or lower extremity regional nerve blockade may be performed as a one-time injection or intermittent blockade via a catheter (i.e., continuous axillary catheter). An interpleural catheter may be used for prolonged intercostal nerve blockade. A femoral nerve block can reduce pain and opioid requirement following total knee replacement.

30. **Name some adjuvant drugs (nonopioids) and techniques that may be used in conjunction with opioids for postoperative analgesia.**
NSAIDs are often used in conjunction with opioids for postoperative analgesia and can act to reduce opioid requirement and improve pain relief. Ketorolac is an example of a popular NSAID that may be administered intravenously. Acetaminophen can be administered orally, intravenously, or rectally. Antiemetics such as hydroxyzine and droperidol have been shown to reduce opioid requirement, possibly as a result of their sedative effect. Transcutaneous nerve stimulation (TENS) has been shown to be effective to some degree after less painful operations.

31. **Are there other pharmacological methods of reducing postoperative pain?**
As well as acetaminophen and NSAIDs, there are some other treatment modalities that can be used with good effect. Examples are the use of lidocaine-containing patches (Lidoderm), which have a local analgesic effect and should therefore be placed over the postoperative wound, and topical glyceryl trinitrate (GTN) patches. GTN has analgesic and antiinflammatory effects as well as a tendency to improve local tissue perfusion. Topical GTN can be considered for use on a postoperative wound and has particular value in the patient in whom NSAIDs are contraindicated. Neither GTN nor Lidoderm has a Food and Drug Administration indication for use in postoperative pain.

32. **Are special considerations required when using patient-controlled analgesia in the older person?**
Many of the same recommendations that apply to PCA in other patient groups apply to PCA in the older person. Drugs should be initiated at a low dose (e.g., 1.0 to 1.5 mg of morphine with a lockout period of 5 to 7 minutes), and close monitoring is required to check for signs of delirium. Assess the patient prior to institution of PCA, to check that he or she has adequate cognitive abilities to understand the use of the system.

KEY POINTS

1. Untreated postoperative pain can impede recovery from surgery.

2. Pain is a predictable consequence of surgery and therefore analgesia should be provided before it reaches its expected postoperative level as a matter of routine.

3. Spinal opioids decrease the dose of opioid needed to give pain relief when compared to other modes of administration.

4. Delayed respiratory depression can complicate epidural and spinal opioid use.

5. Postoperative analgesia should use a multimodal approach, with combinations of opioids, NSAIDs, and local anesthetics, to optimize pain relief.

BIBLIOGRAPHY

1. Bailey PL, Rondeau S, Schafer PG, et al: Dose response pharmacology of intrathecal morphine in human volunteers, *Anesthesiology* 79:49-59, 1993.

2. Ballantyne JC, Carr DB, deFerranti S, et al: The comparative effects of postoperative analgesic therapies on pulmonary outcome: cumulative meta-analysis of randomized, controlled trials, *Anesth Analg* 86:598-612, 1998.

3. Basbaum AI: Spinal mechanisms of acute and persistent pain, *Reg Anesth Pain Med* 24:59-67, 1999.

4. Brodner G, Pogatzki E, Van Aken H, et al: A multimodal approach to control postoperative pathophysiology and rehabilitation in patients undergoing abdominothoracic esophagectomy, *Anesth Analg* 86:228-234, 1998.

5. Christopherson R, Beattie C, Frank SM, et al: Perioperative morbidity in patients randomized to epidural or general anesthesia for lower extremity vascular surgery: the perioperative ischemia randomized anesthesia trial study group, *Anesthesiology* 79:422-434, 1993.

6. deLeon-Casasola OA, Parker BM, Lema MJ, et al: Epidural analgesia versus intravenous patient controlled analgesia, *Reg Anesth* 19:307-315, 1994.

7. Etches RC: Patient-controlled analgesia, *Surg Clin North Am* 79(2):297-312, 1999.

8. Frank ED, McKay W, Rocco A, Gallo JP: Intrapleural bupivacaine for postoperative analgesia following cholecystectomy: a randomized prospective study, *Reg Anesth* 15:26-30, 1990.

9. Gottschalk A, Smith DS, Jobes DR, et al: Pre-emptive epidural analgesia and recovery from radical prostatectomy, *JAMA* 279:1076-1082, 1998.

10. George KA, Chisakuta AM, Gamble JA, Browne GA: Thoracic epidural infusion for postoperative pain relief following abdominal aortic surgery: bupivacaine, fentanyl, or a mixture of both? *Anaesthesia* 47:388-394, 1992.

11. Lavand'Homme P, De Kock M: Practical guidelines on the postoperative use of the patient-controlled analgesia in the elderly, *Drugs Aging* 13(1):9-16, 1998.

12. Liu SS, Allen HW, Olsson GL: Patient-controlled epidural analgesia with bupivacaine and fentanyl on hospital wards, *Anesthesiology* 88:688-695, 1998.

13. Loper KA, Ready LB, Downey M, et al: Epidural and intravenous fentanyl are clinically equivalent after knee surgery, *Anesth Analg* 70:72-75, 1990.

14. Lotsch J, Skarke C, Tegeder I, Geisslinger G: Drug interactions with patient-controlled analgesia, *Clin Parmacokinet* 41(1):31-57, 2002.

15. McDonald AJ, Cooper MG: Patient-controlled analgesia: an appropriate method of pain control in children, *Pediatr Drugs* 3(4):273-284, 2001.

16. Moiniche S, Kehlet H, Dahl JB: A qualitative and quantitative systematic review of preemptive analgesia for postoperative pain relief: the role of timing of analgesia, *Anesthesiology* 96(3):725-741, 2002.

17. Raja SN, Dougherty PM: Reversing tissue injury-induced plastic changes in the spinal cord: the search for the magic bullet, *Reg Anesth Pain Med* 25:441-444, 2000.

18. Rawal N: 10 years of acute pain services: achievements and challenges, *Reg Anesth Pain Med* 24:68-73, 1999.

19. Ready LB, Loper KA, Nessly M, Wild L: Postoperative epidural morphine is safe on surgical wards, *Anesthesiology* 75:452-456, 1991.

20. Slappendel R, Weber EW, Bugter ML, et al: The intensity of preoperative pain is directly correlated with the amount of morphine needed for postoperative analgesia, *Anesth Analg* 88:146-148, 1999.

21. Todd MT, Brown DL: Regional anesthesia and postoperative pain management, *Anesthesiology* 91:1-2, 1999.

22. Urmey WF: Femerol nerve block for the management of postoperative pain, *Tech Reg Anesth Pain Manage* 1:88-92, 1997.

CHAPTER 26

CANCER PAIN SYNDROMES

Gilbert R. Gonzales, MD, and Charles E. Argoff, MD

1. **What are the most common causes of pain in patients with cancer?**
   Pain in patients with cancer may be due to tumor involvement of pain-sensitive structures, to complications of therapy, or to processes not directly related to the cancer. The most common cause of pain in cancer is bone metastases. This is a nociceptive pain syndrome. Having said that, cancer patients can suffer from those pain conditions that patients without cancer develop. Because of abnormal posture, muscle wasting, malnourishment, unsteadiness and immobility, to name but a few, cancer patients can develop mechanical problems that generate pain. Therefore, it is important that a diagnosis is made of the cause of the pain, defining whether it is cancer related or not and which pain-sensitive structure is irritated and causing pain.

2. **Is it common for patients with cancer to have more than one painful site?**
   Yes. In a large study of patients with severe cancer pain, 25% reported pain in two or more sites. Another survey, not limited to severe pain, showed an even higher prevalence of multiple painful sites. Furthermore, multiple sites may have multiple etiologies. For example, a patient with lung cancer could conceivably have postthoracotomy pain from the original surgery, multiple bone metastases, and a painful peripheral neuropathy from chemotherapy.

3. **Name some neuropathic pain syndromes commonly seen in patients with cancer.**
   Tumor invasion of the brachial or lumbosacral plexus is common in patients with cancer. Chemotherapy-related neuritis, postherpetic neuralgia, phantom limb pain, and peripheral neuropathy also occur frequently.

4. **How common is neuropathic pain in patients with cancer?**
   Pain that can be inferred to be due to neurological lesions accounts for approximately 40% of severe pain syndromes. Although the somatic nociceptive pain syndromes are most common overall, patients with neuropathic pain are more likely to be referred to a pain specialist, presumably because of the inherent difficulty in treating these syndromes.

5. **Which factors predispose a patient to develop postherpetic neuralgia (PHN)?**
   Advancing age is the most important factor that predisposes a patient to develop postherpetic neuralgia (PHN). The incidence of PHN rises exponentially after age 70. It is also more common in cancer and immunosuppressed patients than it is in the normal population. PHN commonly occurs in irradiated parts of the body. The trigeminal nerve (ophthalmic division) may also be predisposed to PHN.

   Unfortunately, none of these factors can be controlled. There is some evidence to suggest that the severity of the rash and pain during the acute outbreak may predispose to later pain, so early and aggressive treatment may cut down the incidence of PHN. Also, the administration of analgesic antidepressants during the acute outbreak has been shown to be helpful.

6. **Are opioids known to increase the risk of acute herpes zoster eruptions? Are opioids known to increase the subsequent development of PHN in patients who get acute zoster eruptions?**
Opioids are not known to increase the risk of acute zoster eruptions nor do they increase the risk of postherpetic neuralgia. In fact, good pain control during the acute phase may lessen later pain.

7. **Describe the pain syndrome associated with metastases to the clivus.**
Pain associated with metastases to the clivus is characterized by a vertex headache and exacerbated by neck flexion. There may be associated abnormalities of the lower cranial nerves, most commonly dysphagia from involvement of the glossopharyngeal nerve (IX). Occasionally, there is weakness of the trapezius from involvement of the spinal accessory nerve (XI).

8. **Which types of malignancies are least likely to be painful?**
Leukemia malignancies are least likely to be painful. In general, solid tumors of viscera and metastatic, invasive, destructive, and nerve-compressing cancers are more painful than leukemias. Bone metastases are the most common cause of pain in patients with cancer.

9. **Is phantom limb sensation common after amputation?**
All amputees, including those with cancer-related amputations of limbs and some other parts (i.e., breast, penis, rectum, nose, ears), almost invariably experience phantom sensations the day after surgery. These sensations are not always painful and may not be reported spontaneously. A small proportion of these patients go on to experience phantom limb pain. The rest have sensations that may or may not subside.

10. **What is meant by incident pain?**
Incident pain is when a mass, metastatic lesion, or pathologic fracture causes pain on movement, such as repositioning, deep breathing, or ambulation. This can be a very difficult pain to control, and it may be necessary to immobilize the injured structure. Anesthesiologic or ablative procedures may be required if analgesics are not helpful. Also, medication can be given before the precipitating event on an as-needed basis (e.g., before radiation therapy or physical therapy). Incident pain can also be related to therapy: cannula insertion, venipuncture and physical therapy can all be associated with incident pain.
    Breakthrough pain may occur at the end of a dosing interval. It is easier to overcome, simply by shortening the dosing interval or increasing the amount of each dose.

11. **What is the postthoracotomy pain syndrome?**
There are two types of postthoracotomy pain: (1) immediate postoperative pain, which clears in 3 months and is associated with sensory loss in the area of scar, and (2) postoperative pain that lasts longer than 3 months or recurs in the surgical area following resolution of the initial postoperative pain. When pain recurs after a pain-free interval, suspect tumor recurrence or infection. When these are not found, the pain is most likely neuropathic.

12. **True or false: cancer patients with new onset of progressive headaches should undergo imaging studies, even if there are no objective findings on exam.**
True. Headache is the most common symptom in patients with brain metastasis, and it is the most common neurologic complication or symptom of systemic cancer and carcinomatous meningitis. Headaches may appear to be of the tension type, but tend to progress in duration and severity (see Chapter 14, Brain Tumor Headaches). Eventually, focal neurologic deficits develop in most patients.

13. **What are the clinical differences between radiation injury to the brachial plexus and tumor involvement of the plexus?**
A woman with breast cancer treated with mastectomy and radiation of the brachial plexus region may develop ipsilateral pain with arm and hand weakness (a brachial plexopathy) after her treatments. If the symptoms are referable to the lower brachial plexus (i.e., lower trunk), it is most likely due to tumor recurrence. Radiation is more likely to cause a panplexopathy (i.e., involvement of all three trunks of the brachial plexus).
Horner's syndrome is more common in tumor involvement. Electrophysiologically, myokymia is more commonly seen with radiation injury than with direct tumor involvement.

14. **Why do women treated with radical mastectomy have a numb area just distal to the axilla on the inner upper part of the arm?**
Injury to the intercostobrachial nerve is common in mastectomy patients and results in numbness in this specific area (Fig. 26-1). In some patients, neuropathic pain develops in the same location.

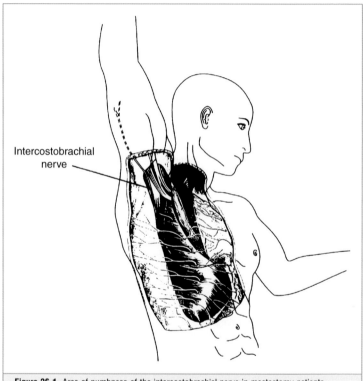

Intercostobrachial nerve

Figure 26-1. Area of numbness of the intercostobrachial nerve in mastectomy patients.

15. **Painful peripheral neuropathies can be seen with which of these agents: cisplatin, vinca alkaloids, procarbazine?**
All of the listed agents and several others can produce a painful peripheral neuropathy. Less often, motor and autonomic dysfunction also occur. With cisplatin and the vinca alkaloids, neuropathy seems to be dose-related. Only about 10% to 20% of patients treated with procarbazine (a monoamine oxidase [MAO] inhibitor) develop neuropathy.

16. **What is steroid pseudorheumatism?**
    Steroid pseudorheumatism can occur after either slow or rapid withdrawal of steroid medication in patients taking these medications for any length of time. It is characterized by arthralgias, diffuse myalgias, muscle and joint tenderness on palpation, and diffuse malaise without objective inflammatory signs on examination. These symptoms revert with reinitiation of the steroid medication.

17. **What is the most common cause of lumbosacral plexopathy?**
    Direct tumor extension into the plexus (by lymphoma or colon carcinoma) is a more common cause of lumbosacral plexopathy than metastatic involvement or radiation injury. Pain radiates down the leg in a radicular distribution.

18. **Mucositis pain from chemotherapy or radiation therapy may be exacerbated by which of the following: secondary fungal infections, secondary viral infections, lack of saliva secretion, secondary bacterial infections, nonopioid analgesics?**
    Except for the nonopioid analgesics, all of the listed conditions may exacerbate mucositis-induced pain. Nonopioid analgesics, such as acetaminophen and the topical anesthetics, are used to treat mucositis pain along with opioid analgesics. Infections and dry mucous membranes may exacerbate the mucositis and the pain.

19. **In what percentage of patients with cancer is the pain unrelated to cancer or its treatment?**
    Ten percent of patients with cancer pain have a preexisting, painful condition such as degenerative arthritis, diabetic peripheral neuropathy, migraine, or other nonmalignant pain condition.

20. **List the pain-sensitive structures in bones and joints.**
    The periosteum and all joint components, except cartilage, are pain sensitive. Articular cartilage is not a pain-sensitive structure. In the intervertebral discs, the annulus fibrosus has nociceptors, but the nucleus pulposus does not.

21. **Do nonsteroidal antiinflammatory drugs (NSAIDs) have direct tumor effects?**
    Yes. The NSAIDs are useful for tumor-induced pain partially because of their effects on the margins of the tumor and the inflammation that can exist there. Furthermore, bone metastases require prostaglandin E_2 for growth, and the NSAIDs inhibit prostaglandin synthesis.

22. **What is the most common site for tumor infiltration of the brachial plexus?**
    The most common site for tumor infiltration of the brachial plexus may vary somewhat by tumor type, but the lower plexus is most commonly involved. This leads to hand weakness and pain in a C7-T1 distribution. A Horner's syndrome is often present. The classic example is Pancoast tumor.

23. **What is the first sign of metastases to the base of the skull?**
    Pain is the first symptom of metastases to the base of the skull. Cranial nerve dysfunction occurs later and depends on which part of the base is involved. Metastases to the occipital condyles are characterized by pain at the nape of the neck, radiating up the back of the head. It is often unilateral and reproduced by local pressure over the occipital condyles.

24. **What symptoms and signs characterize parasellar metastases?**
Most often, patients with parasellar metastases show unilateral, supraorbital, or frontal headache and ocular paresis without proptosis. The facial nerve is not affected by a parasellar metastasis, because it is not anatomically located in or near the parasellar region (it leaves the cranium by way of the internal acoustic meatus). Cranial nerves III, IV, V, and VI (oculomotor, trochlear, trigeminal, and abductus) pass through the cavernous sinus, adjacent to the sella. The mandibular division of cranial nerve V exits before the sinus.

25. **What signs or symptoms characterize the jugular foramen syndrome?**
Hoarseness, dysphagia, glossopharyngeal neuralgia, syncope, and multiple lower cranial nerve abnormalities are the most common abnormalities associated with jugular foramen syndrome. Cranial nerves IX, X, and XI (glossopharyngeal, vagus, and accessory spiral) pass through the jugular foramen.

26. **What are the five cancer pain groups?**
Cancer patients are grouped into the following five categories to help health care workers manage the multidimensional issues that can occur in these patients.
Group I: Patients with acute cancer-related pain
- Associated with the diagnosis of cancer
- Associated with cancer therapy (surgery, chemotherapy, radiotherapy)
Group II: Patients with chronic cancer-related pain
- Associated with cancer progression
- Associated with cancer therapy (surgery, chemotherapy, radiotherapy)
Group III: Patients with preexisting chronic pain and cancer-related pain
Group IV: Patients with history of drug addiction and cancer-related pain, including patients that:
- Are actively involved in illicit drug use
- Are in a methadone maintenance program
- Have a past history of drug abuse
Group V: Dying patients with cancer-related pain

27. **Does increased education improve cancer pain management?**
The answer is not straightforward. Better education does, indeed, produce better practices in pain management. However, a number of surveys have shown that these practices may improve patient satisfaction but do not necessarily decrease pain intensity.

28. **What characterizes the sphenoid sinus syndrome?**
Severe bifrontal headache, nasal stuffiness, diplopia, and intermittent retroorbital pain are characteristics of the sphenoid sinus syndrome.

29. **What is the most dangerous complication of tumor invasion of the brachial plexus?**
Tumor of the brachial plexus commonly spreads along the nerve root into the epidural space. As it does so, pain worsens, and epidural spinal-cord compression can produce paraparesis and bowel and bladder dysfunction.

30. **What are the initial signs and symptoms of epidural spinal-cord compression?**
Epidural tumor from infiltration of bone, causing spinal cord compression, causes pain in the vast majority of patients (95% have pain as the initial symptom). There is local back pain with tenderness to percussion (most commonly in the thoracic region), and there may be radicular radiation of pain. Myelopathic signs appear later. Any patient with cancer and back pain

should be considered to have epidural extension of tumor until proven otherwise. Note that 30% of patients with cancer, back pain, and a normal neurologic examination will still show epidural extension. The epidural veins form a portal circulation with the intracranial veinous system, which accounts for the tendency of pelvic and intraabdominal malignancies to produce cerebral metastasis.

31. **What are the characteristics of lumbar vertebral metastasis?**
Dull, aching midback pain exacerbated by lying or sitting and relieved by standing is the usual complaint. Benign pain is usually relieved by recumbency. Percussion tenderness of the spine is common in prepubertal metastases but uncommon in disc disease.

32. **What are the radiologic differences between vertebral metastases and vertebral abscesses?**
In general, metastases spare the disc space, and infections obliterate the disc space.

33. **What is the usual clinical presentation for tumor infiltration of a peripheral nerve?**
A patient with tumor infiltration of a peripheral nerve may have constant burning pain, hypesthesia, dysesthesia, or sensory loss. There also may be motor dysfunction. Lancinating pains are more common with nerve root involvement.

34. **The World Health Organization (WHO) has developed the cancer pain relief program and has advocated a three-step approach to the pharmacologic treatment of cancer pain. What are these three steps?**
    Step 1: Nonopioids with or without adjuvant medications (mild pain)
    Step 2: Weak opioids with or without nonopioids and adjuvant medications (moderate pain)
    Step 3: Strong opioids with or without nonopioids and adjuvant medications (severe pain)
Therapy may be initiated at any step, depending on the severity of the pain. However, the WHO ladder may not be the best approach in some pain conditions, such as cancer-related neuropathic pain, which are more likely to be controlled by use of tricyclic antidepressants, serotonin-norepinephrine reuptake inhibitors (SNRIs), antiepileptic drugs, and membrane-stabilizing drugs.

35. **In the terminally ill patient with a malignancy considered nonresponsive to radiation, may radiation still be used in some cases to reduce pain caused by the malignancy?**
Yes. A tumor that is not radiosensitive may still be radioresponsive if the response sought is pain reduction. Size reduction is not always necessary to provide analgesia.

36. **Hypophysectomy has been used in the terminally ill patient for pain control in which types of cancers?**
Metastatic bone pain caused by estrogen-positive breast cancer and prostate cancer has been treated with hypophysectomy, although this procedure is rarely used today in the United States. Other types of cancer pain may respond to this dramatic therapeutic modality as well.

37. **What are the most common primary tumors that cause painful vertebral metastases?**
Lung, breast, and prostate are the most common primary tumors that cause painful vertebral metastases. Colon and lymphoma are also seen frequently.

38. **What is the first step in assessing pain?**

The first step in assessing pain is to believe the cancer patient's complaints of pain! Although social and cultural factors and psychologic influences can affect pain experiences, the complaint of pain in the cancer pain patient can rarely, if ever, be assigned to psychologic influences alone. The physician and nurse caring for the patient must start with a belief in the patient's complaint of pain.

39. **What is an opiate? What is an opioid?**

An opiate is a product such as morphine and codeine historically derived from the juice of *Papaver somniferum,* the opium poppy.

An opioid, on the other hand, is a compound that possesses morphinelike characteristics but may not necessarily be derived from the juice of *Papaver somniferum.* These drugs act by having an effect on opioid receptors, of which there are three of clinical relevance (mu, delta, and kappa). Opioids that act at the mu receptor are antagonized by naloxone. An example is meperidine, which is a synthetic morphinelike analgesic. Morphine is, by definition, both an opioid and an opiate (see Chapter 34, Opioid Analgesics).

40. **How does codeine work?**

Codeine has no intrinsic analgesic effect but requires a metabolic step to occur (which converts it to morphine) for analgesia to be produced. Around one in eight patients lack the enzyme required for this process; those patients will get no pain relief when codeine is used, although they may get pain relief if other strong opioids, other than codeine, are used. Dihydrocodeine does not require activation and has intrinsic analgesic effects.

41. **List the three primary groups of opioids (Offermeier's classification). Which are used in cancer pain patients?**
    - Opioid agonists—the mainstay for the treatment of cancer pain. Morphine is the prototypical agonist and is the preferred drug for severe cancer pain.
    - Opioid agonist-antagonists—used for patients with cancer pain in some parts of the world where pure agonists are not available because of governmental restrictions. They are rarely, if ever, used for chronic cancer pain.
    - Opioid antagonists—Narcan (naloxone) is not used for management of cancer pain except to reverse an opioid agonist intoxication, i.e., it reverses respiratory depression, sedation, and analgesia.

42. **Are nonopioid analgesics useful for patients with mild cancer pain? Are they useful for moderate and/or severe cancer pain?**

The nonopioid analgesics are used in cancer patients whose pain is mild or moderate, but they can also be used as an adjunct to a strong opioid to enhance the opioid's effects. Tolerance and physical dependence do not occur with the nonopioid analgesics, but ceiling effects do.

43. **Are opioids always the best analgesics to use in patients with cancer pain?**

No, opioids are not always the best analgesics to use in patients with cancer pain. Just as one would try to define which structure is being irritated (e.g., muscle, bone, joint, nerve, ligament, visceral structure etc.) in a patient with noncancer pain and use the most effective pain-relieving technique or drug for that pain, one should do the same with the cancer pain patient. For example, painful muscle spasm caused by tumor irritation or due to mechanical causes related to abnormal posture in the cancer patient may be best treated with a muscle relaxant drug. Similarly, if neuropathic pain is evident, analgesic antidepressants, antiepileptic drugs, and membrane stabilizing drugs may be a better first choice than opioids.

KEY POINTS

1. Cancer patients develop pain from their cancer but can also develop pain unrelated to their cancer.

2. Phantom awareness is common after any amputation (leg, arm, breast, penis, rectum, etc). Phantom pain is less common, but is still a significant and distressing symptom.

3. Chemotherapy-induced mucositis pain can be exacerbated by secondary bacterial and fungal infection.

4. Back pain in the cancer patients should rouse suspicion of vertebral metastasis or epidural tumor formation.

5. Codeine has no intrinsic analgesic effect and requires metabolism to morphine by a cytochrome enzyme to become active. Around one in eight of the population lack this enzyme and so derive no pain relief from codeine.

CHAPTER 27

PAIN IN RHEUMATOID ARTHRITIS AND OSTEOARTHRITIS

David S. Pisetsky, MD, PhD, and Gary McCleane, MD

1. **What are the causes of pain in rheumatoid arthritis?**

   Pain in rheumatoid arthritis (RA) is multifactorial and varies in origin with duration and severity of disease. In the initial phases of RA, pain results from inflammation, as evidenced by tenderness and swelling of the joint as well as laboratory findings (e.g., increased C-reactive protein, anemia, thrombocytosis). The presence of a rheumatoid factor is also consistent with inflammation. As RA progresses, the damaging effects of erosion of cartilage and bone also cause pain. Patients with this disease may also experience pain from fibromyalgia and complications such as osteoporosis, with fracture of vertebral bodies leading to acute symptoms. When the inflammatory process settles, the joint involved may be damaged so that it is mechanically unstable and more likely to undergo degenerative changes that further contribute to pain.

   When pain in RA occurs disproportionately in a single joint, it is important to exclude septic arthritis, because preexisting arthritis predisposes to joint space infection.

2. **What is synovitis?**

   Synovitis is inflammation of the synovium, which is the lining tissue of the joint. It is the clinical hallmark of RA and produces pain, swelling, and tenderness of the joint. Other signs of inflammation (e.g., heat and redness) occur less prominently in RA than in other forms of arthritis, such as crystal-induced disease. In RA, dramatic proliferation accompanies synovitis, with a variety of cell types including lymphocytes, fibroblasts, and macrophages forming a dense cellular infiltrate that increases the synovium to many times its normal size, producing a structure called the pannus. Cells of the pannus, at the junction with cartilage and bone, cause erosion by the action of toxic products such as proteases. The end-result of this process can be deformity. Although the synovium in RA is filled with various cell types, joint space effusions have a predominance of neutrophils and are turbid and almost purulent in appearance. In advanced RA, synovium can expand so much that it is visible and easily palpable.

   Synovial inflammation and proliferation can occur discordantly in RA. Thus, some patients may have exquisitely painful joints without palpable synovium, whereas others show marked tissue proliferation in the absence of tenderness and pain. In patients with longstanding disease that has "burnt out," synovial tissue may be only minimally tender.

3. **How is RA diagnosed?**

   RA is diagnosed on the basis of history and physical findings. The disease is usually insidious in onset and affects both large and small joints in a symmetric pattern. Characteristic sites of inflammation include the small joints of the hands and feet, wrists, elbows, shoulders, hips, knees, and ankles. The cervical spine is also a prominent location of disease and is generally the only part of the axial skeleton that is affected by RA.

   The diagnosis of RA is supported by the presence of a rheumatoid factor that is an immunoglobulin M (IgM) antiimmunoglobulin G (anti-IgG) antibody. Note, however, that only about 80% of patients with RA display a rheumatoid factor, and that rheumatoid factor can also occur in other clinical settings. The presence of nodules and characteristic deformities (e.g., ulnar deviation, swan neck, and boutonniere deformities of the hands and fingers) substantiate the diagnosis, although these findings indicate more advanced disease and are not invariable.

4. **What are the radiographic findings of RA?**
The usual radiographic findings of RA are soft tissue swelling, juxtaarticular osteopenia, symmetric joint space narrowing, and bony erosion. Radiograph studies are performed to substantiate the diagnosis of RA, evaluate sources of pain, and stage disease to determine therapy. However, findings may be minimal in early disease. Bony erosions are indicative of tissue destruction and signify serious prognosis. Radiographs of joints in RA may also show evidence of osteoarthritis, which can occur secondary to joint destruction. With sustained disease activity, impaired mobility, and corticosteroid therapy, osteoporosis also occurs. It can be demonstrated by radiographic examination and by bone densitometry.

5. **What is a flare?**
RA, like other rheumatic diseases, varies in intensity over time and includes periods ("flares") during which signs of inflammation increase dramatically. Flares can occur without cause, or may follow infection and other stresses. They are associated with increased joint pain and swelling; symptoms such as prolonged morning stiffness, weakness, malaise, and weight loss; and laboratory findings of inflammation. Because RA is a systemic disease, flares are usually polyarticular. The sudden onset of severe pain and swelling in a single joint should raise the suspicion of infection.

6. **How is morning stiffness significant in RA?**
Morning stiffness is a very common complaint of patients with RA and is experienced as soreness and restricted movement upon awakening. This feeling is generalized in distribution and does not simply affect the joints. Although it is a form of pain, patients may not describe it as such.

The duration of morning stiffness is a good indicator of disease activity, and physicians should record this value as part of the clinical assessment. Many patients take a hot shower to relieve the sensation. The "gel phenomenon"—stiffness and soreness that develops after a period of immobility (e.g., sitting in a chair)—is a related symptom.

7. **Differentiate rheumatoid arthritis and osteoarthritis.**
RA and osteoarthritis (OA) are the two most common forms of arthritis. They are sometimes confused with each other because of their predilection for similar joints. The underlying pathophysiology of these diseases is distinct, however.

RA is inflammatory, and it initially involves the synovium and secondarily involves the cartilage. In contrast, OA primarily affects the cartilage, with this structure losing its mechanical properties from degeneration or degradation. Although cartilage in OA lacks the usual signs of inflammation such as an inflammatory cell infiltrate, chondrocytes in the cartilage may produce inflammatory mediators such as interleukin-1 (IL-1) and nitric oxide that cause breakdown of the cartilage matrix. Although OA can be polyarticular in nature, many patients have involvement of only single joints such as the knee or hip. The usual course of RA is symmetric involvement of multiple joints.

In RA, joint fluid is inflammatory and contains neutrophils in abundance (up to 50,000/ml), whereas in OA joint fluid shows few cells ($\leq$1000/ml).

Another difference between these two diseases concerns the impact on bone. In OA, hypertrophic changes cause bony enlargements called spurs or osteophytes. Inflammation in RA lacks a bony reaction.

8. **Give two alternate names for osteoarthritis.**
OA is also called degenerative joint disease or hypertrophic arthritis because of the pattern of cartilage and bone involvement.

9. **What are Heberden's and Bouchard's nodes?**
Heberden and Bouchard's nodes are osteoarthritic bony enlargements in the hands.

10. **Describe primary and secondary osteoarthritis.**
When OA occurs in the absence of a known predisposing cause, it is termed primary. If a contributing factor can be identified, e.g., congenital hip disease, fracture, or excessive motion or use, OA is termed secondary.

11. **What are the demographics of RA and OA?**
Both RA and OA occur more commonly in women than in men for reasons that are unknown. RA usually begins in the fourth and fifth decade of life, while OA starts later and is almost invariable among people in their 80s and 90s. Both diseases run in families, although the etiology is complex and likely multifactorial. Among genetic risk factors for RA, certain human leukocyte antigen (HLA) genes seem to predispose to disease; because disease occurs only occasionally among people genetically at risk, an environmental factor (e.g., infection) may be implicated in pathogenesis.

12. **What is inflammatory OA?**
Some patients with OA have especially prominent inflammation, with joint pain, tenderness, and redness. These patients are considered to have inflammatory or erosive osteoarthritis. This condition can be distinguished from RA on the basis of joint distribution, radiographs, and laboratory signs of inflammation.

13. **What are the radiographic findings of OA?**
The typical radiographic findings of OA are asymmetric joint space narrowing, subchondral sclerosis, cysts, and spur formation. Spurs or osteophytes represent bony outgrowths around the joint. OA and RA can be distinguished radiographically because RA causes symmetric joint space narrowing and lacks hypertrophic changes. Note that pain in arthritis can be referred; thus, a painful joint may show only limited change, necessitating radiographic study of a nearby joint to establish the cause. Knee pain, for example, may be referred from the hip.

14. **Compare joint distribution in OA and RA.**
OA and RA involve many joints in common (e.g., proximal interphalangeal joints of the hands, hips, knees, and cervical spine), but there are important differences that have diagnostic significance.
   - Affected by OA
     ○ Distal interphalangeal joints of hands
     ○ Lumbar spine
   - Affected by RA
     ○ Metacarpophalangeal joints of hands
     ○ Wrists, elbows, shoulder, ankles, small joints of feet
The distribution of joints in OA suggests that this disease is not simply the result of joint use or weight bearing, but reflects particular mechanical or biochemical properties of joints.

15. **What are the classes of drugs used to treat rheumatoid arthritis?**
Pharmacologic therapy for RA can be divided into four main categories: (1) nonsteroidal antiinflammatory drugs (NSAIDs); (2) corticosteroids, which are antiinflammatory and immunosuppressive; (3) analgesics; and (4) disease-modifying antirheumatic drugs (DMARDs). Therapy in RA frequently involves the simultaneous administration of drugs from more than one category, and there is considerable discussion concerning the timing and duration of therapy, as well as relative toxicity and efficacy of different agents.

16. **Discuss the role of disease-modifying antirheumatic drugs in RA.**

DMARDs are drugs that reduce the signs and symptoms of rheumatoid arthritis and can influence the progression of tissue destruction, usually as assessed by radiographs. These drugs may also improve mobility and quality of life, as measured by various indices of patient self-report. The actions of these agents are diverse and in many instances unknown. The term DMARD is confusing, because in some patients an NSAID or corticosteroid can lead to sustained improvement. Furthermore, there is evidence that corticosteroids can also modify radiographic progression.

DMARDs include methotrexate, leflunomide, tumor necrosis factor (TNF) blockers (etanercept and infliximab), IL-1 receptor antagonist (anakinra), gold salts, penicillamine, hydroxychloroquine, and azathioprine. More potent immunosuppressants such as cyclosporine and cyclophosphamide are rarely used in RA, but are placed in this category. Sulfasalazine, which has both antiinflammatory and antibiotic potential, is also in this group.

17. **What determines the selection of a DMARD over other agents?**

Factors pointing to the need for DMARD therapy include the following:
- Clinical evidence of persistent disease activity (e.g., number of painful and tender joints and duration of morning stiffness)
- Inadequate response to NSAIDs
- Laboratory evidence of inflammation (e.g., sedimentation rate or C-reactive protein)
- Erosive changes on radiograph*
- Progressive deformity
- Nodules
- Titer of rheumatoid factor

*DMARDs are used widely in the setting of persistent disease activity even in the absence of radiographic evidence of joint changes, because of the potential for long-term joint damage in RA.

DMARD use is individualized for the patient depending on disease severity and activity, patient preferences, and concerns about toxicity. Methotrexate is frequently the first DMARD tried, because of its well-established efficacy.

18. **What is "early aggressive" therapy of RA?**

Early aggressive therapy refers to the early use of DMARDs, recognizing that erosive damage is irreversible and can begin soon after the onset of disease. In the past, DMARD therapy typically was administered only after the occurrence of erosion. This practice reflected concerns over the toxicity of the more commonly used drugs at that time (e.g., gold salts) and the risk-benefit ratio. Current DMARDs show a much more favorable profile with respect to toxicity, leading to their more widespread and earlier use. In general, DMARD therapy is indefinite, but there is evidence that the earlier they are started, the better the clinical outlook in the long term.

Recently, some clinicians have recommended an even more aggressive approach with combinations of DMARDs in association with high-dose corticosteroids as initial therapy. In this approach, sometimes called the step-down approach, steroid doses are lowered and DMARDs withdrawn gradually as disease stays quiescent. Despite evidence for the utility of the step-down approach, most clinicians start with one DMARD and gradually add others to form a combination that adequately suppresses disease activity.

19. **How do NSAIDs work?**

NSAIDs inhibit the enzyme cyclooxygenase and thus block the generation of prostaglandins from arachidonic acid. Because of the physiological actions of prostaglandins, NSAIDs are antiinflammatory, analgesic, and antipyretic. These activities make the NSAIDs among the most commonly used drugs in all of medicine, whether by prescription or over-the-counter purchase. As now recognized, there are two cyclooxygenase enzymes, denoted COX1 and COX2.

COX1 is constitutively produced, whereas COX2 is inducible. COX1 mediates such effects as platelet aggregation and maintenance of the stomach lining. COX2 mediates inflammation and pain. Currently available NSAIDs have different side effects and also differ in their relative activity against COX1 and COX2.

20. **What are coxibs?**
Coxibs are NSAIDs that are highly selective for the COX2 enzyme. Because the COX2 enzyme mediates prostaglandin production responsible for inflammation and pain, coxibs are analgesic and antiinflammatory, but they lack the side effects related to inhibiting the COX1 enzyme (e.g., bleeding and gastrointestinal irritation). Like nonselective NSAIDs, which affect both COX1 and COX2 enzymes, coxibs are used in both OA and RA. The three currently approved coxibs are celecoxib, rofecoxib, and valdecoxib. Examples of nonselective NSAIDs are indomethacin, ibuprofen, and diclofenac.

Some patients respond to one NSAID or coxib but not to another; the reasons for this remain unclear. It is recommended that more than one of these drugs be tried before considering this type of therapy unsuccessful. The use of some coxibs have been restricted because of their propensity to cause increases in blood pressure and because their use is associated with a higher incidence of myocardial infarction.

21. **What are the side effects of NSAIDs?**
The side effects of NSAIDs relate to their inhibition of the COX enzymes, with activity against COX1 and COX2 leading to predictable side effects because of the distribution of these enzymes and their physiological effects. Inhibition of COX1 can lead to bleeding (especially gastrointestinal), gastric irritation, and ulceration. In contrast, inhibition of COX2, which is found in the kidney, can lead to fluid retention, hypertension, edema, and renal impairment. Coxibs are thus expected to have fewer gastrointestinal complications than nonselective NSAIDs, but both drugs share the potential for renovascular complications.

22. **Which patients are at greatest risk for renal side effects of NSAIDs?**
Patients at risk for renal side effects of NSAIDs have reduced renal blood flow and therefore produce prostaglandins via the action of COX2 as compensation. With prostaglandin production blocked by NSAIDs or coxibs, these patients can suffer from deterioration in renal function. The common settings associated with this complication include chronic renal insufficiency, congestive heart failure, diuretic use, and cirrhosis of the liver. In general, older patients have reduced renal function and are also prone to these side effects. Coxibs must be used with the same caution as nonselective NSAIDs in the setting of renal insufficiency.

23. **How does aspirin differ from other NSAIDs?**
Aspirin was the first NSAID developed. It blocks both COX1 and COX2 enzymes. In contrast to nonselective NSAIDs and coxibs, aspirin irreversibly inactivates these enzymes by acetylation. As a result, the actions of aspirin can be long lasting, particularly for the platelets.

24. **What is the therapeutic dose of aspirin?**
The pharmacologic actions of aspirin vary with dose. A low dose (e.g., a single 325-mg tablet or even a baby aspirin) can produce antiplatelet effects. In contrast, analgesic effects are usually achieved with two 325-mg tablets four times a day. Antiinflammatory effects occur at a blood level of 20 to 25 $mgdl^{-1}$, which requires titration for each patient and verification by determination of a serum salicylate level. For most adults, at least twelve 325-mg aspirin tablets are required for a therapeutic level, although sometimes more than 20 tablets are needed. Because the metabolism of aspirin involves a pathway that becomes saturated, small increases in aspirin dose can be reflected in large changes in salicylate levels and occurrence of side effects.

25. **What is salicylism?**

Aspirin (acetylsalicylic acid) is an NSAID with characteristic side effects that are not present during use of other NSAIDs. These side effects are termed salicylism and are manifest initially by tinnitus (ringing and roaring in the ears) at blood levels that overlap the therapeutic levels. As blood levels increase further, metabolic acidosis, respiratory alkalosis, disturbances in consciousness, coma, and death may ensue.

Aspirin remains a leading cause of drug-related death because of intentional (suicidal) ingestion as well as inadvertent overdosing from simultaneous use of more than one aspirin-containing product. There are hundreds of over-the-counter preparations with aspirin as an ingredient. In a patient on a full salicylate program, additional ingestion of aspirin can lead to toxic levels. Note that in older patients, aspirin can cause reversible deafness and should be avoided in those with hearing impairment.

26. **What is Samter's syndrome?**

Samter's syndrome is marked clinically by asthma, nasal polyps, and sensitivity to salicylates. A proposed mechanism is the shunting of arachidonate metabolites through the lipoxygenase pathway when the cyclooxygenase pathway is inhibited by aspirin.

27. **Describe NSAID gastropathy.**

Prostaglandins produced by COX1 enzymes promote the integrity of the gastric lining, and when their production is inhibited by NSAIDs, bleeding, superficial irritation, and erosion ensues. These lesions are frequently transient, small, and asymptomatic; endoscopy is required for their detection. This condition, known as gastropathy, should be distinguished from peptic ulcer disease, which can also occur in patients on NSAIDs. Many patients on NSAIDs also experience dyspepsia in the absence of other signs of erosion.

28. **How is NSAID gastropathy prevented?**

The frequency of this complication appears to differ among available nonselective NSAIDs, although it occurs with all. To reduce gastric complications these drugs should be taken with food or antacids. If aspirin is used, a buffered or enteric-coated preparation may be less toxic for the gastrointestinal (GI) tract. Other preventive measures include the use of H2 blockers such as cimetidine or ranitidine, as well as misoprostol. Misoprostol is a synthetic prostaglandin approved for use in patients who have had documented GI complications with NSAIDs. Misoprostol should not be used in women of child bearing potential as it can cause, and has been used to induce, abortion.

29. **Do coxibs have fewer GI side effects than nonselective NSAIDs?**

Overall, coxibs have fewer GI side effects than nonselective NSAIDs. As shown by endoscopic studies, the number of lesions is greatly reduced with coxibs; this is expected, on the basis of their selectivity for COX2.

However, the situation with respect to serious peptic ulcer problems is somewhat more complicated. Because these events are much less common than gastropathy, very large studies are required to show a difference between nonselective NSAIDs and coxibs in their effect on complications such as hemorrhage, perforation, or obstruction. In addition, the frequency of these events may differ among nonselective NSAIDs, making studies dependent on the comparator. With these caveats, it is likely that coxibs cause fewer serious ulcer complications than do nonselective NSAIDs; the data for rofecoxib is clearer than that for celecoxib at this time.

Nevertheless, NSAIDs are still widely used in part because of cost issues. Additionally, the safety gain from use of coxibs depends on the clinical setting and patient characteristics such as age and previous history of peptic ulcer disease.

30. **Can aspirin be combined with a coxib? With an NSAID?**
Coxibs do not affect platelet function because they do not inhibit COX1; therefore, they lack benefits in the prevention of cardiovascular or cerebrovascular disease. For patients at risk for these vascular events, a low dose of aspirin can be added to a coxib, although the effect on the GI tract is uncertain. Thus, in the patient with arthritis and a risk for heart disease, aspirin may be used in combination with a coxib.

The cardioprotective effects of nonselective NSAIDs have not been clearly defined, leading to concomitant use of low-dose aspirin with a nonselective NSAID. However, this combination can be problematic because prior administration of a nonselective NSAID may limit the ability of aspirin to acetylate COX1 in the platelet.

31. **What are the differences between acetaminophen and NSAIDs?**
Acetaminophen is an analgesic without antiinflammatory effects. Its mode of action is unclear, although it appears to act centrally and may inhibit the COX enzymes at higher doses. Although acetaminophen may have hepatic toxicity, it appears to lack the gastrointestinal complications of NSAIDs at ordinarily used doses. Acetaminophen is commonly used in the treatment of OA when an antiinflammatory effect may not be essential. In RA, acetaminophen is prescribed as an adjunct to other measures to reduce pain.

32. **How is methotrexate administered? What are its side effects?**
Methotrexate is an antifolate and antimetabolite originally developed to treat malignancy. In the setting of RA, it is given at much lower doses than when given as an anticancer agent. The usual dose is 7.5 to 25 mg per week given as a single dose orally. Some patients respond better when this drug is used parenterally. Methotrexate can be used alone or in combination with another DMARD.

The major side effects of methotrexate are mucositis, mouth sores, and hepatic toxicity, including fibrosis and cirrhosis. Hepatic complications appear low in the setting of RA; routine monitoring of liver function tests including albumin are advisable. Daily folic acid is commonly prescribed to reduce side effects.

33. **Describe the role of tumor necrosis factor-α (TNF-α) in rheumatoid arthritis.**
TNF-a is a potent proinflammatory molecule that is produced by macrophages and is a key regulator of inflammation in RA. Among DMARDs, etanercept and infliximab are biological agents or genetically engineered proteins that bind TNF-α and dramatically reduce signs and symptoms of RA. Etanercept is a fusion protein of the TNF receptor with the Fc portion of the IgG molecule. Infliximab is a chimeric monoclonal antibody. Etanercept is given by subcutaneous injection; infliximab is an intravenous infusion. In addition to their effects on disease activity, both etanercept and infliximab reduce the rate of erosion progression shown by radiograph. TNF-blocker effects are frequently rapid, and their administration is associated with decreased pain and increased sense of well-being within days.

34. **What is the IL-1 receptor antagonist?**
IL-1 is a proinflammatory cytokine that plays an important role in RA inflammation and damage. Its production is stimulated in part by TNF-α. Among molecules downregulating the action of IL-1, the IL-1 receptor antagonist (IL-1Ra) binds to the receptor for IL-1 and prevents its activation by IL-1.

Anakinra (IL-1Ra) is a biological agent that has been approved for the treatment of RA. It is given by subcutaneous administration, although significant doses are required because it must compete with naturally produced IL-1 for effectiveness. Anakinra reduces the signs and symptoms of RA and also can affect radiographic progression. Studies in animals suggest that blockade of TNF-α affects inflammation, whereas IL-1Ra slows the process of cartilage and bone destruction.

35. **What are the complications of DMARD therapy?**

Each of the DMARD agents is associated with toxicity that necessitates surveillance for safety. Common side effects include the following:

- Methotrexate: mucositis, hepatic toxicity
- Hydroxychloroquine: retinal toxicity
- Injectable gold salts: rash, cytopenias, proteinuria
- Leflunomide: hepatic toxicity
- Azathioprine: immunosuppression

The TNF blockers have been in use for only a few years, but there is concern about an increase in the incidence of infection, including tuberculosis, as well as a demyelinating condition. The biological agents can cause injection site reactions.

36. **Describe the effects of corticosteroids on RA.**

Corticosteroids have potent antiinflammatory and immunosuppressive actions by which they effectively reduce joint pain and swelling in RA. They interfere with the inflammatory process at various steps. An important action appears to be blockade of the release of arachidonic acid from the cell membrane, limiting substrate for both the lipoxygenase and cyclooxygenase pathways and reducing leukotrienes as well as prostaglandins. Modulation of leukocyte function, including inhibition of cytokine production, contributes to the therapeutic effect.

37. **How are corticosteroids administered in RA?**

Corticosteroids are administered in RA via three routes:

- Administration of high doses with rapid tapers to treat flares and reduce inflammation (bridge therapy while DMARD therapy is instituted)
- Chronic low-dose administration for treatment of active synovitis that does not respond adequately to NSAIDs or DMARDs
- Intraarticular administration to reduce persistent synovitis in single joints

Prednisone is the most commonly prescribed corticosteroid, and a high dose is 0.5 to 1 mg/kg daily. A low dose is 5 to 7.5 mg daily. Intraarticular injection involves crystalline preparations of triamcinolone that are long acting. Such intraarticular treatment can produce a "chemical synovectomy" and lead to prolonged reduction in pain.

38. **List the side effects of corticosteroids.**

Therapy with corticosteroids is complicated by hypertension, glucose intolerance, cushingoid features, adrenal suppression, osteoporosis, weight gain, infection, cataracts, and central nervous system changes such as depression and psychosis. Intraarticular steroids can lead to infection and cartilage damage. Because of the effects of corticosteroids on bone, chronic administration should be accompanied by the use of calcium and vitamin D as well as a bisphosphonate to reduce fracture risk.

39. **What is the role of opioid analgesics in the therapy of RA?**

The goals of therapy in RA are to decrease inflammation, reduce pain, prevent deformity, promote general health, and increase quality of life. When pain persists and detracts from quality of life despite conventional therapy, opioid pain relievers are prescribed. In general, patients take these medications as needed. Be sure to clarify with the patient the potential for opioid-related side effects as well as the need to use these medications as prescribed. Opioids are frequently used in patients awaiting joint replacement or for whom joint replacements are indicated but cannot be performed because of comorbid conditions.

40. **How can assistive devices reduce pain in arthritis?**

Assistive devices are valuable adjuncts in the care of patients with all forms of arthritis. They can decrease pain and facilitate activities of daily living. Devices include splints, canes, and walkers, as well as a variety of implements that allow activities such as buttoning a shirt, opening a jar, reaching items in a cupboard, and eating. Canes, used in the hand opposite the affected joint, can decrease pain on ambulation and forestall the need for surgery. Note that consultation with a physical or occupational therapist is an essential component in the total management of a patient with advanced arthritis.

41. **What are the surgical procedures for reducing pain in arthritis?**
Although total joint replacement is performed frequently for both RA and OA, it is actually only one of several procedures available in the treatment of these diseases. In RA, synovectomy can reduce pain and delay total joint replacement. This procedure involves removal of proliferated synovium; arthroscopy is increasingly used for this purpose to avoid the greater trauma of arthrotomy. A useful procedure in osteoarthritis is an osteotomy in which a wedge of bone is removed to correct joint alignment and improve biomechanics. Joint fusions are performed for both OA and RA; this procedure reduces pain but sacrifices motion.

42. **What are the indications for total joint replacement surgery in RA?**
Pain is the major consideration for replacement of large joints such as the hip or knee. Among the indicators of pain that require surgery are pain that lasts all day, pain that awakens the patient from sleep, and pain that requires frequent or continuous narcotics. In advanced disease, radiographs can demonstrate joint destruction with coexistent changes of both RA and OA.
   Although functional improvement accompanies total joint replacement, surgery of large joints is usually not performed for this indication alone.

43. **How does the surgical approach to RA of the hands differ from that for large joints?**
In contrast to total joint replacement of the knees or hips, surgery of the hands in RA is undertaken to prevent or correct deformity and improve function. Pain is less often the primary indication for hand surgery, which entails synovectomy and rerouting of tendons in addition to joint replacement.

44. **What are the complications of total joint replacement?**
The major complications of joint replacement are infection, dislocation, fracture, and loosening. Infections of prosthetic joints differ from ordinary joint space infections in their more indolent course and less dramatic signs of inflammation. Loosening causes pain and can be diagnosed by radiographs.

45. **How do cemented and noncemented total joints differ?**
Total joint replacement was pioneered using methylmethacrylate as a cement to secure the joint in place. Over time, inflammation occurs at the interface of the bone and cement, producing lucency on x-ray and causing loosening. The insertion of a new prosthesis is then complicated by the need to remove the old cement.
   A noncemented joint, in contrast, has a highly porous or textured surface, which allows the ingrowth of new bone to keep the prosthesis in place. Whether noncemented joints last as long as cemented joints and eliminate the problem of loosening is still under investigation. Some surgeons believe that cemented joints have better performance and lifespan, even in younger patients.

46. **Describe the treatment of foot pain in RA.**
RA commonly affects the small joints of the feet, causing erosive synovitis and deformity similar to the involvement of the small joints of the hand. The metatarsophalangeal (MTP) heads become subluxed, leading to exquisite pain on walking, callus formation, and ulceration on the soles of the foot. This condition can be treated by use of metatarsal bars on the bottom of shoes to reduce the impact of walking on the MTPs; extra-depth, extra-width shoes and molded shoes to accommodate the deformities and reduce the likelihood of ulceration; and surgery.

47. **What is the surgical approach to RA of the feet?**
The most commonly used surgical procedure is resection of the metatarsal heads, which removes the painful joints and shortens the foot. Frequently, corrective surgery of the feet is the initial procedure performed for a patient with RA with serious involvement of lower extremity joints.

48. **What is the treatment for a painful ankle in RA?**
The ankle is commonly involved in RA, with both tibial-talar and subtalar joints subject to erosive damage. Rather than using a prosthesis, ankle disease is usually treated with fusion, which can be accomplished by either prolonged immobilization or surgery. A triple arthrodesis can eliminate motion in the ankle and thereby reduce pain on walking.

49. **What is a "constrained" prosthetic joint?**
The success of total joint replacement reflects the biomechanical properties of the joint. Hip surgery is very successful because the hip is a ball-and-socket joint with inherent stability. In contrast, the knee joint has a more complicated motion. Although it has features of a hinge, it also allows gliding and rotary movement. A totally constrained prosthetic allows motion in a single plane and mimics a hinge. Prostheses that allow greater motion in other planes are considered to be less constrained.

50. **What is the difference in outcome of total joint replacement in OA and RA?**
Patients with OA, although they may be older and have comorbid conditions, are not systemically ill with their arthritis and often require replacement of only an isolated joint. The bone stock of patients with OA is frequently good. Results of surgery are excellent because of these favorable factors.

   Patients with RA have polyarticular involvement; are systemically ill; and frequently have low bone reserves because of their disease, immobility, and use of medications like corticosteroids. Surgery can eliminate pain and increase mobility in the replaced joint, but patients still experience the consequences of the disease in their other joints. Not surprisingly, although patients with RA may benefit greatly from surgery, they do not show comparable restoration of function.

51. **Describe the pseudothrombophlebitis syndrome.**
Acute pain and swelling in the calf can result from rupture or dissection of a Baker's cyst and can mimic thrombophlebitis. A Baker's cyst is an expansion of the synovial space posterior to the knee joint. It can be appreciated by palpation with the patient standing. The usual cause is RA, although effusions in OA can produce the same lesion. Diagnostic evaluation includes studies to exclude deep vein thrombosis (e.g., venogram or Doppler flow) as well as ultrasound or arthrogram to demonstrate the cyst. The usual treatment is injection of intraarticular steroids into the knee joint.

52. **What are the causes of head pain in RA?**
Headache is common in patients with RA and usually results from arthritis of the cervical spine, which is the only region of the axial skeleton involved in this disease. Patients with RA can also have pain originate in the temporomandibular joints, which are diarthrodial joints subject to erosive synovitis. Inflammatory disease of the eyes can cause ocular pain. Arthritis of the cricoarytenoid joint is associated with sore throat and hoarseness.

53. **What is C1-C2 subluxation?**
The joints of the cervical spine, like other synovial joints, can undergo erosive damage and instability, especially as ligaments are destroyed. Subluxation of the C1-C2 joint (atlantoaxial subluxation) occurs commonly in patients with erosive disease and can be demonstrated by flexion-extension x-ray studies of the spine, with a separation of 2.5 to 3 mm considered

significant. This condition is associated with neck pain, headache, shooting pains in the arms and legs and, when advanced, myelopathy with long tract signs.

In the presence of progressive lower extremity weakness and disturbances of bowel and bladder function, fusion of the spine is performed emergently to stabilize the spine and prevent cord damage. In the vast majority of cases, however, treatment is symptomatic, including collars for immobilization.

54. What is spinal stenosis?

Spinal stenosis refers to narrowing of the spinal canal, which is usually a consequence of degenerative disease. This condition can produce lower extremity pain, which is termed neurogenic claudication. Pain from spinal stenosis is worsened by walking and an upright stance and can be relieved by bending forward, causing a characteristic posture of these patients. Treatment can involve surgery.

55. What is disseminated idiopathic skeletal hyperostosis (DISH)?

Disseminated idiopathic skeletal hyperostosis (DISH) is an exaggerated form of osteoarthritis characterized by prominent spine involvement in association with exuberant spur formation. The spine shows calcification of the anterior longitudinal ligament that appears to flow from one vertebra to another in a pattern called "toothpaste" calcification. In this condition, the disc spaces are preserved. Although DISH is commonly associated with back pain, it can also be an incidental finding of chest x-ray.

56. Which conditions are associated with atypical degenerative osteoarthritis?

OA uncommonly involves joints such as the metacarpophalangeal (MCP) joints, wrists, elbows, and ankles. In the absence of a history of trauma or excessive joint usage, OA of these joints suggests the presence of calcium pyrophosphate dihydrate deposition disease (CPPD). This condition can be demonstrated by radiographic findings of chondrocalcinosis or calcification within the articular cartilage. The presence of CPPD suggests an underlying metabolic problem such as hemochromatosis, hyperparathyroidism, or acromegaly. Indeed, degenerative disease of the MCP joints is a classic presentation of hemochromatosis.

57. What are the findings in pseudogout? How is this condition treated?

Pseudogout is one of the presentations of CPPD. It causes acute monoarticular arthritis, which, like gout, is extremely painful. Pseudogout is diagnosed by the presence of inflammatory joint fluid containing rhomboid-shaped crystals that are positively birefringent by polarizing microscopy; in contrast, monosodium urate crystals in gout are needle-shaped and negatively birefringent. This condition can be treated by joint aspiration, NSAIDs, and sometimes intraarticular steroids. Attacks of pseudogout can be provoked by metabolic changes and occur commonly after stressful events such as surgery.

58. What is polymyalgia rheumatica (PMR)?

PMR is a painful condition that is frequently acute in onset and causes pain in the shoulder and limb girdles in the absence of other signs of arthritis. It occurs in older individuals (>50 years), shows signs of inflammation with an elevated sedimentation rate (>50 mm/hr), and responds dramatically to low-dose corticosteroids. Because RA and systemic lupus erythematosus (SLE) can present with a similar pattern, these conditions must be excluded by appropriate serological tests (rheumatoid factor and antinuclear antibody) before the diagnosis of PMR is made. Many patients with PMR have an underlying temporal arteritis or giant cell arteritis, necessitating biopsy of the temporal arteries especially if symptoms of vessel involvement of the cranial circulation are present.

59. What is fibromyalgia?

Fibromyalgia is characterized by chronic widespread pain in the absence of synovitis and other signs of inflammation. Tender points are the cardinal feature of this disease; pressure on these areas elicits pain. Patients with fibromyalgia, who are usually women, frequently report other symptoms such as fatigue, poor exercise tolerance, headache, irritable bowel, and restless legs. Sleep disturbance is common among patients with fibromyalgia and may reflect a neuropsychological disturbance.

Fibromyalgia may occur alone or be secondary to another condition such as RA, OA, or SLE. The diagnosis of fibromyalgia in the setting of another musculoskeletal disease is based primarily on the presence of tender points.

Therapy for fibromyalgia may involve pregabalin, duloxetine, NSAIDS, tricyclic antidepressants (often at low doses to promote sleep), SSRI agents, and aerobic exercises.

60. Which conditions cause a painful shoulder?

The shoulder is one of the most complex joints in the body and is a frequent site of pain. In addition to inflammatory diseases such as RA, SLE, and PMR, pain in the shoulder can result from degenerative disease, tendonitis, bursitis, adhesive capsulitis, and impingement syndromes. Nerve root entrapment from cervical spine arthritis can also elicit pain. Because pain in the shoulder can also be referred from intrathoracic lesions, evaluation of this condition may necessitate a chest x-ray to rule out malignancy, for example.

61. What is complex regional pain syndrome (type 1) (CRPS)?

Complex regional pain syndrome (type 1) (CRPS; formerly reflex sympathetic dystrophy or shoulder-hand syndrome) is a neurovascular condition characterized by upper extremity pain in association with signs of vasomotor instability such as swelling, blue-red discoloration, and excessive sweating of the affected limb. Allodynia can be elicited. CRPS can occur in isolation or following an injury or illness such as a stroke or myocardial infarction. Indeed, it is common in those with CRPS that the severity of pain experienced is of a severity greater than the initiating noxious stimulus. Sympathetic nerve blocks (e.g., stellate ganglion, lumbar sympathetic, and intravenous regional sympathetic blocks) can be helpful, as can antiepileptic drugs such as gabapentin and pregabalin. Topical treatments including capsaicin and topical lidocaine can be of symptomatic benefit. All drug therapies are "off label."

62. What is avascular necrosis?

Avascular necrosis (AVN) or ischemic necrosis of the bone results from vascular insufficiency to bone and causes painful infarction. AVN can occur in the setting of other forms of arthritis (e.g., SLE or RA), although more commonly it results from the effects of corticosteroids, which may increase marrow fat and impede blood flow. The femoral head is the usual site of involvement, but other bones can be affected. Alcohol can produce a similar condition, sometimes called alcoholic osteonecrosis.

X-ray films in AVN demonstrate collapse, fracture, and bone irregularity, although early diagnosis of this condition requires magnetic resonance imaging. Treatment involves surgery with total joint replacement in more advanced disease.

63. What is the rheumatoid arthritis pain scale?

The rheumatoid arthritis pain scale is an attempt at a valid and reliable clinical instrument for measuring pain in patients with rheumatoid arthritis. It is meant to be a quantitative, single score, self-report of pain. It takes into account physiological, affective, sensory-discriminative, and cognitive factors.

64. **What other treatments can be used for pain relief in patients with OA and RA?**
Acetaminophen, opioids, and NSAIDS form the main oral treatments for pain in patients with
OA and RA. Topical therapy can be with NSAIDs or capsaicin. "Off-label" topical treatments
include the use of lidocaine 5% patch and topical nitrates (which reduce pain and inflammation).
Muscle spasm and spasticity can complicate joint pain and can be treated with skeletal
muscle relaxants such as baclofen, dantrolene, and cyclobenzaprine.

65. **What type of joint injections can be given to treat OA and RA?**
Mention has already been made of intraarticular corticosteroid injection for RA. These injections
can also be given to patients with OA. "Viscosupplementation" involves the injection of
hyaluronic acid on a repeated basis into an osteoarthritic joint; such injections can give
prolonged pain relief.

66. **Has glucosamine any role in the management of OA pain?**
A number of studies have shown that glucosamine, when taken on a long-term basis, can reduce
the pain and increase the mobility of patients with symptomatic osteoarthritis. Its use is
associated with a small increase in the depth of joint cartilage. The effect of glucosamine
may not be evident for up to 6 months.

KEY POINTS

1. Multiple rheumatologic disorders are associated with chronic pain. More than one such
    disorder may exist in the same patient.

2. Both disease-modifying and symptomatic treatments should be considered for patients.

3. The choice of treatment should be individualized and based on the needs of the patient's
    past response to treatment, the adverse effects of the treatment, and other factors.

BIBLIOGRAPHY

1. Anderson DL: Development of an instrument to measure pain in rheumatoid arthritis: Rheumatoid Arthritis
    Pain Scale, *Arthritis Rheum* 45(4):317-323, 2001.
2. Arend WP, Dayer JM: Inhibition of the production and effects of interleukin-1 and tumor necrosis factor a in
    rheumatoid arthritis, *Arthritis Rheum* 38:151-160, 1995.
3. Bradley JD, Brandt KD, Katz BP, et al: Treatment of knee osteoarthritis: relationship of clinical features of
    joint inflammation to the response to nonsteroidal anti-inflammatory drug or pure analgesic, *J Rheum*
    19:1950-1954, 1992.
4. Brandt KD: The role of analgesics in the management of osteoarthritis pain, *Am J Ther* 7(2):75-90, 2000.
5. Buckelew SP, Parker JC: Coping with arthritis pain: a review of the literature, *Arthritis Care Res* 2:136-145,
    1989.
6. Felson DT, Anderson JJ, Meenan RF: The efficacy and toxicity of combination therapy in rheumatoid arthritis,
    Arthritis Rheum 37:1487-1491, 1994.
7. FitzGerald GA, Patrono C: The coxibs, selective inhibitors of cyclooxygenase-2, *N Engl J Med* 345:433-442,
    2001.
8. Gerber LH, Hicks JE: Surgical and rehabilitation options in the treatment of rheumatoid arthritis resistant to
    pharmacological agents, *Rheum Dis Clinics North Am* 21:19-39, 1995.
9. Gonzales GR, Portenoy RK: Selection of analgesic therapies in rheumatoid arthritis: the role of opioid
    medications, *Arthritis Care Res* 6:223-228, 1993.
10. Harris WH, Sledge CB: Total hip and knee replacement, *N Eng J Med* 323:801-807, 1990.

11. Lefebvre JC, Keefe FJ: Memory for pain: the relationship of pain catastrophizing to the recall of daily rheumatoid arthritis pain, *Clin J Pain* 18(1):56-63, 2002.

12. Moreland LW, St. Clair EW: The use of analgesics in the management of pain in rheumatic diseases, *Rheum Disease Clin North Am* 25:153-191, 1999.

13. Pisetsky DS, St. Clair EW: Progress in the treatment of rheumatoid arthritis, *JAMA* 286:2787-2790, 2001.

14. Wolfe F: When to diagnose fibromyalgia, *Rheum Dis Clin North Am* 20:485-501, 1994.

15. McCleane GJ, Smith H, editors: *Clinical management of bone and joint pain*, Binghamton, NY, Haworth Press, 2007.

CHAPTER 28

NEUROPATHIC PAIN

Russell K. Portenoy, MD, Ricardo Cruciani, MD, PhD, and Charles E. Argoff, M

1. **What is neuropathic pain?**

   The term neuropathic pain is applied to any acute or chronic pain syndrome in which the mechanism that sustains the pain is inferred to involve aberrant somatosensory processing in the peripheral or central nervous system (PNS/CNS). Neuropathic pain is commonly distinguished from two other inferred pathophysiologies, nociceptive pain and psychogenic pain. The sustaining mechanisms of nociceptive pain are inferred to involve ongoing activation of pain-sensitive afferent peripheral nerves. This activation may be caused by injury to either somatic (known as somatic pain) or visceral (known as visceral pain) structures. Psychogenic pain is a generic term used to refer to those pains that have sustaining mechanisms related to psychological processes. Other descriptive terms, such as those codified in the American Psychiatric Association's *Diagnostic and Statistical Manual (DSM-IV-R)*, can be used to classify the latter pain syndromes.

2. **Why do the definitions of neuropathic pain, nociceptive pain, and psychogenic pain refer to these disorders as "inferred" pathophysiologies?**

   This classification by pathophysiology is inferred because there is no way to prove or disprove that any particular mechanism is operating in the clinical setting to maintain a chronic pain syndrome. The type of pathophysiology that may be involved is conjectured on the basis of the pain description and associated findings on examination and ancillary tests. Because the diagnosis is inferred, there is the potential for imprecision and oversimplification when labeling patients. Indeed, it is likely that patients often have more than one set of pathophysiology and that each type of pathophysiology actually refers to multiple specific mechanisms. Nonetheless, a pathophysiologic classification has become widely accepted by clinicians, who have observed that it may be useful in defining the type of evaluation that may be needed, selecting appropriate therapies, and determining the prognosis for improvement.

3. **What findings on clinical evaluation suggest that a pain is neuropathic?**

   Neuropathic pain is suggested when patients use terms to describe their pain that are consistent with a dysesthesia, which is defined as an abnormal pain complaint. Pain may be described as burning, electric-like, or shooting. Patients often say that the pain is unfamiliar, unlike any pain experienced before. The examination may reveal allodynia (pain created by a normally non-painful stimulus), hypalgesia or hyperalgesia (relatively decreased or increased perception of a noxious stimulus, respectively), hypoesthesia or hyperesthesia (relatively decreased or increased perception of a nonnoxious stimulus, respectively), or hyperpathia (exaggerated pain response).

   There may be other focal neurologic deficits, such as weakness or focal autonomic changes. Focal autonomic phenomena may include swelling and vasomotor instability (observed as color changes, livedo reticularis, and focal temperature changes). There may also be trophic changes, including alterations of the skin and subcutaneous tissues or the hair and nails.

   Ancillary tests, such as electrodiagnostic studies (electromyogram and nerve conduction velocities), can sometimes be helpful in confirming the existence of a neurologic lesion. Tests such as thermography are occasionally useful to confirm autonomic dysregulation. Quantitative sensory testing (QST) may also be used to aid in the diagnosis.

4. **What are some of the challenges inherent in diagnosing neuropathic pain?**
   When a dysesthesia occurs in the setting of an overt neurologic lesion, the diagnosis of
   neuropathic pain may be straightforward. Even in this setting, however, it may be difficult to
   exclude a contribution to the pain of coexisting processes, such as damage to somatic
   structures sufficient to produce nociceptive pain or psychological processes that exacerbate
   the pain. Furthermore, neuropathic pain can occur without an overt neurologic deficit (for
   example, complex regional pain syndrome type 1 can follow minor soft-tissue injury, and pain
   may be the first and only manifestation of a small fiber polyneuropathy). Finally, neuropathic
   pain can be nondysesthetic, such as the deep aching that commonly occurs from nerve or nerve
   root compression. All of these factors can complicate the diagnosis of neuropathic pain.

5. **The clinical diversity of neuropathic pain suggests that the mechanisms
   responsible are both numerous and complex, presumably involving
   interactions between the PNS and CNS. Is there a useful model for
   conceptualizing these interacting mechanisms?**
   Three decades of basic research have shown that neuropathic pain may result from any of a
   variety of mechanisms that interact in complex ways. The normal response of the PNS and
   the CNS following exposure to a noxious stimulus can become disturbed at multiple levels
   concurrently (Fig. 28-1). This process may involve altered peripheral input (e.g., from

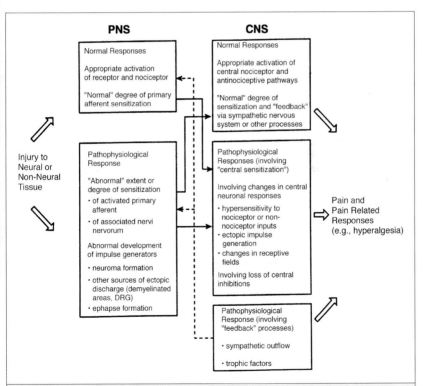

Figure 28-1. Model demonstrating the complex processes that may be involved in the pathophysiology of neuropathic pain. PNS = peripheral nervous system; CNS = central nervous system; DRG = dorsal root ganglion.

sensitization of primary afferent neurons) or central processing (e.g., any of the mechanisms involved in so-called central sensitization; see Question 9), changes in efferent activity in the sympathetic nervous system, and shifts in pain modulatory processes in both the PNS and CNS. Further research is needed to determine the specific processes that result in these pathologic distortions of normal nociception.

6. **From the clinical perspective, what is a useful classification of the heterogeneous population with chronic neuropathic pain?**
Although patients with neuropathic pain are traditionally categorized on the basis of diagnosis (e.g., painful diabetic polyneuropathy) or site of the precipitating lesion (e.g., peripheral nerve), it may be most useful to extend the classification based on inferred pathophysiology, and to suggest that some patients with neuropathic pain have disorders that are primarily sustained by processes in the CNS, whereas others have disorders sustained by processes in the PNS. This distinction is suggested by both clinical and experimental data (Fig. 28-2). For example, a predominant peripheral pathophysiology is suggested by the observation that some patients with neuropathic pain precipitated by nerve injury are cured by a local intervention, such as resection of a neuroma. A predominant central pathophysiology is obvious in those patients whose neuropathic pain is precipitated by stroke.

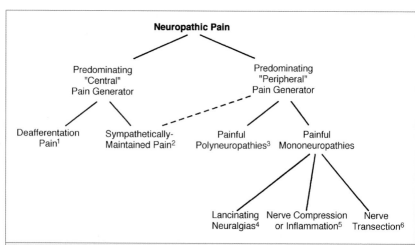

Figure 28-2. Classification of neuropathic pains by putative predominating mechanism. 1. Response to either peripheral or central nervous system injury. 2. Associated with focal autonomic dysregulation (e.g., edema, vasomotor disturbances), involuntary motor responses, and/or trophic changes that may improve with sympathetic nerve block. 3. Multiple mechanisms probably involved. 4. The patterns of peripheral activity or peripheral and central interaction that yield the lancinating quality of these pains are unknown. 5. Nociceptive nervi nervorum (small afferents that innervate larger nerves) may account for neuropathic pain accompanying nerve compression or inflammation. 6. Injury to axons may be followed by neuroma formation, a source of aberrant activity likely to be involved in pain.

7. **What neuropathic pain syndromes are presumably sustained by aberrant somatosensory processing in the CNS?**
Neuropathic pains that are inferred to have sustaining mechanisms in the CNS can be broadly divided into two groups: (1) disorders known as the deafferentation pains, and (2) disorders collectively known as complex regional pain syndromes (previously known as reflex sympathetic dystrophy and causalgia; see Question 50). The deafferentation pains include a large number of specific syndromes, such as central pain (pain following injury to the CNS), pain resulting

from avulsion of a plexus, pain resulting from spinal cord injury, postherpetic neuralgia, phantom pain, and others. Complex regional pain syndrome is presumably sustained by a number of different mechanisms. One such mechanism is believed to involve efferent activity in the sympathetic nervous system and produces a pain known as sympathetically maintained pain.

8. **Which pain syndromes are presumably sustained by aberrant somatosensory processing in the peripheral nervous system?**
Neuropathic pains that are inferred to have sustaining mechanisms in the PNS can be divided into a group of painful polyneuropathies and a group of painful mononeuropathies. Each of these groups, in turn, subsumes many specific syndromes.

9. **Describe the specific CNS mechanisms likely involved in the various types of deafferentation pain.**
Studies in experimental models and humans suggest that a state of "central sensitization" may be relevant to all deafferentation syndromes. Although peripheral input may be important in some syndromes (as suggested by the transitory relief of deafferentation pain that is commonly observed following interruption of proximal somatosensory pathways), the sustaining pathophysiology presumably relates to changes in the response characteristics of central neurons that are at least partly independent of this input.

Central sensitization may involve functional and structural changes in CNS pathways involved in nociception (see Fig. 28-1 and Table 28-1). Each of these changes presumably occurs as a consequence of specific mechanisms, which have only begun to be elucidated. Recent studies, for example, have indicated the importance of an interaction between excitatory amino acids (specifically glutamate) and the N-methyl-D-aspartate receptor in producing sensitization of nociceptive neurons in the dorsal horn of the spinal cord. Although the relationship of these functional and structural changes to chronic pain in humans is conjectural, the range of phenomena underscores the plasticity of central connections and suggests a focus for future research targeted at the prevention or treatment of neuropathic pain.

TABLE 28-1. CHANGES THAT MAY BE INVOLVED IN NEUROPATHIC PAINS SUSTAINED BY ABBERRANT PROCESSES IN THE CENTRAL NERVOUS SYSTEM	
Functional Changes	**Structural Changes**
Lowered threshold for activation	Transsynaptic degeneration
Exaggerated activation	Transganglionic degeneration
Ectopic discharges	Collateral sprouting
Enlarging receptive fields	
Loss of normal inhibition	

10. **Phantom pain is commonly considered to be a type of deafferentation pain. What is phantom pain?**
Although the prototype phantom pain follows limb amputation, the term is applied to pain following amputation of any body part. For example, surveys have described phantom pain following mastectomy and tooth extraction. Some authors also use the term to describe pain in regions of the body that are completely denervated (rendered anesthetic) but not amputated,

such as the area below a transected spinal cord or the area supplied by a severely injured peripheral nerve. This usage may be confusing, however, and it would be preferable to use the term "central pain," or one of its subtypes (see Question 35), to describe a pain that occurs in an area denervated as a result of a CNS lesion, and to use either the generic term "deafferentation pain" or the older term "anesthesia dolorosa" to describe a pain that is inferred to have a central mechanism induced by a severe peripheral nerve injury.

11. **What is known about the specific mechanisms that may result in phantom pain?**
The specific mechanisms that cause phantom pain are not known. One conceptualization suggests that phantom pain is a somatosensory "memory" that does not reside in a specific region of the CNS, but instead involves complex interactions of neural networks in the brain. Recent studies have suggested that the "shrinkage" of the somatosensory cortical representation of an amputated limb correlates with the development of pain. It has also been suggested that pain management with opioids results in reexpansion to its original representation and that this change correlates with pain reduction. The precise pathophysiology underlying these associations is not known.

12. **What is the epidemiology of phantom pain?**
Epidemiologic surveys of phantom pain must distinguish this phenomenon from both nonpainful phantom sensations and stump pain. Failure to be precise may be the cause of variation in older surveys, which have reported transitory or occasional discomfort in the phantoms of 25% to 98% of amputees. Although some surveys suggest that about half the patients with phantom pain continue to experience pain for a period of at least 1 to 2 years, others indicate that a large majority experience resolution of pain (though not necessary all phantom sensation) within 1 year of amputation.

Several studies have attempted to define predisposing factors for the development of phantom pain. Phantom limb pain is rare in congenital amputees or children who lose a limb before the age of 6. This observation suggests that some degree of CNS maturation is required before phantom pain can occur. The experience of pain in the limb prior to amputation has been noted to predispose to the development of phantom pain in some, but not all, surveys. A recent study observed that 57% of patients who experienced pain immediately before amputation developed phantom pain that resembled the preexisting pain in quality and location. A strong association between stump pain and phantom pain has also been reported. Other surveys have suggested that older age, proximal amputations, upper limb lesions, sudden amputations, and preexisting psychological disturbances may increase the likelihood of phantom pain, but these factors have not been confirmed in more recent studies.

13. **What is the natural history of phantom pain?**
Although most patients develop phantom sensations and phantom pain soon after the nerve injury, symptoms may develop at any time after denervation. Most surveys observe that the pain substantially declines over time.

14. **How is phantom pain different from phantom sensation?**
Phantom pain is one element among many phantom sensations. Pain has been termed an exteroceptive sensation, a description that has also been applied to the perception of touch, temperature, pressure, itch, and other sensations. Kinesthetic sensation, which involves the perception of posture, length, and volume, and kinetic sensations, including the perceptions of willed movements and spontaneous movements, also occur. Among the more common kinesthetic sensations are unusual or bizarre postures, foreshortening of a limb ("telescoping"), or distortions in the size of body parts (usually reduction in proximal regions and expansion of distal regions). All these sensations are usually most vivid immediately after amputation. Over time, the size of the phantom often shrinks, and the intensity of all sensation gradually fades.

15. **How is phantom pain different from stump pain?**
    In contrast to phantom pain, in which the inferred "generator" of the pain is in the CNS, stump pain is a peripheral neuropathic pain presumably related to the development of a neuroma at the end of a severed nerve. Patients usually report some combination of aching, squeezing, throbbing, stabbing, and electrical discomfort localized to the distal stump. The onset of the pain is usually delayed for months, and the incidence is lower than that in phantom pain. Following limb amputation, many patients have both stump pain and phantom pain.

16. **Can phantom pain be prevented?**
    Phantom pain may be difficult to treat, and prevention would clearly be ideal. The possibility of prevention has been highlighted by a small trial that demonstrated the efficacy of a 72-hour preoperative epidural infusion of local anesthetic and/or morphine in reducing postoperative phantom pain among patients with preamputation limb pain. Although the data are too limited to recommend regional anesthesia prior to all amputations, this approach should be considered in a selected group of patients who have intense preexisting pain.

17. **What initial management strategies are used for phantom pain?**
    Patients with established phantom pain should be evaluated for the existence of potentially treatable factors that may be exacerbating the pain, such as stump neuroma or depression. Management of these factors may improve outcome. Although there is no compelling evidence that the use of a prosthesis or physical therapy yields analgesic effects in patients with phantom pain, such rehabilitative therapies can have salutary effects on function and should be considered on this basis alone. For the phantom pain itself, a large number of potentially analgesic treatments can be tried in an effort to improve comfort and facilitate functional gains.

18. **Which analgesic agents are most effective in treating phantom pain?**
    There have been very few analgesic clinical trials in patients with phantom pain, and trials of adjuvant analgesic drugs are generally offered in a manner identical to that in other types of neuropathic pain (see Chapter 37, Adjuvant Analgesics). A placebo-controlled trial suggested that calcitonin (200 IU via brief intravenous infusion) may be effective, at least in patients with relatively short-lived phantom pain, and a trial of this drug by intranasal or subcutaneous administration should be considered early. The long-term use of opioids can sometimes be effective in treating phantom pain.

19. **Are nerve blocks helpful to the patient experiencing phantom pain?**
    Although sympathetic nerve blocks usually produce minimal or transitory benefit, rare patients appear to do well, and this small potential for long-term favorable effects warrants a trial of sympathetic blockade in selected patients with refractory pain. Prolonged relief from sensory nerve blocks appears to be even more rare than benefit from sympathetic blocks, and cases have been described in which sensory blockade paradoxically increased the pain.
    Chemical or surgical neurolysis of proximal somatosensory pathways has more risk than temporary nerve blocks, including the potential to worsen pain, and these procedures are not used to manage phantom pain. The dorsal root entry zone lesion has had promising results in a specific type of deafferentation pain syndrome, plexus avulsion (see Questions 47-49), but results have not been favorable in phantom pain. Local injection into the stump, which may be useful for stump pain, also has very limited efficacy in the management of phantom pain.

20. **Describe the role of neurostimulatory approaches in phantom pain.**
    Neurostimulatory approaches are safer than neurodestructive procedures and have been used in the management of phantom pain. Although the results are usually disappointing with transcutaneous electrical nerve stimulation (TENS), its inherent safety warrants a trial in most patients. A large experience with invasive neurostimulatory procedures, including dorsal

column stimulation and deep brain stimulation, has yielded mixed results. These approaches should not be considered until conservative treatments have failed, and the patient has undergone a comprehensive evaluation by experienced clinicians.

21. **True or false: Psychological approaches are unlikely to be successful in the treatment of phantom pain.**
False. The value of psychological interventions as part of a multimodality approach to phantom pain deserves emphasis. In the case of phantom pain, disfigurement and physical impairments may compound the distress related to pain, making psychological intervention all the more important.

22. **Postherpetic neuralgia (PHN) is another common deafferentation pain syndrome. What is the definition of PHN?**
Although it is axiomatic that postherpetic neuralgia (PHN) is defined solely by the experience of prolonged pain following acute herpes zoster infection, the specific time criterion used to diagnose this condition is a matter of debate. In the medical literature, various reports have defined PHN as pain that persists beyond the crusting of lesions, or pain that continues beyond 1, 1.5, 8, or 24 weeks following resolution of the rash. For research purposes, it is probably most reasonable to require a criterion of 4 months from onset of the lesion (1 month for healing of the lesion followed by 3 months of pain). This criterion is used to define an early period, during which therapies for acute herpes zoster are appropriate, and an open-ended period that follows, during which treatments appropriate for PHN should be implemented.

23. **What is known about the mechanisms that result in postherpetic neuralgia?**
Following resolution of a systemic varicella infection, which usually occurs in childhood, the virus maintains a dormant phase in dorsal root ganglia. Herpes zoster is the segmental recrudescence of the varicella virus, the appearance of which presumably involves some type of breakdown in immune surveillance.
    Herpes zoster produces diffuse inflammation of peripheral nerve, dorsal root ganglion, and, in some cases, the spinal cord. Long after the acute infection resolves, the pathology reveals chronic inflammatory changes in the periphery, neuronal loss in the dorsal root ganglion, and a reduction of both axons and myelin in affected nerve. Quantitative sensory nerve testing has suggested that this injury produces different types of damage, which in turn, results in pathophysiologic subtypes of PHN. In one type, destruction of peripheral nerve leads to deafferentation, and in another, small peripheral nerve fibers are present and involved in the pathophysiology of the pain. Some studies have suggested the relatively selective loss of large peripheral nerve fibers in several patients, which could underlie reduced peripheral inhibitory processes mediated by these fibers.

24. **What is the epidemiology of herpes zoster and postherpetic neuralgia?**
The incidence of herpes zoster, which overall is approximately 1.3 to 4.8 cases per 1000 person-years, increases in the older person and the immunocompromised (e.g., patients with cancer or AIDS). Some reports have suggested that the incidence may also be influenced by various systemic insults, such as surgery, toxic exposures, and infections, and focal pathologic processes affecting the spine or nerve roots.
    Although only 10% of all those with acute herpes experience pain for more than 1 month, the incidence rises steeply with age. In one survey, the prevalence of pain 1 year after the eruption was 4.2% in patients 20 years old and younger and 47% in those older than 70. PHN also is relatively more likely among those with severe zoster eruptions and those with a high level of distress.

25. **What is the natural history of postherpetic neuralgia?**
PHN gradually improves in most patients, and clinical experience suggests that the best predictor of future improvement is the course during the recent past. Given this natural history, the interpretation of uncontrolled therapeutic trials must be very cautious, particularly if the

treatment was administered to patients relatively soon after the acute herpes zoster infection. Many ineffective treatments for PHN have been introduced on the basis of "favorable" effects observed during uncontrolled trials. Clinical studies of treatments for PHN should be controlled, if possible, and include a stringent time criterion, such as 4 months from onset of the lesion.

26. **What are the important clinical features of PHN?**
Herpes zoster erupts in the thoracic dermatomes in more than 50% of patients. The trigeminal distribution (usually V1) is next most common. Lumbar and cervical zosters each occur in 10% to 20% of patients. Regardless of location, the pain of PHN is usually complex, described as some combination of deep aching, superficial burning, and paroxysmal pain. Itch is also commonly reported. Allodynia or hyperpathia is variable; in some patients, the sensitivity to touch is the most distressing component. About 10% of patients with herpes zoster infection experience pain without the concomitant presence of skin lesions. The course of this syndrome—zoster sine herpetum—and the incidence of PHN thereafter is believed to be comparable to the more typical herpes zoster presentation. PHN in the ear can follow the so-called Ramsay-Hunt syndrome, a frequently misdiagnosed disorder in which varicella spreads from the geniculate ganglion and produces facial paralysis, hearing loss, vertigo, and pain in the ear. Vesicles in the tympanic membrane may be the only observable sign of the latter disorder.

27. **Can postherpetic neuralgia be prevented?**
With the advent of the varicella vaccine, primary prevention of PHN is now feasible. A reduction in the incidence of this lesion presumably will be observed many years after its use becomes widespread. A recent large trial also has determined that repeat vaccination during late adulthood reduces the incidence of PHN. This treatment may soon become widespread. Studies of antiviral treatment, such as famcyclovir and valacyclovir, have shown that early treatment shortens the time of pain associated with the acute attack, in essence reducing the incidence of PHN (see Question 29).

28. **What about studies of other medications?**
There is no good evidence that any of the other currently available therapies for acute herpes zoster prevent PHN. Corticosteroids and early sympathetic nerve block can have valuable analgesic effects during acute zoster, but do not prevent PHN. Finally, one study suggested that the use of low-dose amitriptyline during acute zoster reduces PHN, but this finding requires confirmation.

29. **What is an appropriate management strategy for acute zoster?**
Antiviral therapy is the first issue to consider when developing a strategy for the treatment of acute herpes zoster. The threshold for using antiviral therapy in the hope of reducing the likelihood of prolonged pain has been lowered as the result of recent studies. Antiviral therapy certainly should be used if patients are at significant risk for tissue injury from the virus itself or if patients are immunocompromised. Those who have overt or imminent injury to the cornea or evidence of damage to motor nerves or nerves supplying viscera (such as the bladder) are in this category. Patients at relatively higher risk of PHN—including older patients (≥60 years), those with intense cutaneous eruptions, and those with very severe pain—are also candidates for antiviral therapy. In the nonimmunocompromised patient, the use of a systemic corticosteroid, such as prednisone, can reduce the acute pain. The same response is likely in those who undergo sympathetic nerve block. The latter procedure is believed by some to reduce the incidence of PHN, but this has not been adequately confirmed. Similarly, the use of low-dose amitriptyline during the acute phase was suggested to reduce the incidence of PHN in one trial and requires confirmation. In all patients, the pain should be aggressively managed with some combination of local measures and analgesic drugs (nonsteroidal antiinflammatory drugs [NSAIDs] or opioids).

30. **Both topical and systemic analgesic drugs are commonly used in the treatment of PHN. What are the topical therapies for this condition?**

    Studies have established that a 5% lidocaine patch (Lidoderm) can be an effective therapy. Some patients benefit from application of the eutectic mixture of lidocaine and prilocaine (EMLA) or from a 5% or 10% lidocaine gel or cream. Although EMLA and high-concentration lidocaine can produce dense cutaneous anesthesia if applied thickly under an occlusive dressing, it may not be necessary to do so, and most patients initiate this therapy using a thin application several times per day. If this is not helpful, and the area of pain is small enough, cutaneous anesthesia can be produced to determine the effect.

    Some data support the use of topical antiinflammatory drugs, such as aspirin in chloroform. Clinical experience with this approach has not been very favorable, and it is seldom used.

    Another topical therapy, capsaicin cream, has been advocated. Capsaicin is a naturally occurring compound that selectively depletes peptide neurotransmitters (such as substance P) from small-diameter primary afferent neurons. Current experience suggests that an adequate trial of this drug, which is generally believed to require three to four applications daily for approximately 4 weeks, will identify a small proportion of patients who report substantial pain relief. Some patients develop local burning and are unable to proceed with a trial.

31. **What systemic analgesic therapies have been used for PHN?**

    Systemic drug therapy for PHN follows the same general approach recommended for other types of neuropathic pain (see Chapter 37, Adjuvant Analgesics). Although the usual first-line approach comprises one or more adjuvant analgesics, consider a trial of an opioid if the pain is severe. Controlled trials have recently been completed and have demonstrated the potential efficacy of opioid therapy in this disorder.

    Among the so-called adjuvant analgesics that have been specifically evaluated for PHN, the most important are the antidepressants and anticonvulsants. Experience is greatest with the anticonvulsants gabapentin and pregabalin and the tricyclic antidepressants, such as amitriptyline, desipramine, and nortriptyline. Newer antidepressants, such as duloxetine, venlafaxine, paroxetine, and maprotiline, also may be tried. Other anticonvulsants are considered as well. Older drugs, such as carbamazepine, have been studied in various types of neuropathic pain and may be considered, but the newer drugs, such as topiramate, lamotrigine, and levetiracetam, are better tolerated in general. These drugs have not been specifically studied in PHN, but are often considered for neuropathic pain of any type. The alpha-adrenergic agonist clonidine also has been studied in PHN and may be considered in refractory cases, as may other drugs used empirically for neuropathic pain, such as the oral antiarrhythmics, some cannabinoids, and baclofen. Sequential trials with these adjuvant analgesics are the major approach to the pharmacotherapy of PHN. Occasional patients benefit from an NSAID or long-term opioid therapy.

32. **Describe the role of anesthesiologic therapy for postherpetic neuralgia.**

    A recent study evaluated the administration of methylprednisolone and local anesthetic into the intrathecal space. A sequence of several injections was found to yield a high rate of favorable responses in a population with prolonged PHN. This approach has raised some safety concerns and, as yet, has not been widely adopted. The data suggest, however, that it should be considered for severe cases.

    Other anesthesiologic approaches that have been specifically advocated for PHN include skin infiltration with local anesthetic or local anesthetic and steroids, intravenous local anesthetic, temporary or permanent blocks of peripheral nerves or nerve roots, sympathetic blocks, epidural steroid administration, and application of a cryoprobe to painful scars. With the exception of intravenous lidocaine, all the clinical reports of these procedures describe anecdotal experience.

33. **What can be done for severe, refractory neuralgic pain?**

Patients with severe refractory pain are often offered empirical trials of intravenous lidocaine (e.g., 2 to 4 mg/kg over 30 minutes), temporary nerve blocks with local anesthetic (including sympathetic nerve blocks), or techniques that involve subcutaneous instillation of local anesthetic or local anesthetic plus a corticosteroid. Neurolysis is not considered except in the most extreme situations, because of the uncertain nature of the results and concern about the possible adverse effects of increased denervation.

In a similarly empirical manner, a trial of a noninvasive neurostimulatory approach, usually TENS, or a trial of acupuncture is often attempted in cases of refractory neuralgia. The use of an invasive neurostimulatory therapy, specifically dorsal column stimulation, is supported by a small number of favorable case reports, and such an approach is sometimes suggested for patients with severe pain refractory to conservative approaches.

Physiatric and psychological approaches are often recommended to patients with refractory PHN in an effort to improve function and, in some cases, alleviate pain. Especially consider these techniques for patients whose pain leads to immobilization of a limb, general inactivity, or maladaptive behaviors.

34. **True or false: A variety of surgical procedures can successfully treat postherpetic neuralgia.**

False. Although patients with PHN have been reported to benefit from a very diverse group of surgical procedures, including neurectomy, rhizotomy, sympathectomy, cordotomy, trigeminal tractotomy, mesencephalotomy, mesencephalothalamotomy, and thalamotomy, the accumulated clinical experience with these techniques has been disappointing and none is recommended routinely.

35. **What is central pain?**

The existence of central pain syndromes provides strong evidence for the concept that changes in the CNS can result in chronic neuropathic pain. The term "central pain" generically describes the large number of deafferentation pain syndromes that can occur following injury to the CNS. These syndromes are variably named by the location of the lesion (e.g., thalamic pain), the inciting injury (e.g., poststroke pain), or the underlying disorder (e.g., pain related to multiple sclerosis). Syndromes associated with uncommon lesions (e.g., syringobulbia) or common lesions that rarely produce pain (e.g., brain tumors) are usually simply described generically as central pain.

36. **Describe the specific mechanisms that may result in central pain.**

Although it is assumed that any of the changes that may be associated with "central sensitization" (see Questions 5 and 9) could be involved in the development of central pain, little is known of the specific processes involved. Clinical observations suggest that damage to spinothalamocortical pathways is a fundamental element in the development of central pain following a lesion at any level of the neuraxis. Possibly, deafferentation or disinhibition of central nociceptive neurons in the thalamus can follow such a lesion and result in the pathophysiologic changes that underlie the phenomenology of central pain.

37. **What is the epidemiology of pain following spinal cord injury?**

Central pain following damage to the spinal cord has been best characterized in patients with traumatic or demyelinating lesions. Following acute spinal cord injury, 10% to 49% of patients develop chronic pain. A variety of syndromes have been described, including a deafferentation, or central, pain syndrome. The epidemiology of this specific subtype of pain resulting from spinal cord injury is unknown.

38. **What characteristics suggest the diagnosis of central pain caused by spinal cord injury?**

    Central pain caused by spinal cord injury is inferred to exist when dysesthesias occur in a nonsegmental distribution below the injury. The clinical features are highly variable. Spontaneous and evoked dysesthesias may be associated with uncomfortable paresthesias described as tingling, numbness, or squeezing. Painful areas may be small or large, unilateral or bilateral, and stable or fluctuating in size and location. Pain may increase spontaneously or in response to changes in climate, stress, smoking, or other factors. Flexor or extensor spasms, which may be spontaneous or precipitated by movement or by distension of the bladder or bowel, can contribute significantly to the pain. Ill-defined visceral pains, which are usually experienced in the lower abdomen or pelvis, are occasionally reported.

    Because the spinal cord ends at or above the L1 vertebral body, central pain can be diagnosed only if an injury is rostral to this level. If chronic neuropathic pain occurs following a spinal injury below L1, the classification is more complicated. In some cases, the pain is segmental or multisegmental, and the pathophysiology is believed to be sustained by peripheral processes. In other cases, the pain is believed to be sustained by processes in the CNS that are induced by injury to the peripheral nerve. This type of pain can be labeled a deafferentation syndrome fundamentally similar to phantom pain (see Question 10).

39. **Can central pain resulting from demyelinating lesions of the spinal cord occur in the setting of established multiple sclerosis? What are the characteristics of this pain?**

    Chronic pain occurs in 23% to 80% of patients with multiple sclerosis. Central pain, which is the most prevalent type, usually occurs in patients with disease of long duration. The pain is usually described as continuous burning. It is sometimes associated with other types of dysesthesias or lancinating pains and may fluctuate in intensity spontaneously or in response to activity, stress, or change in weather. The location of the pain is most often the distal legs and feet, but patients occasionally present with pain of similar quality in a dermatomal distribution or asymmetric nondermatomal region of the trunk or extremity.

40. **What other types of spinal cord pathology have been associated with central pain?**

    Central pain has been described in association with vascular lesions of the spinal cord, syringomyelia, intramedullary and extramedullary neoplasms, cervical spondylosis, inflammatory lesions (e.g., syphilitic myelitis), subacute combined degeneration, and a toxic myelopathy. Central pain can also be iatrogenic, occasionally complicating spinal surgery or cordotomy.

41. **True or false: Central pain can also result from lesions in the brainstem.**

    True. The prototype syndrome of central pain resulting from lesions in the brainstem is thalamic pain following ischemic or hemorrhagic vascular lesions.

42. **What are the characteristics of thalamic pain?**

    Thalamic pain usually occurs months to years after the injury. The pain is usually dysesthetic (continuous burning, often with intermittent stabbing) and may be associated with uncomfortable paresthesias (e.g., squeezing, gnawing, crawling, or tingling). Allodynia is common, and some patients experience dramatic hyperpathia, with diffuse radiation of the pain, pain that continues for a prolonged period after a stimulus is removed from the skin, and extreme distress. The pain can be experienced in the entire hemibody or be localized to a small region. Occasional patients have a pseudoradicular distribution or a so-called cheiro-oral distribution (perioral region and ipsilateral hand).

43. **Describe the psychological and neurologic deficits associated with thalamic pain.**

Psychological and neurologic deficits associated with thalamic pain are diverse. Patients often become withdrawn, inactive, and profoundly depressed. The examination usually demonstrates an obvious sensory disturbance in some part of the affected hemibody. A deficit in pain and temperature sensation appears to be a constant. Patients may or may not have associated hemiparesis or choreoathetoid movements. Some patients demonstrate unilateral dysmetria or a Horner's syndrome.

44. **Can central pain occur following injury to the cerebrum?**

Central pain may complicate trauma, vascular lesions, or neoplasm in the cerebral hemisphere. This observation provides evidence that the cerebral cortex is important in the experience of pain. Other evidence includes the observation of disturbed pain perception from suprathalamic lesions, the identification of nociceptive cortical neurons in primates, the description of occasional patients who report pain following stimulation of parietal regions during cortical mapping experiments, and the rare occurrence of central pain in association with epileptiform cortical activity.

45. **What management strategies are used for central pain?**

The management of central pain is challenging. Like other chronic neuropathic pains, a multimodality approach that focuses on both comfort and function is ideal. A controlled trial of amitriptyline and carbamazepine demonstrated clear analgesic effects from the former drug and equivocal effects from the latter in patients with central poststroke pain. Another controlled trial of lamotrigine was also positive. Anecdotal reports have described the use of other tricyclic antidepressants, other anticonvulsants, naloxone (administered as a brief infusion), mexiletine and other sodium-channel blockers, diphenhydramine, propranolol, anticholinesterase inhibitors, chlorpromazine, L-dopa, and 5-hydroxytryptophan. The usual approach involves sequential trials of drugs selected nonspecifically for neuropathic pain, including antidepressants, anticonvulsants, and others. Some patients respond favorably to opioid drugs.

Peripheral stimulation, usually TENS, may be beneficial. Invasive neurostimulatory techniques, particularly deep brain stimulation, are considered if pain is refractory to systemic analgesic therapy.

46. **Aside from deep brain stimulation, what other invasive approaches can be employed for central pain?**

Other invasive approaches play a limited role in the management of central pain. Temporary somatic or sympathetic nerve blocks with local anesthetic, if helpful, provide only short-lived relief, and these procedures are rarely used. Although surgical neurolytic techniques for the treatment of central pain have been supported in case reports and small series, the likelihood of sustained benefit appears to be extremely low; therefore, these procedures cannot be recommended. The only possible exception is the use of a dorsal root entry zone (DREZ) lesion for "end-zone" pain in patients with spinal cord injury (see Question 49).

47. **What is avulsion of nerve plexus?**

The deafferentation pain syndrome known as avulsion of nerve plexus is a rare but potentially devastating complication of limb trauma. Although severe pain can complicate avulsion of a nerve root at any level of the nervous system, the most important clinical entity follows plexus avulsion injuries, which usually affect the brachial plexus and are commonly followed by severe pain in the insensate limb. Chronic pain, usually continuous burning dysesthesias with superimposed paroxysms, has been reported to complicate brachial plexus avulsions in 26% to 91% of patients. The onset of the pain can be immediate or delayed for months. In one series, approximately one third of patients had severe, unrelenting pain more than 2 years after the injury. Stress, intercurrent illness, and changes in the weather have been reported to increase the pain; discomfort is sometimes reduced by distraction or stereotyped maneuvers, such as gripping or swinging the arm, or massaging the neck or shoulder. The limb, or portions of it, are anesthetic; most patients do not experience allodynia or hyperpathia, but paresthesias and other phantomlike phenomena may be experienced.

48. **How is the diagnosis of plexus avulsion made?**
The distinction between injury to the nerve root itself and avulsion of the root is critical, because the former lesion may be amenable to nerve grafting. Diagnosis usually depends on a combination of clinical findings, electrodiagnostic studies, and imaging procedures (the most important of which is magnetic resonance imaging [MRI], which may demonstrate a pseudomeningocele in cases of root avulsion).

49. **Describe management strategies for painful plexus avulsion.**
A multimodal approach should strive to improve both comfort and function in patients with painful plexus avulsion. A specific surgical procedure, the DREZ, plays a special role in this disorder (see Question 46). Although there is a small possibility of major morbidity from this procedure, favorable clinical experience suggests that it may be considered—but only when pain is severe. Other surgical procedures are generally regarded to be ineffective. The favorable outcome associated with the DREZ lesion suggests that the pathophysiology of the pain associated with avulsion resides in the dorsal horn of the spinal cord.

There are no controlled trials of drug therapy in the treatment of pain associated with avulsion injuries. Empirical trials of the adjuvant analgesics and opioids used nonspecifically for neuropathic pain are usually tried. Other therapies that have been used include sympathetic nerve block, TENS and dorsal column stimulation, trigger point injections into associated regions of myofascial pain, and a variety of psychological and rehabilitative therapies. Splinting of the paralyzed arm and intensive physical therapy to retain residual strength and prevent contractures and joint ankylosis are usually important interventions.

50. **What is sympathetically maintained pain?**
Sympathetically maintained pain (SMP) is also inferred to have a predominating CNS pathophysiology. It is a subtype of neuropathic pain that appears to be sustained by efferent activity in the sympathetic nervous system. The specific mechanisms involved are unknown. Historically, SMP was viewed as equivalent to the diagnoses of complex regional pain syndrome (types 1 and 2) or at least a major subtype of these disorders. The finding that some patients without the clinical characteristics of RSD or causalgia improved after sympathetic block contributed to confusion about these diagnoses.

In an effort to clarify the nomenclature, the International Association for the Study of Pain has adopted the term "complex regional pain syndrome (CRPS) type I and II" to refer to disorders that have the clinical characteristics of RSD (no evidence of nerve lesion) and causalgia (secondary to a nerve lesion), respectively. Patients with CRPS are assumed to have a neuropathic pain, which is presumably produced by some constellation of mechanisms that may or may not involve the sympathetic nervous system. Patients with CRPS, therefore, may or may not have SMP. Although there is a clear association between CRPS and SMP, such that the clinical findings indicative of CRPS should immediately suggest the potential value of interventions directed to the sympathetic nervous system, the two disorders are considered independent. Some patients who do not meet criteria for CRPS respond favorably to sympathetic nerve block and, by definition, also have SMP.

51. **What is known about the mechanisms of CRPS and SMP?**
The specific mechanisms responsible for the unique characteristics of CRPS are unknown. Various mechanisms, which may involve processes in the peripheral nervous system or in the CNS, have been proposed to explain SMP, but no one mechanism, or group of mechanisms

has been confirmed. Based on clinical observations (such as the usual failure of peripheral denervation as a treatment for SMP), there is strong suspicion that the essential pathophysiology involves a process in the CNS. However, controversy about the nature of both SMP and CRPS is ongoing. Indeed, some even question whether SMP actually reflects a relationship between pain and sympathetic efferent function (Table 28-2). An alternative hypothesis suggests that SMP is related to the transmission of nociceptive information in visceral afferents that travel with the sympathetics.

TABLE 28-2. MECHANISMS THAT MAY BE INVOLVED IN THE DEVELOPMENT OF SYMPATHETICALLY MAINTAINED PAIN

Peripheral Processes

Activity in nociceptive visceral afferents that travel with sympathetic efferent fibers

Processes involving sympathetic-somatic link

Sympathetic hyperactivity changes peripheral tissues in a way that activates nociceptors ("vicious circle")

Damaged nociceptors have increased sensitivity to catecholamines released by sympathetic nerves

Prostaglandins released by sympathetic nerves may sensitize nociceptors

Sympathetic-nociceptor ephapses may form

Central Processes

Sympathetically driven activity in nonnociceptive afferents could increase firing of sensitized wide-dynamic-range neuron in the spinal cord

---

52. **What is the epidemiology of the disorders now known as CRPS?**
    Reflex sympathetic dystrophy (CRPS type I) can complicate injury to soft tissue, joint, or bone at any site, including head and trunk. Orthopedic injury to an extremity appears to be the most common predisposing factor. The precipitating injury can range from mild to severe, and some cases develop without any prior event. Although systematic epidemiologic studies are lacking, the incidence following even severe injury appears to be extremely small.

    The classic lesion that predisposes to the development of causalgia (CRPS type II) is a high-speed missile injury that causes stretch, but not interruption, of a peripheral nerve. Surveys of veterans suggest that causalgia can complicate 1% to 5% of such injuries. The vulnerability to causalgia varies with the location of the injury: 90% of cases have damage above the knee or elbow, and the order of nerve involvement is sciatic (40%), median (35%), medial cord of the brachial plexus (12%), and other nerves (13%). The cause of this selective vulnerability is unknown.

    There is a variable interval between injury and the onset of dysesthesia and the other clinical findings indicative of a CRPS. Many patients report that the syndrome began immediately or within hours of the event; others state that the onset was delayed by months.

53. **What are the clinical characteristics of the complex regional pain syndrome?**
    CRPS types I and II are distinguished solely by the history of major nerve injury that characterizes the latter disorder. The diagnosis of either type should be made when chronic pain, which typically has a prominent burning component, is accompanied by autonomic dysregulation in the region of the pain. Autonomic dysregulation may be characterized

by swelling, vasomotor instability (e.g., color change or livedo reticularis), or abnormal sweating. Some patients also develop trophic changes and abnormal motor activity. Trophic changes may include skin that becomes thin and shiny, increase or decrease in the growth of hair or nails, focal atrophy of subcutaneous tissue or muscle, or focal osteoporosis. Abnormal motor function may include tremor, other dyskinesias such as myoclonus or chorea, or dystonia. Other findings on the neurologic examination are similarly variable and may include raised thresholds for sensory stimuli (hypesthesia or hypalgesia), exaggerated responses to suprathreshold events (hyperesthesia, hyperalgesia, allodynia, or hyperpathia) or, paradoxically, a combination of these phenomena.

54. How are the clinical characteristics of CRPS discerned?

Occasionally, a patient with chronic neuropathic pain is suspected of having a CRPS, but the clinical manifestations of autonomic dysregulation or trophic changes are so subtle that the diagnosis cannot be made. If it is important to establish the diagnosis, ancillary tests may be useful to identify subtle autonomic or trophic phenomena. Autonomic changes in the painful region may be indicated by thermographic demonstration of asymmetric skin temperatures or by testing of sudomotor function. Trophic changes may be indicated by patchy demineralization on plain radiography or abnormal radionuclide uptake on a bone scintigram. A three-phase bone scintigram is preferred by some clinicians, who believe that it may be a more sensitive indicator of the abnormalities associated with CRPS. None of these tests have been evaluated in terms of sensitivity, specificity, or predictive value.

55. True of false: There is a specific progression pattern associated with CRPS.

False. Although some authors have described the progression of reflex sympathetic dystrophy (CRPS type I) in three well-defined stages characterized by specific constellations of symptoms and signs, large surveys have not confirmed these patterns in most patients. Rather, there is great individual variation in both clinical findings and long-term outcomes. There are many reports of remission following early and intensive therapy, and some patients appear to remit spontaneously. Others remit and relapse or have a course characterized by persistent or worsening pain.

56. What is the first step after diagnosis of CRPS?

The diagnosis of CRPS is usually followed by a procedure to block sympathetic innervation to the painful site. If this procedure relieves pain, it may be both diagnostic (establishing the existence of SMP) and therapeutic.

57. How is sympathetic block performed?

The traditional method to block sympathetic efferent functions is via neural blockade. A variety of procedures can be used. Pain in the head and upper extremity is usually approached by injection of local anesthetic into the region of the cervical sympathetic chain (the stellate ganglion block), and pain in the lower extremities is typically approached by injection of anesthetic into the region of the lumbar sympathetic chain.

Sympathetic blockade in a limb can also be accomplished using a regional intravenous technique, in which a drug that depletes adrenergic transmitters from sympathetic nerve endings, such as guanethidine or bretylium, is injected into a vein while the venous outflow from the extremity is interrupted with a compression cuff. Although the sympathetic block produced by this procedure can be prolonged, there have been very few trials of the procedure, and a recent metaanalysis of published data failed to demonstrate any benefit. Nonetheless, a regional intravenous infusion is still considered for those patients with suspected SMP who are unable or unwilling to undergo neural blockade.

The final approach to sympathetic blockade is via the intravenous injection of the alpha-adrenergic blocking agent phentolamine. This approach has become widely used as a diagnostic test, and repeated procedures are sometimes employed therapeutically.

However, there have been few studies of the technique, and it is still uncertain that it can fully substitute for sympathetic nerve block.

Most patients undergo a trial period during which at least several sympathetic blocks are performed before the diagnosis of SMP is rejected. The standard approach varies from clinician to clinician. Some recommend the procedure daily, whereas others perform it weekly or less often during this initial period. In some severe cases, continuous sympathetic blockade using local anesthetic infusion is attempted.

58. How is the response to sympathetic block in CRPS interpreted?
The interpretation of a patient's response to sympathetic block can be complicated by technical problems (e.g., how effectively sympathetic outflow was interrupted), the placebo response, and the limitations in the scientific literature about this procedure. Clinical reports of sympathetic nerve block, for example, usually do not apply placebo controls, identical techniques, or standardized criteria for a favorable outcome. Neither these reports nor studies of the phentolamine test provide sufficient information to clearly establish criteria for a positive outcome, or determine the long-term implications of an outcome that appears positive at the time of the test. Most provide no clear indication of the degree or acceptability of pain relief, response of associated phenomena, overall improvement in the functional capacity of the patient, or ability of the procedure to predict long-term outcome.

Despite these difficulties, clinicians still hold to the view that a diagnosis of CRPS should generally be followed by a trial of sympathetic block to determine whether an SMP also exists. The patient's response is usually considered positive if substantial relief is experienced for a period that exceeds the duration of the local anesthetic by many hours or days.

59. What is the management strategy for a patient with CRPS who has a favorable response to sympathetic block and, therefore, coexisting SMP?
Patients with CRPS who have a favorable response to sympathetic block and, therefore, coexisting SMP are usually offered a therapeutic strategy that incorporates repeated or ongoing interruption of sympathetic outflow to the painful area. The approach varies among clinicians and may involve any of the aforementioned procedures on a rigid schedule, or on a schedule based on the clinical course of the patient.

A variety of responses is observed, as shown in the following list. The size of each of these groups relative to the entire population with SMP is unknown.

- Transitory relief after each block that outlasts the duration of local anesthetic effect and lengthens with each block
- Transitory relief that outlasts the duration of the local anesthetic effect, but does increment with subsequent blocks
- Transitory relief that gradually diminishes with each block, until the block is ineffective
- A prolonged favorable response after one or a few blocks

A pattern of response to sympathetic blockade characterized by repeated short-lived periods of analgesia develops in a minority of patients. Traditionally, these patients have been considered for permanent sympathetic interruption via chemical or surgical sympathectomy. Reported response rates for these procedures vary greatly.

60. Describe systemic pharmacotherapy for a suspected or established CRPS or SMP.
The usual approach to systemic pharmacotherapy for a suspected or established CRPS or SMP is based on sequential trials of the adjuvant analgesics and opioids used nonspecifically for neuropathic pain. If a SMP is suspected, therapy also may include repeated intravenous phentolamine infusions. Orally administered drugs have also been used empirically in this case, including sympatholytic (clonidine, prazosin, and various beta-adrenergic blockers, such as propranolol) and nonsympatholytic drugs (calcitonin, nifedipine, and corticosteroids). The medical literature that describes the use of these drugs is very limited. A bisphosphonate

has been studied in a population with RSD, as has calcitonin. Trials of these types of drugs should be considered. Clonidine is a nonspecific analgesic and would presumably be effective in some patients with CRPS, irrespective of the coexistence of SMP. The information about the other drugs is limited to anecdotes or small surveys.

61. **What is the role of physical therapy in treatment of CRPS and SMP?**
Clinicians generally agree that an effort to normalize the function of the painful part using intensive physical therapy is an essential aspect of the therapeutic approach to CRPS and SMP. Patients with SMP who attain pain relief with sympathetic block should capitalize on periods of increased comfort by focusing on these function-oriented therapies. Rehabilitative approaches also can potentially prevent dysfunction in joints and muscles produced by disuse and trophic changes, optimize function at any given level of impairment, and improve psychological well-being.

62. **What is the management strategy for a patient with CRPS who does not have coexisting SMP?**
Management for patients with CRPS who do not have coexisting SMP is similar to that for other patients with chronic neuropathic pain. All patients require a comprehensive assessment that identifies adverse psychological and behavioral phenomena and the extent of disability associated with the pain. A multimodality therapeutic plan that attempts to optimize both comfort and function can be developed from this assessment. The most common approach combines sequential trials of analgesic drugs (nonopioid, opioid, and adjuvant analgesics) with intensive rehabilitative and psychological interventions. Noninvasive neurostimulatory approaches, such as TENS, are also used.

   Recent studies have confirmed the efficacy of dorsal column stimulation in the population with CRPS type 1. This approach is generally considered if noninvasive approaches do not achieve substantial benefit. The use of other neurostimulatory approaches, including acupuncture, percutaneous electrical nerve stimulation, and deep brain stimulation, is anecdotal. Procedures to isolate the painful part from the CNS, either temporarily using somatic nerve blocks or more permanently using chemical or surgical neurolysis, have yielded disappointing results and are not accepted.

63. **True or false: Some types of neuropathic pain are inferred to have a sustaining peripheral pathogenesis.**
True. Some types of neuropathic pain are inferred to have a sustaining peripheral pathogenesis.

64. **What mechanisms may be involved in pain syndromes that are presumably sustained by aberrant somatosensory processing in the peripheral nervous system?**
On theoretical grounds, the varied processes that could lead to peripheral neuropathic pains may be broadly divided into those characterized by activation of normal nociceptors and those characterized by pathologic processes precipitated by axonal injury and attempts at regeneration. The inciting events that lead to these various mechanisms and the linkages between such mechanisms and clinical phenomena are largely unknown. The ability to infer a specific mechanism is limited and rarely changes clinical practice. The exception to this may be the development of a neuroma, recognition of which suggests a variety of peripheral therapeutic interventions targeted specifically to this pathology.

65. **What are the characteristics of a neuroma?**
Neuromas may form at the end of a cut nerve or develop along the course of a successfully regenerated nerve (neuroma-in-continuity). These regions, which appear pathologically as tufts of regenerating small nerve fibers, generate spontaneous discharges, both locally and at the level of the dorsal root ganglion. Once these regions of aberrant activity are established, ectopic

discharges can be evoked by mechanical stimulation and changes in the local environment, including increased concentration of catecholamines, ischemia, and electrolyte disturbances. As illustrated by Tinel's sign, these evoked discharges can be associated with pain.

66. **How are neuropathic pains inferred to have sustaining mechanisms in the peripheral nervous system divided?**
They are divided into a group of painful polyneuropathies and a group of painful mononeuropathies.

67. **Is anything known about the mechanisms responsible for painful polyneuropathy?**
There are many types of painful polyneuropathy, and the variety of etiologies and differences on pathologic examination suggest that the mechanisms responsible for the pain are diverse. Some neuropathies involve predominant injury to the myelin sheath (myelinopathy), and some involve a generalized injury to the neuron itself (axonopathy). Most painful polyneuropathies are axonopathies. Examples include the neuropathies associated with diabetes and nutritional deficiencies.

Many studies have attempted to relate the pain associated with some axonopathies to selective fiber type dysfunction. It has been proposed, for example, that the pain from some polyneuropathies is related to ectopic activity originating from injured small fibers. Studies in patients with painful diabetic neuropathy appear to support this hypothesis. Other studies, however, indicate that all painful polyneuropathies cannot be attributed to this type of mechanism. Some painless neuropathies have selective small fiber loss, and some painful neuropathies have either no selective damage or damage limited to large fibers. The occurrence of pain in several neuropathies with selective large fiber loss suggests an alternative hypothesis, namely that pain may relate to the loss of peripheral inhibition, which may be mediated by activation of large-diameter peripheral nerves. This hypothesis, however, fails to account for the existence of painless neuropathies with selective large fiber loss. Together, these data suggest that selective fiber type dysfunction may be involved in some painful polyneuropathies, but other mechanisms must be involved as well.

68. **What are the characteristics of painful polyneuropathy?**
Complaints about pain are relatively uniform among those disorders characterized by a generalized axonopathy. Patients usually report burning or other dysesthesias of the feet and distal legs (and the hands, when the lesion is advanced); paroxysmal lancinating pains that may be spontaneous or provoked; deep aching in the feet and legs; and muscle cramping. Some patients have allodynia or hyperpathia, and many describe accompanying paresthesias. Some patients find these paresthesias, such as tingling, "crawling" sensations, sensations of heat or cold, or a sense of swelling, to be very unpleasant.

Pain associated with myelinopathy, specifically the acute inflammatory polyneuropathy of Guillain-Barré syndrome, is generally aching and occurs in both the back and limbs. Muscle cramps occur as well.

69. **Painful polyneuropathies are associated with many types of medical illness. What implications does this have?**
The diseases associated with painful polyneuropathy are extremely diverse (Table 28-3). Elucidation of those factors that precipitate or sustain the neuropathy may allow specific treatment targeted at the underlying cause of the neuropathy. The ability to prognosticate is also improved by knowledge of the associated illness. These benefits underscore the importance of a detailed medical assessment of all patients with painful polyneuropathy. This assessment complements the evaluation of pain-related morbidity that should be performed in patients with neuropathic pain.

TABLE 28-3. PAINFUL POLYNEUROPATHIES
Painful Polyneuropathy Caused by Metabolic Disorders
Diabetes neuropathy
Neuropathy associated with insulinoma
Nutritional deficiency
Alcohol-nutritional neuropathy
Specific vitamin deficiency (e.g., niacin, B_{12}, or pyridoxine)
Hypothyroid neuropathy
Uremic neuropathy
Amyloid neuropathy
Neuropathy associated with Fabry's disease
Painful Neuropathy Caused by Drugs or Toxins*
Painful Polyneuropathy Caused by Neoplasm
Subacute sensory neuronopathy
Sensorimotor neuropathy associated with carcinoma
Sensorimotor neuropathy associated with dysproteinemias
Hereditary Painful Polyneuropathy
Painful Polyneuropathies Associated with Guillain-Barré Syndrome

*Examples include isoniazid, gold, misonidazole, nitrofurantoin, vincristine, cis-platinum, paclitaxel, arsenic, cyanide, and thallium.

70. **Where does painful polyneuropathy fit among the heterogeneous peripheral nerve syndromes caused by diabetes?**

Diabetes may cause a remarkably varied group of neuropathies. The distal symmetric polyneuropathies are usually distinguished from an autonomic neuropathy and various mononeuropathies, which may be focal or multifocal, and predominantly sensory or predominantly motor. These focal and multifocal mononeuropathies (such as femoral neuropathy and lumbar radiculoplexopathy [diabetic amyotrophy]) can be intensely painful. The distal symmetric polyneuropathies can be divided into distinct groups, each characterized by a predominant disorder, either motor or sensory, as well as a mixed group in which all fiber types are affected. Patients who have a polyneuropathy in which sensory fibers are involved can have predominant involvement of large fibers, small fibers, or a mixed syndrome. The pathology associated with painful polyneuropathy is a distal symmetric polyneuropathy with predominant involvement of small-diameter afferent fibers. Studies suggest that the lesion that affects these fibers is both vascular and metabolic.

71. **What are the major painful polyneuropathies associated with nutritional deficiency?**

Painful polyneuropathy complicates a diverse group of nutritional deficiencies. The major syndromes include alcohol-nutritional deficiency polyneuropathy, thiamine deficiency, niacin deficiency, and pyridoxine deficiency.

The pathogenesis of the alcohol-nutritional deficiency polyneuropathy probably involves multiple vitamin deficiencies. With abstinence and vitamin supplementation, symptoms and signs may improve. This neuropathy is indistinguishable from that associated with specific thiamine deficiency. A variety of other neuropsychological (Wernicke-Korsakoff syndrome) and cardiac ("wet" beriberi) manifestations may also develop from a lack of thiamine. Pellagra, the syndrome of niacin deficiency, is also associated with a polyneuropathy clinically similar to that observed in alcoholics. Dermatitis and gastrointestinal disturbances accompany the neuropathy in this condition. The neuropathy associated with pyridoxine (vitamin B6) deficiency almost never occurs as a result of inadequate naturally occurring pyridoxine, which is ubiquitous in food; deficiencies are almost always due to ingestion of pyridoxine antagonists, particularly the antituberculous agent isoniazid.

72. **Describe "burning feet" syndrome.**
"Burning feet" syndrome is an acute syndrome characterized by intense, burning pain in the feet. It is associated with erythema and swelling and develops in a subgroup of alcoholic patients. The syndrome can occur with or without clinical evidence of polyneuropathy, but is presumably neuropathic. Patients with other types of nutritional neuropathy also may experience this syndrome.

73. **What metabolic disturbances can result in painful polyneuropathy?**
Hypothyroidism and uremia produce well-characterized painful neuropathies. Hypothyroidism can cause a predominantly sensory polyneuropathy, which may be complicated by pain and muscle cramping, and is associated with a relative impairment of large nerve fibers. Hypothyroid patients can also develop painful muscle cramping in the absence of a clinical neuropathy and painful mononeuropathies due to entrapment. The most common entrapment neuropathy is due to carpal tunnel syndrome.

A predominantly sensory polyneuropathy, which is often painful, is extremely common among those with chronic renal failure. Occasional patients develop severe dysesthesias, which can mimic the "burning feet" syndrome associated with nutritional deficiencies. Both muscle cramping and "restless legs" (often accompanied by uncomfortable paresthesias) are also common and can occur with or without clinical evidence of polyneuropathy. All of these symptoms may improve with dialysis or renal transplantation.

74. **Which clinical syndrome is associated with amyloid polyneuropathy?**
Amyloid produces a progressive sensory polyneuropathy, which may occur in both primary and secondary amyloidosis and is usually associated with pain, impaired small-fiber function (e.g., loss of pain and thermal sensibility), and signs of autonomic neuropathy (e.g., postural hypotension, impaired sweating, and gastrointestinal dysmotility). On pathologic examination, there is a selective loss of lightly myelinated and unmyelinated axons.

75. **What is Fabry's disease? What clinical syndrome does it produce?**
Fabry's disease (also known as angiokeratoma corpus diffusum) is a rare, lipid storage disorder with sex-lined genetics that results from a deficiency of the enzyme ceramide trihexosidase. The related painful polyneuropathy, which is associated with selective loss of small myelinated and unmyelinated fibers, can cause continuous, burning dysesthesias of the distal extremities and intermittent episodes of severe pain, which may be spontaneous or precipitated by activity or other factors. Other features include a maculopapular rash, angiokeratoma corpuscum, and, in the later phases, dysfunction of the heart, liver, and kidneys.

76. **What clinical syndromes caused by exposure to toxins or drugs are associated with painful polyneuropathy?**
Although scores of drugs and toxins may damage peripheral nerves, relatively few cause a painful polyneuropathy. Knowledge of these syndromes is important because removal of the drug or toxin usually leads to gradual improvement. The drugs clearly associated with painful polyneuropathy include isoniazid, gold, misonidazole, nitrofurantoin, and various chemotherapeutic agents such as vincristine, cis-platinum, and paclitaxel. Pain can also be an uncommon accompaniment of other drug-induced neuropathies, but the prevalence of this

complication cannot be stated reliably. The toxins associated with dysesthesias include arsenic (acute or chronic exposure), cyanide poisoning (chronic ingestion of sublethal doses), and thallium salts (acute and subacute ingestion).

77. **How may nerve injury result in the cancer population?**

Nerve injury is common in the cancer population, and may result from direct compression by tumor, the toxic effects of antineoplastic therapy, associated metabolic disturbances, or poorly understood remote (paraneoplastic) effects.

78. **What are the major paraneoplastic painful polyneuropathies?**

A sensorimotor neuropathy associated with carcinoma is a nonspecific paraneoplastic polyneuropathy that can complicate any tumor type. The clinical features, including the onset and course, are variable. Pain may or may not occur, and the incidence, characteristics, and course of this symptom have not been defined. Sensorimotor neuropathies associated with dysproteinemia are somewhat better characterized. A painful polyneuropathy may complicate multiple myeloma, Waldenstrom's macroglobulinemia, solitary plasmacytoma, and osteosclerotic plasmacytoma. Cryoglobulinemia may also result in a pain syndrome, which can be described as acral pain on exposure to cold. In all cases, symptoms and signs often precede the diagnosis of the underlying neoplasm by many months. The subacute sensory neuronopathy is a well-described subtype of paraneoplastic neuropathy that usually begins with aching pain and dysesthesias and paresthesias in the distal extremities. Small cell carcinoma is the most common associated tumor, but other carcinomas and lymphomas have been reported. Symptoms are progressive and ultimately become associated with severe impairment of sensory functions, particularly those mediated by large fibers. The syndrome often precedes discovery of the tumor by months or years, and the course of the neurologic syndrome is usually independent of the neoplasm. On pathologic examination, this disorder has been associated with degeneration of sensory neurons in the dorsal root ganglia. Although the inciting processes are not known, there is evidence that a humoral immunologic insult mediates this lesion.

79. **Are there other painful polyneuropathies?**

Aching or lancinating pains may be experienced by patients with hereditary sensory neuropathy type I, a rare dominantly inherited neuropathy that predominantly affects small myelinated and unmyelinated fibers. Other acquired disorders that may be associated with painful polyneuropathy include the Guillain-Barré syndrome, which is an acute myelinopathy, and the chronic myelinopathies, such as the disorder known as chronic inflammatory demyelinating polyneuropathy. Porphyria and any of the autoimmune diseases can also have pain as a prominent symptom in some patients. Rarely is an idiopathic neuropathy accompanied by disabling pain.

80. **What management strategies are used for painful polyneuropathy?**

Patients must be carefully assessed to develop a multimodality approach that integrates treatments intended to enhance comfort with treatments intended to enhance function. Assessment must include an assiduous search for the underlying etiology of the neuropathy. Primary treatment, such as improved glycemic control for the diabetic or vitamin repletion for those with nutritional neuropathy, can provide some patients with dramatic symptomatic relief and should be implemented whenever appropriate.

The use of analgesic drugs, including opioids, and many of the so-called adjuvant analgesics parallels the approaches used for other types of neuropathic pain. A trial of topical analgesics also is often considered.

Drug therapies directed at the primary disorder and analgesic drugs are usually combined with physiatric and psychological interventions, as appropriate. Invasive analgesics have a very limited role. There have been favorable anecdotal reports about the use of dorsal column stimulation, but this procedure should be considered only in those patients with refractory, disabling dysesthesias who have been evaluated by experienced practitioners. With the exception of trigger point injections, which appear to benefit some patients who develop secondary myofascial pains in limbs weakened by the neuropathy, anesthetic approaches are rarely useful. There is no evidence that denervation procedures improve painful neuropathy.

81. **What are the lancinating neuralgias?**
In addition to the painful polyneuropathies, neuropathic pains related to aberrant processes in the peripheral nervous system also include mononeuropathies and multiple mononeuropathies. These diverse symptoms have been divided into a few subtypes, including a group of disorders called lancinating neuralgias.

    As typically applied, the term "neuralgia" refers to pain caused by damage to a peripheral nerve and is experienced in the distribution of the nerve. This terminology can be confusing given the varying types of painful peripheral mononeuropathies, and it is useful to clarify it by distinguishing a group of disorders related to nerve injury and described as brief paroxysmal pains (i.e., lancinating pains similar to trigeminal neuralgia).

82. **What is known about the mechanisms that may be specific to the lancinating neuralgias?**
It has been proposed that both a peripheral process and a central process are necessary elements in the pathogenesis of trigeminal neuralgia and, by extrapolation, of the other lancinating neuralgias. In the case of trigeminal neuralgia, the peripheral lesion usually appears to be an aberrant arterial loop that chronically injures the trigeminal nerve at a site just outside the brainstem. Presumably, this focus can both produce ectopic impulses and diminish segmental inhibition. Such processes might predispose to paroxysmal discharges of interneurons in the trigeminal nucleus, which, in turn, cause intermittent paroxysmal firing of trigeminothalamic projection neurons that underlie the experience of pain.

83. **What are the characteristics of the lancinating neuralgias?**
The lancinating neuralgias are characterized by the experience of brief, usually shocklike pains, which may occur in isolation or in runs of variable duration. Some patients also experience a more continuous aching or burning of milder intensity in the region of the neuralgia. The latter pain may occur for a brief period after a severe attack of the lancinating component, or more continuously during periods of frequent attacks.

84. **Describe the common types of lancinating neuralgias.**
Trigeminal neuralgia is the best characterized lancinating neuralgia. This syndrome most often affects the mandibular branch of the trigeminal nerve. Pain is usually precipitated by activation of a trigger zone or sometimes by activities such as chewing. The neurologic examination in idiopathic trigeminal neuralgia is normal. When secondary (e.g., related to multiple sclerosis or a tumor in the middle cranial fossa), the examination may demonstrate findings consistent with trigeminal dysfunction. Large surveys have suggested that most patients with idiopathic trigeminal neuralgia have structural pathology, such as an aberrant arterial loop or a fibrous band, that compresses the trigeminal adjacent to the brainstem.

    Other, uncommon neuralgias of the head and neck have been well characterized, including glossopharyngeal neuralgia, occipital neuralgia, geniculate (or nervus intermedius) neuralgia, and superior laryngeal (or vagal) neuralgia. The variety of these syndromes suggests that any focal nerve injury anywhere in the body can result in predominant lancinating dysesthesias. When this occurs, the resulting disorder can be named according to the nerve affected. For example, intercostal neuralgia refers to lancinating chest pains that may follow injury to the intercostal nerves, and ilioinguinal neuralgia is used to describe intense inguinal stabbing pain that can complicate injury to the ilioinguinal nerve.

85. **If a pain syndrome occurs following injury to a peripheral nerve, will it always have a lancinating component?**

As noted, injury to any peripheral nerve can result in a syndrome in which lancinating pains predominate. Alternatively, injury can result in a neuropathic pain syndrome largely or exclusively characterized as continuous dysesthesias. Although these differences presumably reflect variation in the underlying pathology or pathophysiology, the nature of this variation is unknown. From the clinical perspective, the difference is important because of the therapeutic implications associated with lancinating neuralgias.

86. **What does the diagnosis of a lancinating neuralgia imply for therapy?**

The existence of a structural lesion that distorts or compresses the nerve has been identified in a large majority of surgically managed patients with trigeminal neuralgia. Based on this observation, and a smaller surgical experience in patients with glossopharyngeal neuralgia and other syndromes, such structural lesions are assumed to be prevalent among all patients with idiopathic neuralgias of the head. This potential has justified surgical exploration of patients with intractable neuralgia.

Most patients with lancinating neuralgias benefit from drug therapy. The pharmacologic treatment of trigeminal neuralgia is the model for all the lancinating neuralgias. Conventionally therapy proceeds first with trials of anticonvulsant drugs and a selected group of other drugs, such as baclofen.

Patients with pain syndromes refractory to drug therapy also may be candidates for invasive measures that destroy the offending nerve. The success of these procedures in some patients illustrates the importance of a peripheral pathophysiology for the pain.

87. **Like the lancinating neuralgias, many other types of neuropathic pain can be inferred to have a sustaining peripheral pathogenesis. What are the major similarities and differences among the syndromes that can be classified in this way?**

All painful mononeuropathies are associated with a peripheral nerve injury. The injury to the nerve may be traumatic, vascular, neoplastic, or inflammatory. The timing of the injury (acute, subacute, or chronic) may or may not correlate with the temporal characteristics of the pain, and the pain may precede or follow the overt presentation of the injury. The pain may be the only problem associated with the injury, or pain may accompany other neurologic deficits (motor, sensory, or autonomic) referable to the nerve.

The pain is usually experienced, at least partly, in the distribution of the damaged nerve. The descriptors used by patients with painful nerve injury vary. Some use words that are typically applied to nociceptive pains, such as aching, throbbing, or sharp, and others supply terms consistent with dysesthesia, including burning, electrical, or stabbing.

The diversity of these syndromes extends to the findings on examination of the painful area. There may be an area of sensory loss (that is, a raised threshold to response), with or without accompanying areas of hyperesthesia, hyperalgesia, allodynia, or hyperpathia. Focal tenderness is common, and some patients have a highly localized area of exquisite sensitivity along the course of a nerve, which may suggest the site of neuroma formation or entrapment.

The clinical heterogeneity in the population with painful mononeuropathy presumably reflects the varying mechanisms that may be responsible for the pain. These mechanisms may be broadly divided into those that produce pain as a result of axonal transection (resulting in neuroma or related pathology) and those that produce pain without severe damage to axons.

88. **What types of pain syndromes are associated with nerve trauma?**
The types of painful mononeuropathy that follow nerve trauma exemplify this broad division in the mechanisms that may be responsible for the pain. Trauma that severs axons may be followed by the development of a painful neuroma. The resultant syndromes, which include stump pain, postsurgical pain syndromes, and other traumatic nerve injuries, appear to be fundamentally similar. Nerve compression not severe enough to transect axons also is extremely common, and the pain syndromes that result presumably relate to mechanisms independent of neuroma formation. The latter syndromes, which include cervical or lumbar root compression and entrapment neuropathies, are extremely prevalent.

89. **What pain syndromes are associated with other types of nerve pathology?**
Severe pain can accompany acute inflammation of a peripheral nerve. This pathogenesis is observed in herpes zoster, idiopathic brachial or lumbar plexopathy (also known as plexitis), and local infection.

Nerve ischemia or infarction related to a vascular insult also can be very painful. The prototype disorder is diabetes mellitus, which is associated with many well-defined painful mononeuropathies related to nerve ischemia, such as femoral neuropathy. These disorders typically present a relatively brief progressive phase characterized by pain and evolving weakness; the pain usually improves gradually and strength slowly returns over months. Pain may also accompany a mononeuritis or mononeuritis multiplex caused by vasculitis. Rarely, large vessel occlusion can cause a painful focal neuropathy. The pain in this condition may be resulting from ischemia of muscle and other soft tissue, as well as injury to the nerve.

Tumors originating from peripheral nerves are usually associated with pain. Whereas benign tumors, such as neurofibroma, typically cause modest pain, malignant neoplasms usually produce severe pain.

90. **The diagnosis of a painful peripheral mononeuropathy suggests the potential utility of interventions directed at the site of the lesion. Should invasive approaches be used early in the management of these disorders?**
Although invasive approaches intended to ameliorate focal pathology can provide some patients with dramatic analgesia, there are no assurances that such interventions will be helpful, and all carry substantial risks. In one survey, for example, 31 of 48 patients who underwent surgery for pain owing to nerve injury were unchanged or made worse by the operation; almost half were made worse. The use of local invasive therapies requires sound clinical judgment informed by recognition of the latter possibility.

91. **What noninvasive management strategies should be considered for painful mononeuropathies?**
With few exceptions, the pharmacologic approaches to the treatment of painful peripheral mononeuropathies are nonspecific and similar to those applied in the management of other neuropathic pains. Both systemic and epidural corticosteroid therapy have been specifically advocated for painful radiculopathy, but controlled trials have failed to confirm the value of systemic steroids, and the use of epidural steroids remains controversial. Most experienced clinicians will consider the use of epidural steroid injection in selected patients with painful radiculopathy that has not responded to conservative management. A short course of a systemic corticosteroid has been shown to be beneficial in pain caused by carpal tunnel syndrome, and it is possible this approach may be helpful in other types of compressive neuropathies.

Given the focal nature of the pain, a trial of a noninvasive neurostimulatory approach, such as TENS, should be considered in most cases. Physiatric and psychological interventions may benefit both pain and disability and should also be considered in all patients with painful peripheral mononeuropathies.

92. **What invasive analgesic approaches should be considered for painful mononeuropathies?**
Clinical experience indicates that some patients with painful mononeuropathy, particularly a syndrome consistent with neuroma formation, obtain long-term pain relief following repeated temporary nerve blocks or a prolonged block using a local anesthetic infusion technique. These procedures are relatively benign and could be considered earlier than those intended to produce permanent damage to neural tissue.

Neurolysis is sometimes considered for patients who experience transitory relief after each of many repeated nerve blocks. Cryoblock yields a longer lasting interruption of nerve function than local anesthetic instillation and has a lower likelihood of serious complications than chemical neurolysis. Although very limited data are available, the use of cryoblock may be considered an alternative to chemical or surgical neurolysis in carefully selected patients with painful mononeuropathy.

The focal nature of the painful mononeuropathies also suggests the utility of surgical approaches in some patients. The potential for deterioration exists with all such procedures, and none should be considered until after reasonable conservative measures have been exhausted. Surgery should not be performed unless local anesthetic blocks suggest that the pain could potentially improve if the peripheral focus was eliminated. Unfortunately, pain relief during anesthetic blocks does not predict successful outcomes from surgery.

The surgical approaches applied in the management of peripheral painful mononeuropathies usually address etiologic factors, such as release of entrapment, decompression of a nerve root, or resection of a neuroma. Procedures to denervate the painful part, such as neurectomy or rhizotomy, are rarely considered.

Invasive neurostimulatory approaches, such as dorsal column stimulation, do not damage neural tissue and may be a reasonable step in selected patients with refractory painful mononeuropathy. As with other types of neuropathic pain, the use of invasive neurostimulatory procedures should be considered only by experienced practitioners capable of providing a comprehensive assessment of the patient and expertise in the implementation of the technique.

KEY POINTS

1. Both peripheral and central nervous system mechanisms may be responsible for neuropathic pain conditions.

2. Identifying as specifically as possible the etiology of the neuropathic pain syndrome may lead to more effective treatment.

3. Numerous therapies, including pharmacologic, interventional, and physiatric, are available for the treatment of neuropathic pain.

BIBLIOGRAPHY

1. Gilron I, Bailey JM, Tu D, Holden RR, Weaver DF, Houlden RL: Morphine, gabapentin, or their combination for neuropathic pain, *N Engl J Med* 352:1324-1334, 2005.

2. Oxman MN, Levin MJ, Johnson GR, et al: A vaccine to prevent herpes zoster and postherpetic neuralgia in older adults, *N Engl J Med* 352:2271-2284, 2005.

3. Pappagallo M, editor: *The neurological basis of pain*, New York, 2005, McGraw-Hill.

4. Portenoy RK: Neuropathic pain. In Portenoy RK, Kanner RM, editors: *Pain management: theory and practice*, Philadelphia, 1996, F.A. Davis, pp 83-125.

5. Robinson JN, Sandom J, Chapman PT: Efficacy of pamidronate in complex regional pain syndrome type I, *Pain Med* 5(3):276-280, 2004.

6. Singleton JR: Evaluation and treatment of painful peripheral polyneuropathy, *Semin Neurol* 25:185-195, 2005.

7. Stacey BR: Management of peripheral neuropathic pain, *Am J Phys Med Rehabil* 84(Suppl 3):4-16, 2005.

8. Wilson P, Stanton-Hicks M, Harden RN, editors: *CRPS: current diagnosis and therapy*, Seattle, 2005, IASP Press.

PSYCHOLOGICAL SYNDROMES

Dennis R. Thornton, PhD, and Charles E. Argoff, MD

CHAPTER 29

1. **Which psychiatric disorders are associated with chronic pain?**
   Pain may be the chief complaint in a number of psychiatric disorders; conversely, pain can lead to disturbing psychological symptoms. Pain is often the presenting symptom in somatoform disorders. Most patients experiencing chronic pain report depressive symptoms at some point during the course of their condition. Pain is rarely the presenting symptom of a delusional disorder. Individuals with chronic pain secondary to accidents, often motor vehicle accidents, may exhibit symptoms of posttraumatic stress disorder. Whereas anxiety is the most common concomitant of acute pain, depression is the overriding symptom in chronic pain. Anxiety may also contribute to fixation on symptoms.

2. **What is the DSM-IV?**
   The *Diagnostic and Statistical Manual of Mental Disorders, Fourth Edition—DSM-IV—*is the official manual of the American Psychiatric Association. Its purpose is to provide a framework for classifying disorders and defining diagnostic criteria for the disorders listed. A multiaxial system is employed to foster systematic and comprehensive assessment of the various clinical domains. Five axes are described; the first three relate to clinical diagnoses.
   Axis I: Clinical disorders and other clinical conditions that may be the focus of clinical attention
   Axis II: Personality disorders and mental retardation
   Axis III: General medical conditions
   Axis IV: Psychosocial and environmental problems
   Axis V: Global assessment of functioning
   Of note is the fact that the *DSM* has recently undergone revisions, and some changes are relevant to the field of pain.

DEPRESSIVE DISORDERS

3. **Is there an association between chronic pain and depression?**
   Depression is considered to be the most common emotional response to persistent pain. However, accurate assessment may be difficult. Significant depressive symptoms are present in 30% to 87% of patients with chronic pain, and about 35% of chronic pain patients meet criteria for a major depressive episode. Insomnia, difficulty with concentration, and generalized fatigue are reported in 34% to 53% of patients not meeting stringent criteria for a major depressive disorder. Patients most often ascribe such symptoms as secondary to their pain, rather than as true depression, leading to false negatives in the statistical analysis of incidence of depression.

4. **What is the cause-and-effect relationship between pain and depression?**
   The cause-and-effect relationship between pain and depression is undetermined. Rates of depressive symptoms are consistently higher among populations of chronic pain patients (CPP).

However, there have been few studies comparing the incidence of depressive symptoms in CPP with incidence in other populations of chronically ill medical patients.

Clinicians and researchers continue to debate which comes first, depression or chronic pain. Those adhering to a "pain prone" or "masked depression" (see Question 6) orientation have proposed that underlying depressive symptomatology is expressed through pain behavior. Proponents of the diathesis-stress perspective believe that the physical and psychological stress of the chronic pain experience contributes to the development of depressive symptoms.

One fact is certain: it is difficult to assess depression in patients with pain.

5. **Name some impediments to the accurate assessment of depression in chronic pain populations.**

Several issues lead to underdiagnosis of depressive symptoms. Physicians and patients often ascribe the loss of energy, decreased interest, disrupted sleep pattern, appetite disturbance, and social withdrawal to a normal reaction to severe pain and disability. Prolonged duration of these symptoms, however, may be indicative of a depressive syndrome. Patients may become defensive talking about their feelings because of societal stigmas regarding mental illness and may be reluctant to portray themselves as "weak." Finally, shifting the focus to psychological issues may be threatening for the patient, because of fear that the examiner will conclude that the pain complaints are secondary to depression and not "organic" in nature.

6. **Are chronic pain syndromes a physical manifestation of a "masked depression"?**

Traditional psychoanalytic theory postulated that pain could be a face-saving means of expressing underlying depressive symptomatology; hence, a masked depression. Individuals with such interpsychic dynamics had been labeled as "pain-prone personalities." This has been a pervading construct, and it continues to have supporters.

However, more recent research and literature reviews point to depressive symptoms emerging as a consequence of the experience of chronic pain. The day-to-day burdens of chronic pain have been described as "major fateful events" that result in great psychological distress and significant, negative changes in lifestyle. Individuals with a biological predisposition for depression (the "scar hypothesis") may be more vulnerable to the development of depressive symptoms as their condition worsens. In short, there is movement away from the idea of pain-prone personalities.

7. **Is there a possible physiological construct that would explain the diathesis-stress hypothesis?**

In animal models, chronic pain paradigms are associated with activation of the hypothalamo-pituitary-adrenal axis. Chronic pain acts as an "inescapable stress." The inability to avoid or escape from stress promotes learned helplessness and is associated with depressive symptoms.

8. **What are the diagnostic criteria for a major depressive disorder?**

To be diagnosed with a major depressive disorder, the patient needs to have experienced five of the following over at least a 2-week period, and occurring nearly every day: depressed/sad mood, markedly diminished interest or pleasure, significant weight loss or gain, insomnia or hypersomnia, psychomotor agitation or retardation, fatigue, feelings of worthlessness or excessive or inappropriate guilt, diminished cognitive abilities, recurrent thoughts of death, or suicidal ideation. These symptoms should not be better accounted for by another psychiatric disorder, medical illness, or reaction to medication. There is no history of a manic episode. These symptoms should represent a change from the patient's previous affective state.

9. **How does the *DSM-IV* address psychological symptoms in patients with physical illness?**

In *DSM-III-R* the focus was on psychological disturbance, and symptoms "clearly due to a physical condition" were not included. This stipulation has been eliminated from the *DSM-IV*. Therefore, more individuals with chronic pain syndromes may meet criteria for specific psychiatric disorders.

10. **What is the relationship between chronic pain and suicide risk?**
The relationship between chronic pain and suicide risk is multifaceted. Consider the following:
   - Chronic pain and illness contribute to depressive symptoms.
   - Chronic medical illness has been labeled a motivating factor in approximately 25% of all suicides. The experience of chronic pain is likely to be a significant factor in promoting suicide ideation and attempts.
   - Depressive symptoms and suicide are strongly associated.
   - 45% to 70% of completed suicides have a history of mood disorder.
   - Concomitant psychiatric syndromes can impair adjustment to the impact of chronic pain.
   - 25% of patients with at least one general medical illness report suicidal ideation, and 9% are reported to have made a suicide attempt.
   - Some surveys have suggested that up to 50% of patients with chronic nonmalignant pain have contemplated suicide at some point.
   - Pain that is either inadequately controlled or poorly tolerated further increases risk.
   - The duration of pain may increase risk.
   - Lack of social supports also increases vulnerability to suicidal ideation and attempts.
   - A personal and/or family history of substance abuse puts the patient at greater risk.
   - Passive and other maladaptive coping strategies are reflective of, and contribute to, a greater sense of helplessness and hopelessness.
   - Because many pain patients view themselves as disabled by their pain, often with little hope for improvement, they are at risk for affective disorders and suicidal potential.
   - Good work status decreases suicidal risk, whereas the loss of employment increases vulnerability.

11. **Do chronic pain patients acknowledge their depression and suicidal feelings?**
Willingness of any individual to confide depression, suicidal feelings, or other disturbing emotions depends on a variety of factors. One survey, conducted by a pain self-help organization, found that patients with nonmalignant pain reported that depression was among the most disturbing aspects of the chronic pain experience. Fifty percent of these individuals commented that profound feelings of hopelessness had led them to consider suicide.
   Clearly, the development of trust within the doctor-patient relationship is a key factor in providing the patient with a sense of personal safety to acknowledge feelings of desperation. The degree of depression will mediate both suicidal intent and willingness to disclose. Research has documented that suicide intent among chronic pain patients is relatively low in comparison to psychiatric populations. Should a patient express intent, it is essential that immediate action be taken to prevent self-injury.

12. **Are there data on suicide completion within the chronic pain population?**
Although it is generally felt that the chronic pain population is at significant risk for suicide, there is a dearth of literature on the subject. White men and women, aged 35 to 64 years and receiving workers' compensation for pain, were shown to be at two to three times greater risk for suicide than the general population. However, this rate was significantly lower than that seen in a psychiatric population. Despite the study limitations, the authors concluded that CPP are at significant risk for suicide.

13. **What depressive symptoms are seen in patients with chronic pain, even without true depression?**
CPPs commonly experience a significant decrease in their level of energy. Pain is physically and psychologically wearing, and analgesic, antidepressant medications and a more sedentary lifestyle can contribute to fatigue. Sleep disturbances are also quite common, with individuals experiencing difficulty falling asleep or being awakened during the night because of pain.

Pain and/or medication may impair concentration and decrease energy. Irritability, frustration, and dysphoria can parallel the level of pain.

14. **What is dysthymia?**
Dysthymic disorder refers to persistent, low-level, depressive feelings. It appears to be fairly common among chronic pain patients. These individuals tend to view the "glass as half empty" and describe their mood as "blue" or "down in the dumps" more often than not. Characteristics of dysthymia include long-standing lack of interest in anything, low self-esteem, and a propensity for self-criticism. Dysthymic patients describe their pessimistic outlook as normal for them (egosyntonic). Major depressive episodes are a marked departure from the patient's normal euthymic mood. Depressed patients describe their pessimistic outlook as abnormal (egodystonic).

15. **List the diagnostic criteria for dysthymic disorder.**
The following are the diagnostic criteria for dysthymic disorder:
- Over at least a 2-year period, a depressed mood is present more often than not, i.e., most of the day and most days.
- While depressed, two or more of the following occur:
  - Poor appetite or overeating
  - Insomnia or hypersomnia
  - Low energy or fatigue
  - Low self-esteem
  - Poor concentration or difficulty making decisions
  - Feelings of hopelessness
- Over the 2-year period, symptoms have not been absent for more than 2 months.
- The syndrome is not better accounted for by a major depressive episode, nor has such an episode occurred during the first 2 years of the symptoms.
- No history of a manic episode.
- Symptoms do not occur during the course of a psychotic disorder.
- Symptoms are not better accounted for by medication effects or secondary to a general medical condition.
- Significant occupational, social, or other impairment results from the symptoms.

16. **What are adjustment disorders?**
The term "adjustment disorder" applies to patients who do not meet criteria for dysthymia or major depressive disorder, but seem to be having significant difficulty coping. The diagnostic criteria are as follows:
- Emotional or behavioral disturbance developing in reaction to an identified stressor and occurring within 3 months of the onset of the stressor.
- The syndrome is of clinical significance as noted by:
  - Distress excessive to that expected by exposure to such a stressor, and/or
  - Impairment in social, occupational, or life sphere functioning
- Stress-related disturbance not better accounted for by another Axis I diagnosis or is an exacerbation of a preexisting disorder.
- Symptoms do not represent bereavement.
- Upon cessation of the stressor, symptoms resolve within a 6-month period.

ANXIETY DISORDERS

17. **What is the association between anxiety and pain?**
Anxiety is most closely associated with acute injury and pain. Autonomic signs (the "flight-or-fight" response) and emotional distress commonly appear together. Anxiety may also be associated with chronic pain and is often mixed with depressive symptoms.

18. **How can anxious and depressive feelings influence the clinical presentation of pain complaints?**

The emergency department (ED) is a setting in which anxiety symptoms and other disorders play a significant role in the patient's presentation. In one study, 35% of patients with acute chest pain to an urban ED were identified as displaying significant signs of panic (17.5%) or depression (23.1%). No difference in the prevalence of panic was observed between those with or without acute cardiac ischemia. Both panic and depression increased the likelihood of previous ED visits, and the authors concluded that about one in three patients going to the ED with acute pain reports symptoms consistent with a psychiatric disorder.

19. **What are the core features of a panic disorder?**

The quintessential feature of a panic disorder is the unanticipated panic attack, often described as coming "out of the blue." At least two attacks are needed to meet criteria for panic disorder, and they are followed by protracted concern about experiencing additional attacks or the implications of the attacks. The concern continues for at least 1 month. Patients may seek medical reassurance, request tests, and report that they feel like they are "going crazy." If significant avoidance behaviors develop, the patient may meet criteria for panic disorder with agoraphobia.

20. **Is general anxiety disorder (GAD) also associated with the pain experience?**

Yes. GAD has been associated with the presentation of somatic complaints, pain in particular. A fairly high incidence of anxiety has been noted within chronic pain inpatient programs. However, little work has been done to assess the prevalence of anxiety disorders among CPPs being treated on an outpatient basis.

21. **What are the primary diagnostic criteria for GAD?**

Patients with GAD experience persistent and excessive worry or nervousness. Symptoms continue for 6 months and are present nearly all the time. The patient is unable, or finds it difficult, to control these concerns. To be diagnosed as GAD, anxiety must be accompanied by at least three of the following: restlessness, fatigue, difficulty concentrating, irritability, muscle tension, or sleep disturbance. Symptoms are not better ascribed to another Axis I diagnostic category nor a consequence of an underlying medical condition. Distress and any associated physical symptoms result in significant disruption of functioning.

POSTTRAUMATIC STRESS DISORDERS

22. **Is there an association between posttraumatic stress disorder (PTSD) and chronic pain syndromes?**

Posttraumatic stress disorder (PTSD; previously called "shell shock" or "battle fatigue") was a sequela of intense combat and war situations. However, increasing evidence shows that civilians can be subject to symptoms of PTSD, which may follow motor-vehicle accidents, work-related injuries, or violent crime. Pain is a common concomitant of the disorder.

23. **What are the essential clinical features of *DSM-IV* diagnostic criteria for PTSD?**

The following are the clinical features of the *DSM-IV* diagnostic criteria for PTSD:
  - Experiencing, being exposed to, or confronted with a traumatic event in which serious harm or the threat of harm was present and the individual experienced an intense emotional reaction of fear, hopelessness, or horror
  - Reexperience of the event through intrusive distressing recollections, disturbing dreams, flashbacks, intense emotional and/or physical distress upon reexposure to symbolic cues
  - Persistent avoidance of symbolic stimuli and general psychic numbing, which manifest in such forms as avoidance of feelings, discussions, or exposure to stimuli related to the

trauma; amnesia for aspects of the trauma; diminished interest or detachment; restricted affect, and foreshortened future
- Symptoms of increased arousal, e.g., sleep disturbance, irritability, impaired concentration, hypervigilance, and an exaggerated startle response
- Symptom duration of more than 1 month
- Significant impairment of functioning

24. What symptoms are likely in patients with both PTSD and chronic pain?
Patients with both PTSD and chronic pain are likely to experience social fears, anxiety, and somatic focus.

25. Do symptoms of PTSD occur commonly among patients with chronic pain?
Yes. Roughly 10% to 33% of chronic pain patients who were involved in motor-vehicle accidents (MVAs) display significant symptoms of PTSD within the first year of their accident. Psychophysiological reactivity, other medical complications, and litigation may retard remission of symptoms. About one third of chronic pain patients who suffered work-related injuries meet criteria for PTSD, and an additional 18% experience some PTSD-related symptoms.

Compared to those without symptoms of PTSD, those meeting criteria had a greater tendency to suppress their anger, were more depressed, and were more likely to have had a premorbid history of headaches. Individuals who had past histories of anxiety or disorders appear more likely to develop driving-related phobias than those without such histories.

26. What are the implications of PTSD in regard to chronic pain?
The early phases of treatment following accidents and injuries are most often focused on the medical and physical aspects, with the assumption that physical healing will allow for full recovery. Psychological trauma may go unnoticed, and functional progress may slow. Closer inquiry may reveal underlying anxieties, painful recollections, and emotional withdrawal. Patients may state that they no longer drive because of physical discomfort, but fail to mention the stress associated with driving. Providing support and informing patients that these psychological sequelae are not uncommon among pain patients will help them convey their fears, so that appropriate support can be provided.

27. Are there specific treatments for pain patients with symptoms of PTSD?
Systematic desensitization is a behavioral technique that is quite successful treating phobias. It has achieved good results when applied to pain patients with PTSD. The underlying premise is that you cannot be relaxed and anxious at the same time. The patient is taught relaxation and other coping strategies to foster a state of physical relaxation and inner calm and self-efficacy. The patient is then gradually exposed to the feared object.

28. Does domestic violence place a woman at higher risk for PTSD or a chronic pain syndrome?
Yes. Domestic violence puts a woman at higher risk for PTSD or a chronic pain syndrome. Battering is an assault on the entire being. Constant fear, degradation, and lack of control and power, coupled with the physical pain and injury, have a devastating effect on self-esteem and sense of identity. This continuous state of siege constitutes a unique trauma that can result in a plethora of psychological and somatic syndromes. Depression and posttraumatic stress disorder are commonly observed in this population. Pain complaints, both acute and chronic, may represent a guarded secret of conflict and a sense of helplessness.

29. What approach should the clinician take when domestic violence is suspected?
Suspected domestic violence is undoubtedly a delicate situation where empathy and communication can go a long way. The most practical and effective way to address this problem is to establish the habit of routinely asking all women patients about their home life and

violence. Systematic questioning eases the process for the clinician and ensures that the necessary questions are posed; such smooth handling then fosters a sense of safety and acceptance in the patient, allowing her to share her experiences. The clinician should avoid insinuating guilt or laying blame.

FACTITIOUS DISORDERS

30. **What is Munchausen syndrome?**
    Munchausen syndrome is the label given to a subpopulation of individuals diagnosed with a factitious disorder (*DSM-IV*). The stereotypic portrait is of a lifelong history of somatic complaints, attempts to be admitted into hospitals, and requests for tests. Pain complaints often include severe right lower quadrant pain associated with nausea and vomiting, dizziness and blacking out, massive hemoptysis, generalized rashes and abscesses, fever of undetermined origin, bleeding secondary to ingestion of anticoagulants, and lupuslike syndromes. Patients often display considerable sophistication in presenting medical facts and treatments. Symptoms may be inconsistent with pathology; additional symptoms may spontaneously emerge during the interview; and symptoms are presented with a dramatic flair. This syndrome is uncommon, and a prevalence of 0.14% has been cited in a series of patients with chronic pain.

31. **List the four types of factitious disorder.**
    The following are the four types of factitious disorder:
    - Predominantly psychological signs and symptoms
    - Predominantly physical signs and symptoms
    - Combined psychological and physical signs and symptoms
    - Factitious disorder not otherwise specified

32. **What are the diagnostic criteria for factitious disorders?**
    The diagnostic criteria for factitious disorders are as follows:
    - The patient intentionally produces or feigns physical or psychological signs or symptoms.
    - The motivation for the behavior is to assume the sick role.
    - External incentives for the behavior (such as receiving economic gain, avoiding legal responsibility, or improving physical well-being, as in malingering) are absent.

33. **What is the major distinction of the factitious disorder?**
    Individuals with factitious disorders intentionally feign either psychological or physical symptoms to assume the sick role. These acts are voluntary in that the behaviors are purposeful and deliberate. However, they are performed with a degree of compulsivity, denoting the underlying psychopathology and an inability to curb such actions.

34. **Differentiate factitious disorder and malingering.**
    The difference between factitious disorder and malingering lies in motivation. Although both are intentional behaviors, the malingerer is motivated by external factors rather than an unconscious need to maintain the sick role. This motivational factor also distinguishes malingering from conversion disorder or other somatoform disorders. Because of the conscious and intentional nature of the behaviors, malingering is not considered a psychiatric disorder.

SOMATOFORM DISORDERS

35. **What are the somatoform disorders? Which are most common in chronic pain patients?**
    Patients with somatoform disorders express their unconscious conflicts as physical complaints (i.e., they "somatize"). In contrast to malingering, the disorders in this category are

considered manifestations of unconscious processes rather than a conscious effort to deceive. These symptoms must be of such severity as to interfere with occupational, social, or interpersonal functioning or prompt the patient to seek and receive medical attention. The most relevant somatoform disorders for chronic pain patients are somatization disorder, conversion disorder, pain disorder, and hypochondriasis.

36. **What essential features do pain-related somatoform disorders share?**
In all pain-related somatoform disorders, pain is the predominant feature and causes distress sufficient to interfere with daily functioning and warrants seeking medical attention. Additionally, the patient usually spends considerable time, effort, and money looking for the physician who will have the "cure," despite the report of negative or minimal findings, failed interventions, or repeated declarations that nothing more can be done to resolve the underlying problem.

37. **What are the *DSM-IV* diagnostic criteria for somatization disorder?**
Somatization disorder was initially based on literature describing Briquet's syndrome. The new criteria are as follows:
   ■ A history of multiple somatic complaints that began prior to age 30 and have persisted over a number of years. Symptoms have resulted in social or occupational dysfunction and prompted the patient to seek medical treatment.
   ■ At some point during the course of illness, the patient must report experiencing the following: four pain symptoms, two gastrointestinal symptoms, one sexual symptom, and one pseudoneurological symptom.
   ■ With the benefit of appropriate medical workup, there is either:
      (a). No known medical explanation for symptoms, or
      (b). If a medical condition is identified, the symptoms, complaints, and impairment are excessive to the norm.
   ■ Symptoms are not feigned as in fictitious disorders or intentionally manufactured as in malingering.

38. **What are the *DSM-IV* diagnostic criteria for pain disorder?**
The *DSM-IV* diagnostic criteria for pain disorder are as follows:
   ■ Pain is the prominent symptom, present in one or more areas of the body and of sufficient severity for the individual to seek medical attention.
   ■ Impairment of clinical significance is experienced in social and occupational life spheres.
   ■ Psychological factors are viewed as instrumental in the onset, course, and/or exacerbation of the pain complaint.
   ■ Pain is not produced intentionally.
   ■ The pain symptom is not better accounted for by another mental disorder.
   Also note that pain disorder may be acute or chronic, and may be associated with psychological factors alone or with both psychological factors and a general medical condition.

39. **What are the *DSM-IV* diagnostic criteria for hypochondriasis?**
The following are the *DSM-IV* diagnostic criteria for hypochondriasis:
   ■ Patient is preoccupied with the belief or fear of having a serious illness, which is assumed because of misinterpretation of body sensations.
   ■ Patient is not dissuaded by appropriate reassurances.
   ■ Belief is not of delusional intensity.
   ■ Significant social and occupational impairment occurs in response to the intense distress.
   ■ Symptoms persist for at least 6 months.
   ■ Preoccupation is not better accounted for by another mental disorder.

40. **Are pain patients likely to display symptoms of a conversion disorder?**
Chronic pain patients may experience nonanatomic sensory symptoms (anesthesias and paresthesias). These symptoms have been noted among individuals said to be suffering from

"compensation neurosis" and are cited as the third most frequent symptom following depression and anxiety. These types of nonanatomic sensory abnormalities have been found in 24% to 50% of injured workers applying for compensation or Social Security disability. Male and female compensation patients appear equally likely to meet criteria for conversion disorder.

41. What are the *DSM-IV* criteria for conversion disorder?
The following are the *DSM-IV* diagnostic criteria for conversion disorder:
- Symptoms affect voluntary motor or sensory modalities, suggesting a neurologic or medical condition.
- Initiation and/or exacerbation of symptoms is associated with stressors or conflicts implicating psychological influence.
- Symptoms are not intentionally produced.
- Symptom pattern is not adequately explained by known medical condition or culturally sanctioned behavior.
- Symptoms cause significant distress and disruption in function and prompt the patient to seek medical attention.
- Symptoms are not limited to pain or sexual dysfunction and are not better described as part of a somatization or other mental disorder.

42. Why is the somatizing patient difficult to treat?
Somatizing patients do not recognize the effect of their emotions. Although the onset of the symptoms may have occurred during a stressful period, this connection tends to be denied or forgotten by the patient. The symptoms may allow the patient to ignore or deny the underlying conflict (primary gain). Individuals with a high degree of conversion are convinced that they are ill (disease conviction), show few signs of dysphoria ("la belle indifference"), and tend to deny and/or minimize life problems while focusing on physical symptoms.

43. Are chronic pain patients vulnerable to dependence on prescribed medications?
Chronic pain patients are no more vulnerable to dependence on prescribed medications than are any other patients. Severe and persistent pain prompts patients to seek virtually any means that will bring relief. Analgesic medications are commonly employed and are appropriate for treating acute pain. There has been controversy regarding the continued use of analgesic medications, particularly opioids, in individuals with chronic nonmalignant pain syndromes. Although a small percentage of pain patients purposefully seek strong analgesics for the euphoric effects, this is not the rule, and true addiction is unusual.

44. What determines substance dependence?
Current diagnostic criteria for substance dependence include a maladaptive use pattern over a 12-month period that results in functional impairment and distress manifested by three or more of the following:
- Tolerance
  - Increasing amounts of the substance are needed to achieve the initial effect.
  - The patient experiences markedly diminished effect from the same amount.
- Withdrawal
  - Characteristic withdrawal symptoms if substance is stopped abruptly.
  - Withdrawal symptoms are eased or eliminated with reinstitution of substance.
- Substance is used in greater amounts or for a longer duration than originally intended.
- Persistent desire or unsuccessful efforts to curb or discontinue use.
- Excessive time is spent in efforts to obtain or recover from the use of the given substance.
- Occupational, social, and recreational activities are sacrificed because of substance use.
- Despite acknowledgment of ill effects, substance use is continued.

KEY POINTS

1. Many different psychological syndromes have chronic pain associated with them, including depressive disorders, anxiety disorders, posttraumatic stress disorders, factitious disorders, and somatoform disorders.

2. A precise causal relationship between depressive disorders and chronic pain has not been established.

3. Patients with chronic pain are no more vulnerable to dependence on prescribed medications than other patients.

BIBLIOGRAPHY

1. American Psychiatric Association: *Diagnostic and statistical manual of mental disorders*, 4th ed, text revision, Washington, DC, 2000, American Psychiatric Association.

2. Asmundson GJ, et al: Posttraumatic stress disorder and work-related injury, *J Anxiety Dis* 12(1):57-69, 1998.

3. Benjamin D, Pincus H: Suicidal ideation and suicide attempts in general medical illness, *Arch Int Med* 160(10):122-1526, 2000.

4. Blackburn-Munro G, Blackburn-Munro RE: Chronic pain, chronic stress and depression: coincidence or consequence? *J Neuroendocrinol* 13(12):1009-1023, 2001.

5. Chibnall JT, Duckro PN: Post-traumatic stress disorder in chronic post-traumatic headache patients, *Headache* 34(6):357-361, 1994.

6. Dohrenwend BP, et al: Why is depression comorbid with chronic myofascial face pain? A family study test of alternative hypotheses, *Pain* 83:183-192, 1999.

7. Fishbain DA, Cutler RB, Rosomoff RS, Rosomoff HL: The problem-oriented psychiatric examination of the chronic pain patient and its application to the litigation consultation, *Clin J Pain* 10:28-51, 1994.

8. Fishbain DA, et al: Chronic pain-associated depression: antecedent or consequence of chronic pain? A review, *Clin J Pain* 13(2):116-137, 1997.

9. Fishbain DA: The association of chronic pain and suicide, *Semin Clini Neuropsychiatr* 4(3):221-227, 1999.

10. Fisher BJ, et al: Suicidal intent in patients with chronic pain, *Pain* 89(2-3):199-206, 2001.

11. Hitchcock LS, Ferrell BR, McCaffrey M: The experience of chronic nonmalignant pain, *J Pain Symptom Manage* 9(5):312-318, 1994.

12. Kuch K, Cox BJ, Evans RJ: Posttraumatic stress disorder and motor vehicle accidents: a multidisciplinary overview, *Can J Psychiatr* 41(7):429-434, 1997.

13. Simmonds MJ, Kumar S, Lechelt E: Psychosocial factors in disabling low back pain: causes or consequences, *Disabil Rehabil* 18(4):161-168, 1996.

14. Smith PH, Gittelman DK: Psychological consequences of battering: implications for women's health and medical practice, *N C Med J* 55(9):434-439, 1994.

15. Wilson KG, Mikail SF, D'Eon JL, Minns JE: Alternative diagnostic criteria for major depressive disorder in patients with chronic pain, *Pain* 91(3):227-234, 2001.

PAIN IN CHILDREN

Patricia A. McGrath, PhD, and Stephen C. Brown, MD, FRCP

CHAPTER 30

1. What types of pain do children experience?

Like adults, children can experience many different types of pain throughout their lives: acute pain caused by disease or trauma; acute pain and heightened emotional distress caused by repeated invasive medical procedures; recurrent episodes of headache, stomachache, or limb pain unrelated to disease; and chronic pain caused by injury, disease, psychological factors, or of unknown etiology.

However, the prevalence of certain types of pain is different for adults and children. For example, chronic back pain is a major problem for adults but not for children. Common pain problems for children include chronic headache, complex regional pain syndrome–type 1, and variants of pain and somatization disorder. Although the prevalence of these pains increases throughout childhood, few epidemiological studies have been conducted on chronic pain in children. Thus, little is known about the pathophysiology and the prevalence of different types of chronic pain; the children most vulnerable to develop chronic pain according to age, sex, ethnicity, personality; and individual risk and prognostic factors.

2. How do children's pain experiences differ from those of adults?

Results from neurodevelopmental studies in animals and clinical studies in humans show clear developmental differences in pain sensitivity because of the increased plasticity of children's nociceptive systems. Newborn infants are more sensitive to painful stimuli than adults. Children report stronger pain for stimuli that evoke moderate tissue damage in comparison to adults.

Also, children's pain perceptions differ from those of adults because of developmental changes in their understanding and previous pain experiences. As children mature they experience a wider diversity of pains varying in location, intensity, and quality. Like adults, the nature and diversity of children's pain experience form their frame of reference for perceiving any new pain and for evaluating its aversive significance. Yet, unlike adults who have generally a wide frame of reference of pain experience, children's frames of reference change considerably as they mature and sustain more diverse types of tissue damage. Thus, even a mild level of tissue damage may evoke strong pain if the type of tissue damage is a new pain experience for a child or the maximum that the child has experienced.

3. What is plasticity?

Like adults, children can experience pain without tissue injury or any apparent injury at all. They can also sustain injury without experiencing pain and can experience very different pains from the same type of tissue damage. Children's nociceptive systems are plastic in that they have the capacity to respond differently to the same amount of tissue damage.

We now know that children's perceptions of pain depend on complex neural interactions. Impulses generated by tissue damage are modified both by ascending systems activated by a noxious stimulus (e.g., touch) and by descending pain suppressing systems activated by various situational factors, such as a child's expectations about what he or she will feel.

4. **What myths have complicated our management of children's pain?**
The following myths have complicated our management of children's pain:
- Infants have immature nervous systems and do not feel pain. (They do.)
- Untreated acute pain has no long-term adverse effects. (It does.)
- Children are at a higher risk of drug addiction when they receive opioids for pain control. (They are not.)
- Health professionals cannot measure pain in children. (They can.)
- Children do not suffer from chronic pain. (They do.)

5. **How do you assess pain in infants?**
From birth, infants exhibit an array of distress behaviors (e.g., cries, facial expressions, withdrawal behaviors) and physiological reactions (e.g., changes in heart rate, blood pressure, oxygen level) in response to tissue damage. Health care providers assess pain by carefully monitoring these distress indices.

Several pain scales that can be used for children, including infants (Table 30-1 and Figs. 30-1 and 30-2), comprised of itemized lists of the various distress behaviors, have been designed to more specifically assess pain intensity. Clinicians complete these scales by observing infants for a specified period, noting which behaviors occur, and ranking their intensity on a 0-4 scale. The greater the number and intensity of distress signals, the greater the pain level.

TABLE 30-1. VERBAL DESCRIPTOR SCALES TO ASSESS PAIN INTENSITY FOR CHILDREN

Pain Intensity for Children 7 Years of Age and Older	Pain Intensity for Children Younger Than 7 Years of Age
No pain	None
Mild pain	A little bit
Moderate pain	A medium amount
Strong pain	A lot
Intense pain	A real lot

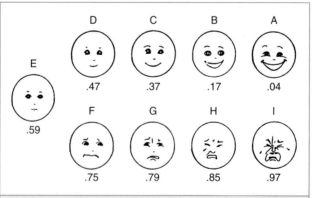

Figure 30-1. Facial affective scale to assess pain affect. (From McGrath PA: *Pain in children: nature, assessment and treatment,* New York, 1990, Guilford Press, with permission.)

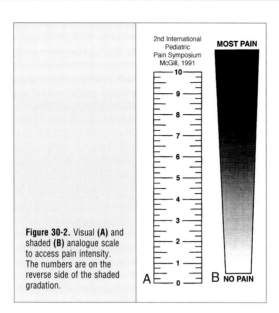

Figure 30-2. Visual **(A)** and shaded **(B)** analogue scale to access pain intensity. The numbers are on the reverse side of the shaded gradation.

6. **How do you assess pain in children?**
Several behavioral pain scales have been designed for children, as well as infants. The majority are more appropriate for use with children aged 6 to 10 than with adolescents, because adolescents usually display different and more subtle distress behaviors. Because a child's pain behaviors naturally vary in relation to the type of pain experienced, different behavioral scales must be used for children with acute, recurrent, and chronic pain. Children who are physically or developmentally impaired can be assessed using behavioral scales composed of the subtle cues that parents recognize; these scales are under development.
   By the age of 5, most children can differentiate a wider range of pain intensities and can use many analogue, facial, and verbal rating scales (see Figs. 30-1 and 30-2) to indicate the strength of their pain. Children choose a level on the scale that best matches the strength of their own pain. These scales are easy to administer, requiring only a few seconds once children understand how to use them. Many of these scales yield pain scores on a scale of 0 to 10.

7. **What role does self-report play in assessing pain in children?**
Self-report pain measures potentially provide the most comprehensive information about children's pain. Children can provide essential information about their pain in their own words. Children begin to understand pain through their own hurting experiences; they learn to describe the different characteristics of their pains (intensity, quality, duration, and location) in the same way that they learn specific words to describe different sounds, tastes, smells, and colors. Toddlers begin to communicate the presence of pain, using words learned from their parents to describe the sensations they feel when they hurt themselves. They can point to its general location. Gradually, they learn to distinguish three different levels of pain intensity, such as "a little," "some or medium," and "a lot." Children under age 5 can use facial scales (children's faces depicting different levels of distress) or concrete physical scales (object graded in size, poker chips that represent one to four pieces of hurt) to show how much pain they have.

8. **Which pain assessment tools should be incorporated into routine clinical practice?**

Pain assessment is an integral component of the diagnosis and treatment for children with pain. A thorough medical history, physical examination, and assessment of pain characteristics and contributing factors are necessary to establish a correct clinical diagnosis. Always ask a child directly about his or her pain experience, and obtain objective information about the pattern, intensity, and quality of pain to facilitate an accurate diagnosis. A few structured questions can be easily incorporated within the regular clinical interview. Children can be asked to describe their pain according to its similarity to other sensations they have experienced. In addition, ask children to rate their pain during the course of their medical treatment, using a simple validated scale.

No one pain measure is equally appropriate for all children or for all types of pain. Health care providers who treat a wide range of children's pain problems need a flexible pain measurement inventory consisting of a brief pain interview for general use, a few pain scales (for younger and older children) that children can use in the clinic and at home, and a comprehensive interview (for children with recurrent and chronic pain) to evaluate the factors that can trigger pain episodes, exacerbate pain, or prolong pain-related disability.

9. **Is there a basic treatment algorithm that covers pain control in children?**

Yes. There is a basic treatment algorithm that covers pain control in children. It provides a brief summary of the steps to controlling pain in children (Fig. 30-3). The first step is to assess the child with pain, evaluating not only the primary sensory characteristics of the pain (its quality, intensity, location, duration, and aversive component) but also the extent to which situational factors (cognitive, behavioral, and emotional) may be influencing the child's pain. Direct appropriate physical and medical examinations not only at the primary source of pain but also at secondary sources.

Once a differential diagnosis has been made, the treatment plan for most pains consists of analgesics, adjuvant analgesics, or anesthetic interventions, plus cognitive, physical, and behavioral interventions, to address all of the factors that contribute to the pain.

Children and parents should receive specific feedback on causes and contributing factors as well as the rationale for the treatments selected. Treatment includes measuring children's pain regularly, evaluating the effectiveness of interventions, and revising the plan as necessary. Because the factors that influence a child's pain are dynamic, not static, adjustments must be made to treatment regimens for children who will be experiencing recurrent or long-term pain.

10. **What are the basic guidelines for selecting and administering traditional analgesic drugs?**

Four simple concepts should be followed when administering analgesics to children: (1) by the ladder; (2) by the clock; (3) by the child; (4) by the mouth.

11. **What does "by the ladder" mean?**

"By the ladder" refers to a three-step approach for selecting progressively stronger traditional analgesic drugs (acetaminophen, codeine, or morphine) according to a child's level of pain (mild, moderate, or strong). The approach is based on our scientific understanding of how analgesics affect pain of nociceptive origins. If the child's pain persists despite use of the appropriate drug and recommended dosing schedule, the clinician moves up the ladder to the next most potent analgesic. Even when children require opioid analgesics, they should continue to receive acetaminophen (or nonsteroidal antiinflammatory drugs, if appropriate) as supplemental analgesics.

Recently, attention has focused on "thinking beyond the ladder" and using adjuvant analgesics as the first step for children whose pain has neuropathic origins. Adjuvant analgesics include a variety of drugs with analgesic properties that were initially developed to treat other health problems, such as convulsions and depression. These drugs more specifically target neuropathic mechanisms and are critical analgesics for certain types of pain.

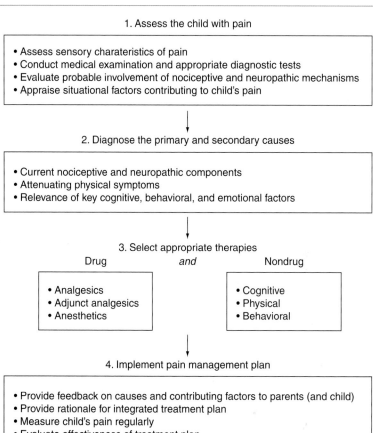

1. Assess the child with pain

- Assess sensory charateristics of pain
- Conduct medical examination and appropriate diagnostic tests
- Evaluate probable involvement of nociceptive and neuropathic mechanisms
- Appraise situational factors contributing to child's pain

↓

2. Diagnose the primary and secondary causes

- Current nociceptive and neuropathic components
- Attenuating physical symptoms
- Relevance of key cognitive, behavioral, and emotional factors

↓

3. Select appropriate therapies

Drug   *and*   Nondrug

- Analgesics
- Adjunct analgesics
- Anesthetics

- Cognitive
- Physical
- Behavioral

↓

4. Implement pain management plan

- Provide feedback on causes and contributing factors to parents (and child)
- Provide rationale for integrated treatment plan
- Measure child's pain regularly
- Evaluate effectiveness of treatment plan
- Revise plan as needed

Figure 30-3. A treatment algorithm for controlling children's pain. (From McGrath PA, Brown SC: Pain control in paediatric palliative care. In Doyle D, Hanks GW, MacDonald N, editors: *Oxford textbook of palliative medicine,* 3rd ed, Oxford, in press, Oxford University Press, with permission.)

12. **Explain the term "by the clock."**

"By the clock" refers to the timing for administering analgesic medications. Analgesics should be administered on a regular schedule, e.g., every 4 or 6 hours, based on the drug's duration of action and the severity of the child's pain, not on an as-needed (PRN) basis, unless a child's episodes of pain are truly intermittent and unpredictable. When PRN dosing is used, children must first experience pain before they can obtain pain relief. These breakthrough episodes of pain can cause serious problems for children who fear that their pain cannot be controlled. Unlike adults, who generally realize that they can demand more potent analgesic medications or demand more frequent dosing intervals, children have little control and little awareness of alternatives, and fear that their pain cannot be controlled. As a result, they may become progressively frightened and upset, so that their pain increases. Moreover, the doses of opioids required to relieve existing or breakthrough pain are higher than those required to prevent the recurrence of pain. Thus, it is essential to establish and maintain a therapeutic window of pain relief for children.

13. **What does "by the child" mean?**
    "By the child" refers to the need to base analgesic doses on each child's individual circumstances. No one analgesic dose will reliably relieve pain for all children who have a similar medical condition or similar level of pain. Instead, children vary with respect to how much of a drug or what type of a drug is required to control their pain. The goal is to select a dose that prevents children from experiencing pain before they receive the next dose. It is essential to monitor a child's pain regularly and adjust analgesic doses as necessary.

    As an example, the effective opioid dose to relieve pain varies widely among different children or in the same child at different times. Some children require massive opioid doses at frequent intervals to control their pain. If such large doses are necessary for effective pain control, and the side effects can be managed by adjunctive medication so that children are comfortable, then the doses are appropriate.

14. **Explain the term "by the mouth."**
    "By the mouth" refers to the oral route of drug administration. Medication should be administered to children by the simplest effective route, usually by mouth. Because children are afraid of injections, they may deny that they have pain or may not request medication. When possible, children should receive medication through routes that do not cause additional pain. Although optimal analgesic administration for children requires flexibility in selecting routes according to children's needs, parenteral administration is often the most efficient route for providing direct and rapid pain relief. Opioid analgesics are less potent when administered orally, rather than parenterally.

15. **Which parenteral routes of administration are relatively pain-free?**
    Because intravenous (IV), intramuscular (IM), and subcutaneous (SQ) routes cause additional pain for children, serious efforts have been expended on developing more pain-free modes of administration that still provide relatively direct and rapid analgesia and on improving the effectiveness of oral routes. Many hospitals have restricted the use of IM injections because they are painful and drug absorption is not reliable; they advocate the use of IV lines into which drugs can be administered directly without causing further pain. Topical anesthetic creams should be applied prior to the insertion of IV lines in children. The use of portacatheters has become the gold standard in pediatrics, particularly for children who require administration of multiple drugs at weekly intervals.

16. **Describe the role of continuous infusion in pain management for children.**
    Continuous infusion has several advantages over intermittent SQ, IM, and IV routes. This method circumvents repetitive injections, prevents delays in analgesic drug administration, and provides continuous levels of pain control without children experiencing increased side effects at peak level and pain breakthroughs at trough levels. Continuous infusion should be considered in the following circumstances: children have pain for which oral and intermittent parenteral opioids do not provide satisfactory pain control; intractable vomiting prevents oral medications; IV lines are not desirable; and children would like to remain at home despite severe pain. Children receiving a continuous infusion should continue to receive "rescue doses" to control breakthrough pain, as necessary.

17. **Can patient-controlled analgesia (PCA) be used in children?**
    Yes. PCA enables children to administer small bolus doses of analgesics when they need extra pain control on top of a background infusion of medication. PCA provides children with a continuum of analgesia that is prompt, economical, and not nurse dependent, and it results in lower overall opioid use. It has a high degree of safety, allows for wide variability between patients, and eliminates delay in analgesic administration.

18. **What is the role of regional techniques in pain control for children?**
Regional techniques (epidural and spinal) for the administration of local anesthetics and analgesics continue to be an integral part of pain control in children. Experience from many centers suggests that these techniques can be extremely useful for children with advanced cancer and resulting pain that may be difficult to control by more conventional means. It is also feasible for children to receive epidural and spinal infusions at home on an extended basis. Although infection is possible, the reported infection rates in several series of cancer patients have been quite low.

Note that when children receive potent analgesics and anesthetics, whether by IV or regional anesthetic techniques, appropriate monitoring is paramount for children's safety. This involves the education and training of staff; immediate availability of resuscitative drugs and equipment; and an accurate and timely pain record consisting of vitals signs and pain and sedation scores.

19. **How do parents know which over-the-counter (OTC) products are safe and effective for children?**
Parents should be advised that many over-the-counter (OTC) analgesic medications have not been specifically evaluated and approved for use in children. The labeling on most drugs states that the product is contraindicated for children less than 16 years of age. Yet, some of these drugs may be extremely beneficial for children. Thus, it is important to consult with physicians who know the differences between prescription and OTC drugs and are able to advise parents on how to use them.

Both the U.S. Food and Drug Administration and the pharmaceutical industry are attending more to the need to develop and evaluate analgesic products specifically for use in infants and children.

20. **How do parents know which complementary and alternative medicines (CAMs) are safe for children?**
An extensive array of nondrug therapies are available to treat children's pain, including counseling, guided imagery, hypnosis, biofeedback, behavioral management, acupuncture, massage, chiropractic manipulation, homeopathic remedies, naturopathic approaches, and herbal medicines. Many such therapies share a "child-centered" focus, addressing the unique causative and contributing factors for each child's pain. Nondrug therapies are generally regarded as safe, with few contraindications for use in healthy children. However, they should not be regarded as equally effective.

21. **How can parents find out about effectiveness of CAMs?**
The evidence base supporting the efficacy of CAMs in pain control varies widely from "unknown" (i.e., they have not been studied) to "promising" (anecdotal reports suggest possible effectiveness for certain children) to "strong and compelling" (consistent positive results have been obtained in several well-designed studies). Strong and consistent evidence supports the efficacy of most cognitive and behavioral therapies for relieving pain in children. However, little pediatric research has been conducted on the other therapies regarded as complementary to traditional medical approaches, despite increasing interest in their use. The evidence supporting efficacy derives primarily from anecdotal and case reports.

The inadequacy of the published information makes it impossible to summarize whether findings are consistently positive. At present, we do not have valid information about the efficacy of most CAMs for children. Note that the lack of evidence about their efficacy does not indicate that these therapies are ineffective, but rather that research is needed.

22. **How are cognitive therapies used in pediatric clinical practice?**

Cognitive therapies are an essential component of pain control because treatment should be directed at all of the causes of children's pain and suffering (Table 30-2). Cognitive therapies are directed at a child's beliefs, expectations, and coping abilities. They encompass a wide range of approaches from basic patient education to formal psychotherapy. Cognitive interventions are the most powerful and versatile nondrug pain therapies for children. A basic cognitive intervention comprises providing children with age-appropriate information about pain and teaching them how to use simple coping strategies. When children receive accurate information about what will happen to them and what they may feel, they can improve their understanding, increase their control, lessen their distress, and reduce their pain. Health care providers should emphasize the sensory aspects (i.e., tingling, cool, sharp) rather than the hurting aspect when they prepare children for invasive procedures.

Distraction and focused attention, as well as guided imagery, are practical tools that health professionals and parents can routinely use when children experience pain. Genuine distraction and attention—when the child's attention is fully absorbed by an activity or topic other than his or her pain—is a very active process that can lessen neuronal responses evoked by tissue damage. Parents and staff members can assist children to concentrate fully on something besides their pain. Music, lights, colored objects, tactile toys, sweet tastes, and other children are effective attention-grabbing stimuli, particularly in young children. Conversation, games, computers, and interesting movies are effective distracters for older children and adolescents.

TABLE 30-2. NONDRUG THERAPIES		
Cognitive	**Behavioral**	**Physical**
Information	Exercise	Massage
Choices and control	Relaxation therapy	Physiotherapy
Distraction and attention	Biofeedback	Thermal stimulation
Guided imagery	Behavioral modification	Sensory stimulation
Hypnosis		TENS
Psychotherapy		Acupuncture

TENS = transcutaneous electrical nerve stimulation.

23. **What is the role of behavioral therapy in pain management for children?**

Behavioral therapies are designed to change either children's own behavior or the behavior of the adults who interact with them. The therapeutic objective is to lessen behaviors that can increase children's pain, distress, and disability, while increasing behaviors that can reduce pain. Progressive muscle relaxation and simple repetitive physical exercise (depending on the patient's preference) are convenient methods for most children to use during painful medical treatments. During stressful treatments, many children seem naturally to tense their muscles and hold their breath. Some children can learn to relax by alternately tightening and loosening their fists, by rhythmically moving a leg, or by deep, paced breathing.

General exercise regimens are an important component of pain management for children experiencing recurrent or persistent pain, as well as for children requiring multiple and repeated painful treatments. The objective is to restore as many of a child's normal activities as possible to provide them with enjoyment, increase their participation in social events, increase their independent pain management, and help them reduce their stress.

24. **What should be done to minimize pain for children experiencing multiple invasive procedures (e.g., bone marrow aspirations, catheter placements, lumbar punctures)?**
It is essential to provide children undergoing invasive procedures with appropriate analgesic or anesthetic treatments, such as topical anesthetic creams before painful needle insertions and sedatives for aversive procedures. However, note that many children prefer not to be sedated, and wish to remain alert and aware. Children can use simple coping strategies to complement the analgesic regimen. Pain can be minimized when children have increased control, increased choice, and accurate information about what will happen. Imagery, distraction, and attention-focusing are valuable tools for many children.

However, the key concept underlying the use of all analgesic and cognitive-behavioral therapies for children is "by the child" (see Question 13). When possible, respect children's preferences for remaining alert or being sedated. Staff can assist the children who prefer to remain alert in learning coping techniques that they can easily use during the procedures.

25. **What are recurrent pain syndromes?**
Like adults, most children—even very young children—experience an occasional headache, stomachache, or diffuse limb pain. However, as many as 40% of otherwise healthy children experience repeated pain episodes. Unlike pain from disease or trauma, the pain itself, rather than an underlying disease, is the problem. After adequate investigation, it is important for parents and children to understand that there is no single source of tissue damage that can be fixed by a single treatment. Instead there are usually multiple causes (Fig. 30-4). Although hereditary factors may predispose certain children to develop pain, other factors may trigger pain episodes, increase pain, prolong disability, or maintain the cycle of repeated episodes.

Typically, several cognitive, behavioral, and emotional factors share a key etiologic role in these pain syndromes. Regardless of some apparent similarity in a child's pain characteristics (e.g., frequency, intensity), certain factors may be primary causes for one child's pain but almost negligible causes for another child's pain. Thus, health care providers must ascertain which factors are relevant for which children.

26. **Describe the treatment approach to recurrent pain syndromes.**
Treatment emphasis in recurrent pain syndromes should shift from a disease-centered focus to a more child-centered focus. The extent to which various cognitive, emotional, behavioral, and familial factors are the primary causes for recurrent pain will determine the particular composition of a multistrategy treatment. Because pharmacologic methods relieve the painfulness of an individual episode but do not generally change the syndrome, an integrated, flexible approach combining physical, behavioral, and cognitive methods should be used. In general, a cognitive-behavioral approach that modifies the primary and secondary contributing factors is most effective for treating children with recurrent pain syndromes.

27. **What is the best approach for treating neuropathic pain in children?**
Neuropathic pain differs from nociceptive pain in that the pain is generated not by ongoing tissue damage, but by changes in the nervous system as a consequence of injury to it (see Chapter 28, Neuropathic Pain). Children's neuropathic pain should be managed from a multimodal perspective, by which they receive appropriate medication, physical therapy, and educational counseling to learn specific pain-reducing strategies. Tricyclic antidepressants and anticonvulsants are the drugs of choice for most children. Sympathetic blocks may be useful for

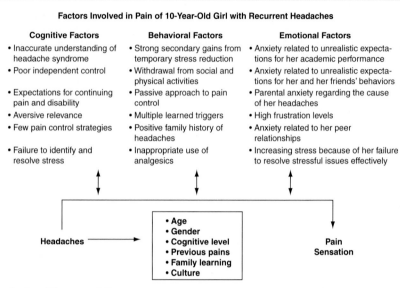

Factors Involved in Pain of 10-Year-Old Girl with Recurrent Headaches

Cognitive Factors	Behavioral Factors	Emotional Factors
• Inaccurate understanding of headache syndrome	• Strong secondary gains from temporary stress reduction	• Anxiety related to unrealistic expectations for her academic performance
• Poor independent control	• Withdrawal from social and physical activities	• Anxiety related to unrealistic expectations for her and her friends' behaviors
• Expectations for continuing pain and disability	• Passive approach to pain control	• Parental anxiety regarding the cause of her headaches
• Aversive relevance	• Multiple learned triggers	• High frustration levels
• Few pain control strategies	• Positive family history of headaches	• Anxiety related to her peer relationships
• Failure to identify and resolve stress	• Inappropriate use of analgesics	• Increasing stress because of her failure to resolve stressful issues effectively

Headaches →
- Age
- Gender
- Cognitive level
- Previous pains
- Family learning
- Culture
→ Pain Sensation

Treatment Recommendations:

1. Assist child in identifying and resolving stressful situations.
2. Teach child to cope more effectively with routine frustrations.
3. Teach parents and child about pain systems, recurrent pain syndromes, and true vs. learned headache triggers.
4. Reduce secondary gains associated with child's pain by providing consistent and nonmaladaptive responses to her pain complaints.
5. Teach child nonpharmacologic methods of pain control, such as muscle relaxation through biofeedback and nonstressful exercise.

Figure 30-4. (From McGrath PA, Hillier LM: Controlling children's pain. In Gatchel R, Turk D, editors: *Psychological treatment for pain,* New York, 1996, Guilford Press, with permission.)

those believed to have sympathetically maintained pain, who fail to progress with a vigorous regimen of physical therapy and cognitive-behavioral treatments.

Many children with neuropathic pain are significantly disabled by pain. They require more specialized therapy to enable them to return to school and to social and physical activities. Their parents will require assistance to understand that the treatment of neuropathic pain is different from that of disease/trauma pain, particularly with respect to the need for children to resume activities rather than wait until the pain, discoloration, or altered sensitivity has resolved completely.

28. **Describe a difficulty particular to neuropathic pain in children.**
Many children develop a disability problem in addition to a pain problem because the protective behaviors appropriate for acute disease or trauma pain can lead to progressive loss of use of the affected limb (e.g., for children with complex regional pain syndrome–type 1) and increasing withdrawal from physical and social activities. When significant disability is present, the pain diagnosis should include both a neuropathic pain condition and a disability problem, so that families understand that they are not inextricably linked. Often families believe that all functional disability is related to the continuing pain, but usually there are distinct factors that are prolonging disability—factors that should be addressed as part of the multimodal pain program. The model (see Fig. 30-3) can be used to list these factors and explain their role to families.

29. **What is the best approach for treating chronic pain in children?**
    Chronic pain generally has multiple causes, often with both nociceptive and neuropathic components, rather than a single cause. Like that of adults, children's chronic pain affects the entire family and must be viewed within a broader context. Pain management is complicated by prolonged emotional suffering, impaired physical functioning, decreased independence, and (often) an uncertain prognosis. Children's chronic pain must be treated from a multidisciplinary perspective.

    Treatment begins with a thorough physical examination, appropriate diagnostic tests, and evaluation of contributing situational factors. Drug therapies, physical therapies, and cognitive-behavioral therapies must be incorporated into a flexible, child-centered program. No single discipline has the expertise to assess and manage chronic pain independently, because the multiple therapies needed to address each of the causes transcend the expertise of any one discipline. Multidisciplinary teams are required to identify the specific causes and to select the best available treatments.

30. **What is pediatric palliative care?**
    A sixteenth-century aphorism defines the essence of pediatric palliative care: "To cure sometimes, to relieve often, to comfort always." The comprehensive care of children includes curative therapies when available, pain and symptom management, and compassionate support for children and their families. It is essential to focus not only on the medical management of children's diseases but also on the psychosocial and spiritual factors that affect children's pain and suffering.

    The goal of palliative care is to achieve the best quality of life for children from the time of diagnosis throughout their life. Pain control is an integral component of pediatric palliative care. Children may experience acute, recurring, or persistent pain caused by invasive procedures, the cumulative effects of toxic therapies, progressive disease, and psychological factors. The pain is often complex with multiple sources, comprised of nociceptive and neuropathic components. In addition, several situational factors usually contribute to children's pain, distress, and disability. Pain control should include regular pain assessments, appropriate analgesics administered at regular dosing intervals, adjunctive drug therapy for symptom and side-effects control, and nondrug interventions to modify the situational factors that can exacerbate pain and suffering. Thus, a multimodal approach is needed to adequately treat pain in children receiving palliative care.

31. **Are there special dosing considerations for neonates and infants?**
    Neonates and infants require the same three categories of analgesic drugs as older children. However, the difference in pharmacokinetics and pharmacodynamics among neonates, preterm infants, and full-term infants warrants special dosing considerations for infants and close monitoring when they receive opioids. Acetaminophen can be safely administered to neonates and infants without concern for hepatotoxicity when given for short courses at the recommended dose (10 to 15 mg/kg) (Table 30-3). The starting doses for opioid analgesics in infants under 6 months of age are one-quarter to one-half the suggested doses. As for children, the dosage and mode of administration of opioids need to be titrated between the degree of analgesia required and a reasonable level of sedation.

32. **What are the guidelines for opioid use in managing pain in children?**
    The following are guidelines for opioid use in managing pain in children:
    1. Pick an appropriate route. For chronic dosing, oral administration is preferred. IV and SQ administration are essentially equivalent. Avoid IM administration because it hurts. Whenever continuous IV infusion is used, hourly PRN rescue doses with short-onset opioids should be available. A rescue dose is usually 50% to 200% of continuous hourly dose. If more than six rescues are necessary in a 24-hour period, increase the hourly infusion rate by the total amount of rescues for the previous 24 hours divided by 24. An alternative is to increase infusion rate by 50%.

TABLE 30-3. NONOPIOID DRUGS		
Drug	Dosage	Comments
Acetaminophen	10-15 mg/kg PO, every 4-6 h	Lacks gastrointestinal and hematological side effects; lacks antiinflammatory effects (may mask infection-associated fever).
Ibuprofen	5-10 mg/kg PO, every 6-8 h	Antiinflammatory activity. Use with caution in patients with hepatic or renal impairment, compromised cardiac function or hypertension (may cause fluid retention, edema), or history of GI bleeding or ulcers (may inhibit platelet aggregation).
Naproxen	10-20 mg/kg/day PO, divided every 12 h	Antiinflammatory activity. Use with caution and monitor closely in patients with impaired renal function. Avoid in patients with severe renal impairment. Dose limit of 1 g/day.
Diclofenac	1 mg/kg PO, every 8-12 h	Antiinflammatory activity. Similar GI, renal, and hepatic precautions as noted above for ibuprofen and naproxen. Dose limit of 50 mg/dose.

GI = gastrointestinal; PO = by mouth.
Note: Increasing the dose of nonopioids beyond the recommended therapeutic level produces a ceiling effect, in that there is no additional analgesia but there are major increases in toxicity and side effects.

2. Pick an appropriate drug.
3. Pick an appropriate dose. If inadequate pain relief and no toxicity at peak onset of opioid action, increase dose in 50% increments.
4. To change opioids: Because of incomplete cross-tolerance, if changing between opioids with short duration of action, start the new opioid at 50% of the calculated equianalgesic dose. Titrate to effect. If changing between opioids from short to long duration of action (i.e., morphine to methadone), start at 25% of equianalgesic dose and titrate to effect.
5. When discontinuing drug or tapering opioids: For anyone receiving opioids for more than 1 week, the dose should be tapered to avoid withdrawal symptoms. Taper by 50% for 2 days, then decrease by 25% every 2 days. When dose is equianalgesic to an oral morphine dose of 0.6 mg/kg/day, it may be stopped. Some patients on opioids for prolonged periods may require much slower tapering.
6. Meperidine is not recommended for chronic use because normeperidine may accumulate. Normeperidine is a toxic metabolite with a long serum half-life that can cause myoclonus, hyperreflexia, and seizures. "Usual" starting doses are often determined empirically.

33. **Discuss opioid-related side effects in children.**
Opioids have no fixed upper dosage limit. The dose can be increased as necessary to maximize pain control, as along as children do not experience dose-limiting side effects (i.e. vomiting, respiratory depression). The goal should be titrating medication either up or down for maximum clinical effect. Side effects must be anticipated and treated aggressively. Because opioids produce physical dependence and tolerance, doses must be increased over time to control

pain. Doses must be adjusted according to the child's need depending on pain severity, prior analgesic medication use, and the bioavailability and drug distribution of the medication.

All opioids have a similar spectrum of side effects. These well-known problems should be anticipated and treated whenever opioids are administered, so that children can receive pain control without suffering untoward effects. Children may not report all side effects (i.e., constipation, dysphoria) voluntarily, so ask them specifically about these problems. Some side effects may resolve within the first 1 to 2 weeks of initiating therapy as the child develops tolerance to them (e.g., nausea, vomiting, and drowsiness). The clinician must educate the patient about these problems and encourage him or her to give the medication an adequate trial. Slow titration may minimize side effects. Other side effects may require aggressive treatment. If side effects persist despite appropriate interventions, conversion to an alternate opioid may be indicated.

34. Are children at particular risk for addiction?
No. The risk of opioid addiction in children has been greatly exaggerated. Although physical dependence—the body's routine and gradual adjustment to the drug so that the body requires the drug on some regular basis—is common, it can be controlled easily by gradual tapering of medication doses. Physical dependence may develop in as short a period as 7 to 10 days. Similarly, tolerance may develop. Tolerance is a pharmacokinetic/pharmacodynamic phenomenon in which progressively higher levels of the drug are required to achieve the same physiologic effect.

Physical dependence and tolerance are very different from addiction. Addiction represents a pattern of drug use in which an individual is wholly absorbed in the compulsive use and procurement of a drug and has a tendency to relapse after withdrawal. Drug dosing continues despite harmful effects. There is no empirical evidence that children receiving opioid analgesics for pain control are at risk for addiction. In contrast, children who do not receive appropriate analgesic medications are probably more at risk for pseudoaddiction by becoming excessively concerned about receiving their next medication dose in the hope that they might eventually relieve their suffering.

35. What is the role of adjuvant medication for children with chronic pain?
Adjuvant medications (see Chapter 37, Adjuvant Analgesics) play a primary role for children suffering persistent pain or pain of neuropathic origins and for children receiving palliative care.

KEY POINTS

1. Pain must be assessed and appropriately treated in children to avoid the consequences of undertreated pain.

2. As many as 40% of otherwise healthy children experience recurrent pain problems such as headache, abdominal pain, and lower limb pain.

3. Special dosing requirements of children need to be considered when treating this population.

BIBLIOGRAPHY

1. Anand KJS, McGrath PJ, editors: *Pain in neonates*, New York, 1993, Elsevier.
2. Apley J: *The child with abdominal pains*, Oxford, 1975, Blackwell Scientific.
3. Bush JP, Harkins SW, editors: *Children in pain: clinical and research issues from a developmental perspective*, New York, 1991, Springer-Verlag.

4. Fitzgerald M, Jennings E: The postnatal development of spinal sensory processing, *Proc Natl Acad Sci* 96:7719-7722, 1999.

5. Galloway KS, Yaster M: Pain and symptom control in terminally ill children, *Pediatr Clin North Am* 47:711-746, 2000.

6. Hansson PT, Fields H, Hill RG, Marchettini P, editors: *Neuropathic pain: pathophysiology and treatment*, Seattle, 2001, IASP Press.

7. Hillier LM, McGrath PA: A cognitive-behavioral program for treating recurrent headache. In McGrath PA, Hillier LM, editors: *The child with headache: diagnosis and treatment*, Seattle, 2001, IASP Press, pp 183-220.

8. Jacox A, Carr DB, Payne R, et al: *Management of cancer pain: clinical practice guideline*, Rockville, MD, 1994, Agency for Health Care Policy and Research, U.S. Department of Health and Human Services, Public Health Service.

9. McGrath PA: Chronic pain in children. In Crombie IK, editor: *The epidemiology of chronic pain*, Seattle, 1999, IASP Press, pp 81-101.

10. McGrath PA: *Pain in children: nature, assessment and treatment*, New York, 1990, Guilford Press.

11. McGrath PA, Brown SC: Pain control in paediatric palliative care. In Doyle D, Hanks GW, MacDonald N, editors: *Oxford textbook of palliative medicine*, 3rd ed, Oxford, in press, Oxford University Press.

12. McGrath PA, Gillespie J: Pain assessment in children and adolescents. In Turk D, Melzack R, editors: *Handbook of pain assessment*, 2nd ed, 2001, New York, Guilford Press, pp 97-118.

13. McGrath PA, Hillier LM, editors: *The child with headache: diagnosis and treatment*, Seattle, 2001, IASP Press.

14. McGrath PA, Stewart D, Koster AL: Nondrug therapies for childhood headache. In McGrath PA, Hillier LM, editors: *The child with headache: diagnosis and treatment*, Seattle, 2001, IASP Press, pp 129-158.

15. McGrath PJ, Finley GA, editors: *Chronic and recurrent pain in children and adolescents*, Seattle, 1999, IASP Press.

16. McGrath PJ, Unruh A: *Pain in children and adolescents*, Amsterdam, 1987, Elsevier.

17. McGrath PJ, Walco GA, Turk DC, et al: Core outcome domains and measures for pediatric acute and chronic/recurrent pain clinical trials: Ped IMPACT recommendations, *J Pain* 9(9)771-783, 2008.

18. Price DD: *Psychological mechanisms of pain and analgesia*, Seattle, 1999, IASP Press.

19. Ross DM, Ross SA: *Childhood pain: current issues, research, and management*, Baltimore, 1988, Urban & Schwarzenberg.

20. Rusy M, Weisman SJ: Complementary therapies for acute pediatric pain management, *Pediatr Clin North Am* 47:589-599, 2000.

21. Schechter NL, Berde C, Yaster M, editors: *Pain management in children and adolescents*, 2nd ed, Baltimore, in press, Williams & Wilkins.

22. World Health Organization: *Cancer pain relief and palliative care in children*, Geneva, 1998, World Health Organization.

CHAPTER 31

PAIN IN THE OLDER PERSON

Ronald Kanner, MD, FAAN, FACP

1. **What is meant by "the older person"?**
   Of interest, most medical dictionaries do not give a definition for "old" or "older person." The *International Dictionary of Medicine and Biology, Stedman's Medical Dictionary,* and the *Mosby Medical, Nursing, and Allied Health Dictionary* omit the word "old" and define "elder" as "sambucus" (the elderberry). The American Association of Retired Persons (AARP) accepts people over the age of 50; most "senior communities" have a minimum age of 55; New York State provides housing help for those over the age of 60. The most commonly used working definition of the older person is over 65. However, most aging studies that began with people 65 and older now have a large cadre of people over 85. New definitions are emerging rather rapidly. "Old" is now generally taken to mean ≥75, and the "old old" is now ≥80. Most physicians, however, see octogenarians who are athletic, fit, and active.

2. **Why is it important to address pain in the older person?**
   The over-85 population is proportionally the fastest-growing segment in American society. Approximately 34 million people in the United States are aged 65 or older. This is expected to increase to 70 million by the year 2030. As older patients represent an increasingly larger proportion of the population, their health care needs assume a much greater role. Furthermore, the prevalence of pain in the older person is probably double what it is in younger adults. This number grows even larger in institutionalized older patients. Some of the common painful diseases, such as arthritis and cancer, are also more prevalent in the older patient. Furthermore, relatively few studies address the needs and specific problems of the aged population.

3. **How common are pain complaints in the older patient?**
   Acute pain occurs with similar frequency in the older patient as it does in the young. However, the incidence of chronic pain appears to increase up to about age 70. After that, it levels off. Older patients are more likely to experience pain in the major joints, back, legs, and feet. Headaches, in general, appear to be less common in the older patient population than in the young. Of older patients living independently, 20% to 50% percent suffer from pain. The incidence of untreated pain may be as high as 85% in long-term care facilities.

4. **An 80-year-old woman complains of pain in both shoulders and hips, as well as a generalized aching feeling. What diagnoses should be considered?**
   Polymyalgia rheumatica is a disease of the older patient characterized by aching pain in the shoulders and hips, along with a general feeling of malaise. The erythrocyte sedimentation rate is elevated (usually >80), and the pain responds readily to low doses of oral steroid medications. This syndrome is sometimes associated with temporal arteritis, which requires much higher doses of steroids and carries the risk of sudden blindness. Although fibromyalgia is usually considered a disease of younger people, rheumatologists have been recognizing it in a progressively older population.

   Whenever an older person experiences a chronic, diffuse pain syndrome, an underlying metabolic or neoplastic cause should be sought.

5. **What are the impediments to accurate pain assessment in the older patient?**
Pain is a truly subjective phenomenon. Its assessment requires careful, detailed communication between sufferer and health care practitioner. Older patients are more likely to underreport pain than are younger patients, possibly because of their desire to be perceived as "good patients." In a study of patients with duodenal ulcer or myocardial infarction, older patients reported milder pain than younger patients. They tend to have more faith in the medical system and more respect for physicians.

Cognitive impairment, a fairly common problem in the older patient, may render patients unable to use appropriate descriptors for pain. Impaired hearing and vision also may cause communication difficulties. In such cases, behavioral signs can be used to assess pain; however, they are often less accurate than good verbal reports. Although the precise severity of pain may be difficult to assess, even patients with significant cognitive impairment can report the presence of pain.

Unfortunately, there are relatively few well-validated scales for the older patient. The verbal and visual analogue scales used in younger patients do not have the same degree of validation in the older person.

6. **What impact does chronic osteoarthritis have on quality of life in the older person?**
Compared to their peers with no chronic illnesses, older patients with osteoarthritis, with and without additional comorbidities, have a significantly worse quality of life. Some of this is due to the pain itself and some is related to analgesia consumption. Interestingly, one study showed that a better quality of life was associated with noncompliance, fewer visits to the physicians, and taking oral nonsteroidal antiinflammatory drugs (NSAIDs).

7. **What scales are available for assessment of pain in patients with dementia?**
The Discomfort Scale for Patients with Dementia of the Alzheimer Type (DS-DAT) is difficult to validate because it was generated from the impressions of nursing staff caring for demented patients. It lists a series of items that, in the staff's opinion, indicate that a patient is in pain. Examples include noisy breathing, negative vocalization, sad versus content facial expression, frightened facial expression, frown, tense versus relaxed body language, and fidgeting. As its name indicates, the DS-DAT is a discomfort scale and may not assess pain directly. It is unclear whether distress, discomfort, or pain is being assessed. Behavioral methods of pain assessment may be valid for the presence or absence of pain, but they do not assess the intensity of pain. Certain facial expressions are common with intense pain, but they are not necessarily graded responses.

8. **Are patients with cognitive impairment capable of using a self-assessment scale?**
Generally, patients with mild to moderate cognitive impairment can still complete some short self-assessment scales. Up to 30% of severely impaired patients can still complete at least one assessment scale. An attempt should always be made to allow an older patient to report pain in his or her own words and to produce a rating of intensity that can be reassessed. Investigators have recently developed a "pain thermometer" to be used not only for older patients but also for very young patients.

9. **Are patients with Alzheimer's disease likely to report more or less pain than cognitively intact patients?**
It appears that patients with Alzheimer's disease tend to experience less intense pain than unaffected patients and may also have less of the affective component associated with pain. However, it is not clear that analgesic intake differs between the groups, and special attention must be paid to the side effects that may occur in a cognitively impaired population.

10. **Are NSAIDs safe in older patients?**

Advancing age greatly increases the risk of side effects from NSAIDs. The incidence of gastrointestinal (GI) bleeding from NSAIDs is nearly twice as high in patients over 65 as in young patients. Older patients are also at greater risk for adverse renal and cardiac effects. However, note that many of the resultant disorders are generally more common in the older person anyway, even without NSAIDs.

The daily dose of NSAIDs is related directly to the risk of GI complications, regardless of age. Unfortunately, because older patients commonly see more than one physician, they may receive multiple prescriptions for NSAIDs. Patients exposed to multiple NSAIDs have a higher risk of GI bleeding than patients taking a single drug.

Changing the route of administration does not seem to offer much benefit in terms of GI bleeding. One study showed that patients receiving rectal forms were more likely to bleed than patients receiving oral forms. Some of this difference may have been because of the mistaken belief that rectal administration was safer; patients given the drug by the rectal route may already have been at risk for GI bleeding. Recent data regarding the cardiovascular risks of NSAIDs and more selective agents raises additional concerns when using these types of agents in the older patient.

11. **What pharmacokinetic factors affect drug dosing in the older patient?**

All phases of pharmacokinetics are affected in aging, including absorption, distribution, metabolism, and elimination. However, effects are often in opposite directions. In general, the older patient tends to require lower doses of medications than younger patients. Absorption is often irregular in the older person because of delayed transit time or malabsorption syndromes. The volume of distribution of most drugs is smaller in the older person than in the young. Older patients tend to have a lower lean body mass. Hepatic metabolism and renal clearance are also diminished.

Such factors lead to relatively higher levels of drug at a given dose. In many instances, increased effects from medications are due to longer duration of action rather than simply higher peaks of concentration.

12. **Are older patients less sensitive to pain than younger patients?**

Both clinical and experimental tests offer conflicting data. Some studies have shown that pain threshold is slightly elevated in older patients. Others have shown no difference between the old and young. Pain tolerance has similarly been reported as either slightly increased or unchanged in the older person. In some large epidemiologic studies, pain complaints are listed as being less frequent in the older than in the young. Some of the difference may be a reporting bias. Joint pain, however, is clearly more prevalent in the older patient population. Older patients suffering from clinical pain syndromes may be less likely to report pain than their younger counterparts.

13. **What is the likelihood that a frail, older patient living in the community will suffer from pain and obtain adequate analgesics?**

A large Italian study showed that 39% to 49% of patients older than 65 suffered from significant daily pain. Twenty-five percent received Step 1 therapy, 6% Step 2 therapy, and 3% Step 3 therapy (see the World Health Organization's Cancer Pain Relief Program, described in Chapter 26, Cancer Pain Syndromes). Patients older than 85 were less likely to receive analgesics than were younger patients. In this study, low cognitive performance was also an independent predictor of failing to receive any analgesics.

14. **What are the clinical implications of the pharmacokinetic changes seen in the older patient?**

Given diminished volume of distribution, longer half-life, and reduced clearance, it follows that plasma levels will be elevated for a longer period after a given dose. Therefore, in the older patient, drugs with a short serum half-life are generally preferable to longer-lasting drugs.

With the opioid analgesics, four or five serum half-lives are required to reach steady-state drug levels, putting patients at greater risk for accumulation. Close monitoring is required after any drug change or increase in dose.

15. **What specific problems are seen with tricyclic antidepressants used for pain in the older patient?**

Most of the troublesome side effects of the tricyclic antidepressants (TCAs) are due to their anticholinergic effects. In patients with cognitive impairment, anticholinergic activity can lead to increased confusion. (One of the major deficits in Alzheimer's disease is a deficit in cerebral acetylcholine.) Narrow-angle glaucoma, another common problem in the older patient, may be markedly exacerbated. Older patients with benign prostatic hypertrophy are at greater risk for urinary retention. Dysautonomia (orthostatic hypertension), which causes slight dizziness on arising and is often present to a mild degree in the older patient, may be markedly exacerbated by the anticholinergic side effects. Finally, cardiac conduction blocks can be worsened by TCAs.

16. **What are the common side effects of opioid analgesics in the older patient?**

Constipation is by far the most common and troublesome side effect of opioids. It is even more prevalent in the older patient, in whom constipation is generally more common.

Respiratory depression is unusual, unless appropriate pharmacokinetic guidelines are disregarded. (Cheyne-Stokes breathing patterns during sleep are not uncommon in the older patient; opioids should not be discontinued solely on the basis of observing this respiratory pattern.)

17. **When is respiratory depression a problem in the older patient?**

There are primarily two situations in which respiratory depression can become a problem:

(1) When drugs with a long serum half-life are used, many days may pass before a steady state is reached. Thus, with drugs such as levorphanol and methadone, serum levels may rise for more than 1 week, despite steady dosing. If older patients are not monitored carefully, this can lead to respiratory depression.

(2) If patients with severe pain receive escalating doses of opioids, they are usually tolerant to such doses. However, if the underlying pain syndrome is relieved, previously tolerated doses of opioids may produce respiratory depression.

18. **What is the most common cause of adverse side effects in the older patient?**

Polypharmacy (the use of more than one drug for a specific problem) is a prescription for disaster in the older patient. In a study of falls in the older patient, prescription of multiple drugs was the single most common cause. Patients taking a combination of analgesics, antidepressants, and sedatives are much more likely to suffer confusion than patients taking a single agent.

19. **What is the basic rule of thumb for analgesic therapy in the older patient?**

Start low, go slow. Initial dosing in the older patient should be started at about half the level that you would use in a younger patient. TCAs should be started at no higher than 10 mg at bedtime. Titration must be gradual and careful. Doses of TCAs should be increased only by the amount at which they were started, and only after 3 or 4 days at each level.

20. **Which pain syndromes are more common in the older patient than in the younger patient?**

Arthritis and other articular complaints leap immediately to mind as pain syndromes that are more common in the older patient. However, trigeminal neuralgia and postherpetic neuralgia are also more common in the older person than in the young. Temporal arteritis and polymyalgia rheumatica are almost exclusively diseases of the older patient. Pure psychogenic pain is seen much less commonly in the older patient than in the young. However, masked depression (see Chapter 29, Psychological Syndromes) may present as a pain syndrome in older patients. The prevalence of cancer also rises with advancing age, bringing with it all of the pain syndromes associated with malignancy.

21. **What are the consequences of poorly controlled pain in the older patient?**
Consequences of poorly controlled pain in the older patient include the following:
- Older patients with pain tend to have reduced mobility. As they become more and more immobile, depression ensues. Lack of functional ability appears to be more of a determinant of depression than severity of disease.
- As with younger patients, chronic pain may lead to decreased socialization, sleep disturbances, and possibly even impaired immunity.
- Inadequate pain control may be a cause of unexplained agitation and restlessness.
- When pain is poorly controlled, physicians tend to prescribe more medications. Polypharmacy can lead to increased confusion and falls.

Most analgesic studies have been conducted in patients between 18 and 65 years of age. The exclusion of the very young and the very old makes it difficult to make firm statements about the analgesic efficacy of drugs in either age group.

22. **What factors lead to the underprescribing of opioid analgesics in older patients?**
Both factual and fictional ideas lead to the relatively low doses of opioids prescribed for older patients. First, older patients tend to respond to lower doses than younger patients. However, they are also less likely to complain about pain and to request analgesic medications. Even when left to their own devices (patient-controlled analgesia), older patients tend to take lower doses of analgesics than younger patients. Second, there seems to be a belief in the medical community that older people require less analgesia than young patients.

23. **Which drugs should be avoided in the older patient?**
Within each class of drug used for pain treatment, certain drugs are more likely to produce side effects in the older person.

Nonnarcotic analgesics (NSAIDs): It is generally a good idea to use nonacetylated drugs with a relatively simple metabolism. Indomethacin and piroxicam have relatively long serum half-lives and tend to produce more GI problems than drugs such as salsalate and ibuprofen. This caution applies to their role as analgesics, not as antiinflammatories.

Opioid analgesics: It is probably best to stay with a pure agonist rather than a mixed agonist-antagonist such as pentazocine or butorphanol. The mixed drugs are more likely to produce psychotomimetic effects in the older patient. In addition, drugs with a long serum half-life, such as methadone and levorphanol, require a greater length of time to reach steady state than drugs with a short serum half-life.

Propoxyphene: This drug can have neurotoxic effects and should be avoided in the older patient.

Antidepressants: The tertiary amine tricyclics are more likely to produce anticholinergic side effects than the secondary amine drugs.

24. **How should the side effects of analgesics be treated in the older patient?**
All patients taking opioid analgesics should be put on a bowel regimen before starting the drug. A simple combination of a senna preparation and stool softener is usually sufficient. Nausea, on the other hand, should not be treated prophylactically. Not all older patients become nauseated on opioids, and the side effects of the antiemetics may be worse than the problems caused by the opioids.

25. **How should analgesics be chosen for older patients in pain?**
The same three-step ladder (WHO; see Question 13) that applies to younger patients applies to the older person. Mild-to-moderate pain should be treated with nonopioid analgesics.

Moderate pain requires minor opioids, possibly in combination with nonnarcotics and adjuvant drugs. Severe pain requires potent opioids. The only differences for older patients are that lower doses should generally be used, and combinations of medications may cause more cognitive impairment.

KEY POINTS

1. Older patients are the fastest growing segment of the U.S. population; thus, an increasing number of patients with chronic pain will be older.

2. Specific pain syndromes may be more likely to occur in the older population; this should be considered when evaluating the older patient in pain.

3. Knowledge of the potential pharmacokinetic and pharmacodynamic changes in the older patient should guide the prescriber's choice of analgesic, as well as specific dosing.

BIBLIOGRAPHY

1. Auret K, Schug SA: Underutilisation of opioids in elderly patients with chronic pain: approaches to correcting the problem, *Drugs & Aging* 22(8):641-654, 2005.

2. Barkin RL, Barkin SJ, Barkin DS: Perception, assessment, treatment, and management of pain in the elderly, *Clin Geriatr Med* 21(3):465-490, 2005.

3. Edwards I, Salib E: Analgesics in the elderly, *Aging Ment Health* 6(1):88-92, 2002.

4. Gowin KM: Diffuse pain syndromes in the elderly, *Rheum Dis Clin North Am* 26(3):673-682, 2000.

5. Helme RD, Gibson SJ: The epidemiology of pain in elderly people, *Clin Geriatr Med* 17(3):417-431, 2001.

6. Herr K, Spratt KF, Garand L, Li I: Evaluation of the Iowa pain thermometer and other selected pain intensity scales in younger and older adult cohorts using controlled clinical pain: a preliminary study, *Pain Med* 8(7):585-600, 2007.

7. Landi F, Onder G, Cesari M, et al: Pain management in frail, community-living elderly patients, *Arch Intern Med* 161(22):2721-2724, 2001.

8. Manz BD, Mosier R, Nusser-Gerlach MA, et al: Pain assessment in the cognitively impaired and unimpaired elderly, *Pain Manag Nurs* 1(4):106-115, 2000.

9. McCarberg BH: Introduction: Special Topic Series: pain and the elderly, *Clin J Pain*, 20(4):205-206, 2004.

10. Morton AH. Inappropriately defining "inappropriate medication for the elderly" [Comment, letter, review], *J Amer Geriatr Soc* 52(9):1580; author reply 1581-1582, 2004.

11. Portenoy RK, Farkash A: Practical management of nonmalignant pain in the elderly, *Geriatrics* 43(5):29-40, 44-47, 1988.

12. Won A, Lapane KL, Vallow S, Schein J, et al: Long-term effects of analgesics in a population of elderly nursing home residents with persistent nonmalignant pain, *Journals of Gerontology Series A-Biological Sciences and Medical Sciences* 61(2):165-169, 2006.

TOPICEUTICALS

Brad Galer, MD

CHAPTER 32

OVERVIEW

1. **What is the history of topicals (topiceuticals) as analgesics?**
   Evidence shows that since the dawn of man humans have been grinding plants and herbs into poultices and liniments to treat ailments such as inflammation, itch, and pain. Ancient cultures from around the world, including Egyptians, Chinese, Romans, Indians, and Native Americans, have utilized plants in their environment to formulate externally applied analgesics. Topical formulations of plant-derived natural products that have been used for centuries and are still used today as analgesics include camphor, capsaicin, and menthol.

2. **How is a topiceutical medication different from a transdermal drug?**
   Medications formulated as either a topical (topiceutical) or a transdermal preparation must be delivered across the skin, the body's largest organ, which is designed to keep out foreign substances (including medications). These types of medications differ in what happens to the medication once it penetrates (absorbs) through the skin.

   Transdermal preparations are formulated to deliver medication across the skin and into the bloodstream; the bloodstream carries the medication throughout the body for a body-wide or systemic effect. Basically, with transdermal drug systems, the body is exposed to medication as if a tablet were swallowed and dissolved in the stomach. These kinds of patches can be applied to any skin area (according to the product instructions) because the medication will eventually find the bloodstream for delivery to the targeted area in the body. An example is the Durogesic patch (Janssen Pharmaceutica, Titusville, N.J.).

   A **topical patch** must be placed directly over the painful area. Medication in a topiceutical does not reach the bloodstream in an amount to produce any meaningful effect. Rather, topical medications penetrate the skin and remain in the upper layers of the skin to produce local effects when used according to the package instructions. Care must be taken when applying topical medications because application of excessive amounts for extended periods of time over a larger area can promote increased medication penetration and result in amounts in the bloodstream that cause side effects. Once the medication crosses the skin, it is where it needs to be and works on tissues (muscles, ligaments, tendons, nerves) that lie directly underneath the skin application area. Examples of topiceuticals include Bengay spa cream (Pfizer, N.Y.), Lidoderm patch (Endo Pharmaceuticals, Chadds Ford, Pa.), and EMLA cream (AstraZeneca, Wilmington, Del.).

   Delivering medications directly to the tissues directly under the skin application area can be an advantage. Topiceuticals can be safely added to an existing pain treatment plan without worry about drug-drug interactions with other body-wide (systemic) analgesics. Because it is not uncommon for pain patients to require several pain medications, the flexibility to add topiceuticals to the mix is helpful. The risk of unwanted body-wide side effects is also significantly reduced.

3. **What are the various topical formulations available for the treatment of pain?**
Topical formulations to treat pain can be obtained as both prescription and nonprescription (e.g., over-the-counter) drugs. Prescription topical pain relievers include creams and skin patches. Skin patches vary in appearance from a soft, felt, white rectangular patch to a pink, flesh-colored, oval patch that heats up when exposed to air. Over-the-counter (OTC) medications include creams, ointments, lotions, rub-on sticks, gels, sprays, and patches.

4. **What are the advantages and disadvantages of using topical medications?**
There are numerous **advantages** associated with delivering medication across the skin with little body-wide activity. Patients are able to place the medication directly at the location where it is needed. This reduces the level to which the entire body is exposed to the medication. Low body-wide exposure leads to reduced body-wide side effects and low risk for drug-drug interactions. Topical products are generally easy to use and begin to work relatively quickly. They are widely available in a number of different dosage formulations both by prescription and over the counter at the pharmacy. These dosage formulations do not require the use of needles and therefore are nonpainful when applied. Topiceuticals offer an alternative for patients who fear needles and who are unable to swallow tablets and capsules (e.g., patients with mouth sores, children, or older persons). Some skin patches can be cut to fit exactly over the painful skin area.

Disadvantages with topical medications depend on the specific dosage formulation. Ointments, creams, and lotions may stain clothing and leave behind an oily residue (especially ointments). Children may remove the medication and accidentally eat it or put it in the ears or eyes. Some formulations require measurement or are dosed according to weight (e.g., for use on children). Skin patches may cause the skin area to become pale, itchy, red, or inflamed. If the skin is oily or hairy, it may be difficult for the patch to stay in place. Showering or swimming may not be possible while wearing a patch. One newly available type of skin patch (Synera) may cause thermal burns if the top cover is removed. Another skin patch requires a device that permits electrical current to run through the patch and skin to enhance the medication delivery and can be applied only by a health care professional at the office, clinic, or hospital.

OVER-THE-COUNTER PAIN RELIEVERS

5. **What topiceuticals are currently available in the united states without a prescription? How are they being used?**
Nonprescription (OTC) topiceuticals for the relief of pain can be divided into the following four broad categories:
- Local anesthetics, such as lidocaine or benzocaine
- Counterirritants, such as menthol and camphor
- Antiinflammatory medications, such as methyl salicylate
- Capsaicin, a medication made from hot chili peppers

In general, all of these medications have similar application instructions (3 to 4 times daily), and patients should wash their hands thoroughly after application of any topical preparation. (See Table 32-1 for more specific information).

Local anesthetics, such as lidocaine (e.g., ELA-Max) or benzocaine (e.g., Lanacane) work to relieve pain by blocking the nerves underneath the skin that send pain signals to the brain, thereby reducing the amount of pain and discomfort felt after an injury or sunburn.

Medications containing menthol or camphor (e.g., Bengay spa cream) are referred to as counterirritants. They essentially work to relieve pain by distracting the brain from receiving pain signals resulting from conditions such as osteoarthritis or injuries such as sprains and strains.

TABLE 32-1. AVAILABLE NONPRESCRIPTION (OTC) TOPICEUTICALS

Example Products (Manufacturer)	Active Ingredient	Use	Information for Proper Use	Common Side Effects	Additional Tips for Use
Local Anesthetic-Containing Products					
ELA-Max (Ferndale)	4% lidocaine in a topical cream	Relief of local pain caused by minor cuts and burns, abrasions, sunburn, insect bites, needle sticks for blood draws, and needle insertion into veins	Apply to affected areas no more than 3 or 4 times per day	Irritation, redness, itching, rash	Not recommended for use on mucous membranes
Xylocaine (Astra)	0.5%-2.5% lidocaine in gels, creams, ointments, depending on the product.		Apply only to intact skin For external use only		Not for use in patients less than 2 years old without consulting a physician
Solarcaine (Schering-Plough)					
DermaFlex (Zila)	Many generic lidocaine products also available.				Avoid contact with eyes, mouth, or nose and inside of ears
Nupercainal (Ciba)	0.5%-1.0% dibucaine				Dressing recommended for children to prevent accidental ingestion
Lanacane (Combe)	5%-20% benzocaine in gels, ointments, creams, lotions, and sprays. Many generic benzocaine products also available.				Do not use in large amounts over raw skin or blistered areas; do not use more often than 3 or 4 times per day
Hurricaine (Beutlich)					

(Continued)

TABLE 32-1. AVAILABLE NONPRESCRIPTION (OTC) TOPICEUTICALS (CONTINUED)

Example Products (Manufacturer)	Active Ingredient	Use	Information for Proper Use	Common Side Effects	Additional Tips for Use
Menthol- or Camphor-Containing Products					
Bengay Spa Cream (Pfizer) Therapeutic Mineral Ice Gel (Bristol-Myers)	1.25-16% menthol in creams, gels, patches	Relief of pain of muscular aches, neuralgia, rheumatism, arthritis, sprains and like conditions	Apply to affected areas no more than 3 or 4 times per day Apply only to intact skin For external use only	Irritation, rash, burning, stinging, swelling	Not recommended for use on mucous membranes Avoid contact with eyes, mouth or nose and inside of ears
Capsaicin-Containing Products					
Capzasin-HP & Capzasin-P (Thompson Medical) Zostrix, Zostrix-HP (GenDerm)	0.025-0.075% capsaicin in creams, gels, lotions	Temporary relief of pain from rheumatoid arthritis, osteoarthritis, and relief of neuralgias such as the pain following shingles or diabetic neuropathy	Apply to affected areas no more than 3 or 4 times per day Apply only to intact skin For external use only	Burning, redness, stinging, cough	Not for use on mucous membranes Avoid contact with the eyes Wash hands immediately after application Use caution when handling contact lenses after application Do not bandage tightly

(Continued)

TABLE 32-1. AVAILABLE NONPRESCRIPTION (OTC) TOPICEUTICALS (CONTINUED)

Example Products (Manufacturer)	Active Ingredient	Use	Information for Proper Use	Common Side Effects	Additional Tips for Use
Salicylate-Containing Products					
Myoflex (Fisons)	Many products available, ranging from 83%–55% methyl salicylate in creams, gels, ointments, and lotions	Relief of pain of muscular aches, neuralgia, rheumatism, arthritis, sprains, and like conditions	Apply to affected areas no more than 3 or 4 times per day	If applied to large areas may cause tinnitus, nausea, or vomiting	Not recommended for use on mucous membranes
Sportscreme (Chattern)			Apply only to intact skin		Avoid contact with eyes, mouth, or nose and inside of ears
Infrarub (Whitehall)			For external use only		
Aspercreme (Chattern)					
Arthritis Formula Bengay (Pfizer)					
Combination Products					
Flexall Ultra Plus Gel (Chattern)	Many different products that combine menthol or camphor with a salicylate or capsaicin in creams, gels, liquids, or patches	Relief of pain of muscular aches, neuralgia, rheumatism, arthritis, sprains, and like conditions	Apply to affected areas no more than 3 or 4 times per day	See information above for each of the various ingredients' side effects	Not recommended for use on mucous membranes
Icy Hot Chill Stick (Chattern)			Apply only to intact skin		Avoid contact with eyes, mouth, or nose and inside of ears
Arthritis Hot Cream (Chattern)			For external use only		
Banalg Lotion (Forest)					

Products that contain antiinflammatory ingredients, such as methyl salicylate (e.g., Myoflex or Aspercreme) work by reducing the inflammation (swelling) at the site of injury. By reducing the inflammation in the affected area, these compounds reduce the ongoing irritation of local nerves. In turn, this reduces the amount of pain signals these nerves send to the brain.

A relatively new group of OTC topical analgesics are made from hot chili peppers. One of the chemicals contained within these peppers (capsaicin) is the main ingredient of products such as Zostrix and Capzasin-HP. They work to relieve pain by emptying the nerves of a chemical that is necessary for the nerve to send pain signals to the brain. Initially, as the medication empties the chemical from the nerve, there may be a temporary increase in pain; this usually subsides within a few minutes after application. These particular medications should be applied carefully, and patients should wash hands thoroughly after application to prevent a burning sensation caused by touching other areas of the body.

Finally, certain OTC topical analgesic products may contain various combinations of the ingredients mentioned above in an attempt to gain added benefit by using together medications that work differently.

6. **What are specific examples of OTC pain relievers?**
Examples of OTC pain relievers can be found in Table 32-1, which includes information about active ingredients, proper use, and side effects.

PRESCRIPTION PAIN RELIEVERS

7. **What are the most commonly prescribed topiceuticals in the United States? How are they used?**
Over the past 5 years, there has been increasing interest in developing topical medications for the treatment of various pain conditions. Table 32-2 lists prescription topiceuticals available in the United States and includes information concerning their use, directions for use, and side effects.

Representative of this subcategory of topiceuticals are the Lidoderm patch and EMLA cream. In 1999, the **Lidoderm patch** (lidocaine 5%) (Endo Pharmaceuticals, Chadds Ford, Pa.) was approved by the Food and Drug Administration and introduced for the relief of pain caused by damaged nerves following a shingles infection. It works to block the formation and movement of pain signals from the injured or affected nerves to the brain. Damaged and affected peripheral sensory nerves are extremely sensitive to the blocking effects of lidocaine; therefore, absorption of the drug into the bloodstream is not necessary for effect. This topical formulation releases an amount of lidocaine sufficient to block pain signals in the local tissues but not enough to cause complete numbness of the area. It reduces pain but does not affect other sensations. Lidoderm is a 10-by-14-cm, white, polyester felt patch that contains an adhesive with 5% lidocaine (700 mg) and is covered with a clear, film-release liner. The liner is removed prior to patch application to the most painful area of intact skin (e.g., no blisters or open skin ulcers). It also can act as a barrier for patients whose painful area may be extra sensitive to touch. Since the Lidoderm patch's introduction, it has been also widely used successfully for pain associated with other nerves, such as diabetic neuropathy, carpel tunnel syndrome, and postmastectomy pain, as well as nonnerve pains such as low back, myofascial, osteoarthritis, and sports injury pains.

EMLA cream (AstraZeneca Pharmaceuticals, Wilmington, Del.) is a cream or a topical adhesive disc system that delivers medications (lidocaine and procaine) for the production of complete skin numbness in the area to which it is applied. This medication is used in newborns, children, and adults and can be applied to normal intact skin for relief of local pain resulting from needle sticks for blood draws and needle insertion into veins and mucous membranes in advance of superficial minor surgery (e.g., circumcision or genital wart removal) or skin procedures (e.g., tattoo removal, biopsies, and laser treatments). Lidocaine and procaine work

TABLE 32-2. AVAILABLE PRESCRIPTION TOPICEUTICALS

	Formulation	Use	Information for Proper Use	Common Side Effects	Additional Tips for Use
Lidoderm Patch (lidocaine patch 5%) Endo Pharmaceuticals (Chadds Ford, Pa.)	Lidocaine 5% in a nonwoven, polyester felt patch	Relief of pain persisting after a shingles infection	Apply up to 3 patches (after removing the protective liner) to the site of pain for 12 hours in a 24 hour period	Mild redness or swelling of skin in area of patch application; generally clears up after patch removal	Avoid contact with eyes Fold the patch onto itself and discard in trash; keep away from children and pets
			Apply only to dry, intact skin		Store in envelopes until use so the patches do not dry out
			Cut the patch if needed to fit the area of painful skin		Do not apply in conjunction with other creams, ointments, lotions, or heating pads
Synera Topical Patch (lidocaine 70 mg and tetracaine 70 mg) Endo Pharmaceuticals (Chadds Ford, Pa.)	Lidocaine 70 mg and tetracaine 70 mg in a patch containing a heating element	Relief of local pain caused by needle insertion into veins, needle sticks for blood draws, or skin procedures of the upper skin layers (e.g., biopsy of the skin where tissue is removed for further examination)	For needle insertion or vein puncture, apply 1 patch for 20 to 30 minutes	Mild redness, swelling, paleness of skin, or abnormal feeling in area of patch application; generally clears up after patch removal	Do not cut the patch or remove the top cover—the patch could heat to temperatures that could cause burns
			For skin procedures involving the upper layers of the skin, apply patch for 30 minutes prior to the procedure	Remove patch if irritation or burning sensation occurs with patch application	Do not block the holes on the top of the patch—the patch may not properly heat
			Apply only to intact skin		Fold the patch onto itself and discard in trash; keep away from children and pets

(Continued)

TABLE 32-2. AVAILABLE PRESCRIPTION TOPICEUTICALS (CONTINUED)

	Formulation	Use	Information for Proper Use	Common Side Effects	Additional Tips for Use
LidoSite Topical System (lidocaine HCl/epinephrine topical iontophoretic patch 10%/0.1%) and the LidoSite Controller B. Braun (Bethlehem, Pa.)	Lidocaine 10% and epinephrine 0.1% in a circular reservoir, single-use patch; the treatment side and return reservoir on the other side complete the electrical circuit	Relief of local pain caused by needle insertion into veins, needle sticks for blood draw, lasers used to burn skin lesions away in upper skin layers	One patch should be applied by a health care professional in a health care setting for 10 minutes Apply only to intact skin	Electric current may cause skin irritation, burning feeling, or burns Skin under the patch may show short-lived skin whitening or redness, rash, or pain/burning sensations	For use in patients 5 years old and older Uses electric current to help the drug cross the skin; not for use in someone with electrically sensitive devices (e.g., pacemakers) Contains a sulfite (sodium metabisulfite) that can pose allergic reactions of varying degrees Not tested for use on mucous membranes

(Continued)

TABLE 32-2. AVAILABLE PRESCRIPTION TOPICEUTICALS (CONTINUED)				
	Formulation	Use	Information for Proper Use	Common Side Effects	Additional Tips for Use
EMLA Cream (lidocaine 2.5% and procaine 2.5%) AstraZeneca (Wilmington, Del.)	Lidocaine 2.5% and procaine 2.5% in a cream (may use with Tegaderm skin dressing)	For use on normal intact skin for local pain relief or on genital mucous membranes for minor surgery involving the upper skin layers and as a pretreatment for more extensive skin numbing procedures	Apply a thick layer of cream and use a dressing to cover the cream	Skin paleness, redness, burning, alternations in temperature sensation, edema, itching, and rash in the area of patch application	Dressings are recommended to keep the cream in place and to protect clothing
			Cream amount required, size of application area, and length of application time vary depending on the type of procedure and the age of the patient (e.g., adult, child, newborn)		Avoid contact with the eye
		Used in adults for blood draw needle sticks, genital wart removal; in children for blood draw needle sticks; in newborns prior to circumcision			Use care when applying cream over large areas or leaving it on the skin for longer than 2 hours
					Acutely ill, debilitated, older, or severe liver disease patients may be more sensitive to body-wide effects of lidocaine/procaine

by blocking nerve signals (pain and other sensation [touch]) to the brain. The cream is applied to intact skin under a dressing that covers the skin and helps the cream from coming off (and also protects children from accidental ingestion). The disc has a backing, a cellulose disc (where the medication is located), and an adhesive tape ring. It covers a relatively small area, and the medication portion is in contact with the skin in an even smaller area (10 cm^2). EMLA cream has been reported to be not as effective for long-term (chronic) pain conditions, including nerve pain.

FUTURE DEVELOPMENTS

8. **What topicals now in development may become available in the United States over the next few years?**
   For many decades, topical nonsteroidal anti-inflammatory drug (NSAID) products have been prescribed in Asian and European countries with good success. Patients may be most familiar with NSAIDs available in tablet form (i.e., ibuprofen) that are swallowed. Anti-inflammatory medications relieve pain by treating the inflammation (i.e., swelling) that often makes pain feel worse. Formulations of several topical NSAIDs are being developed for the U.S. market. In addition, novel formulations of local anesthetics are being developed for the treatment of neuroma (abnormal regrowth of severed nerves) pain and headache disorders. New formulations of NMDA-antagonists, another class of medications, may help treat some neuropathic pain disorders also.

KEY POINTS

1. Unlike transdermal agents, which require a systemic concentration to be effective, topical analgesics exert their effect via a local and not systemic mechanism.

2. Advantages of topical analgesics include a limited risk for drug-drug interactions, a limited risk for systemic side effects, and an analgesic treatment option for patients who cannot swallow pills and/or are fearful of needles.

3. Disadvantages of topical analgesics include accidental eye exposure and subsequent irritation, restriction of activities while using the topical agent (e.g., showering or swimming), and various skin reactions.

4. Future development of topical pain relievers in the United States may include the development of topical nonsteroidal antiinflammatory agents (NSAIDs) as well as NMDA receptor antagonists.

BIBLIOGRAPHY

1. Argoff CE: Topical agents for the treatment of chronic pain, *Curr Pain Headache Rep* 10(1):11-19, 2006.
2. Galer BS, Gammaitoni A: Use of topiceuticals (topically applied, peripherally acting drugs) in the treatment of chronic pain, *Current Drug Therapy* 1:273-282, 2006.
3. Galer BS, Gammaitoni A, Alvaraz N: Pain, *Scientific American Medicine*, Chapter 10, Section XIV, 2001, WebMD.

CHAPTER 33

NONSTEROIDAL ANTIINFLAMMATORY DRUGS AND ACETAMINOPHEN

Robert A. Duarte, MD, and Charles E. Argoff, MD

1. **List the indications for treatment with aspirin, acetaminophen, and nonsteroidal antiinflammatory drugs (NSAIDs)?**
   Aspirin, acetaminophen, and other NSAIDs are generally considered to be the drugs of choice for mild to moderate pain. They represent the first step in the analgesic ladder proposed by the World Health Organization. These agents have a relatively low abuse potential and are primarily used in nociceptive somatic pain syndromes, e.g., arthritis. They do, however, have a ceiling effect. Pure opioid analgesics such as hydromorphone and morphine do not. The ceiling effect refers to the dose after which additional quantities of an analgesic no longer provide additional analgesia. For example, 2000 mg of aspirin does not provide more analgesia than 1000 mg of aspirin and may lead to more side effects.

2. **Describe the mechanism of action of the NSAIDs.**
   The antiinflammatory effect of nonsteroidal antiinflammatory agents is due mainly to inhibition of the enzyme cyclooxygenase (COX), which is required for synthesis of prostaglandins and thromboxanes. There are two COX isoforms: COX1, which is expressed constitutively in most tissues and is thought to protect the gastric mucosa and platelets, and COX2, which is expressed constitutively in the brain and kidney but can be induced at sites of inflammation. Traditional NSAIDs are nonselective COX1 and COX2 inhibitors, whereas celecoxib is a selective COX2 inhibitor.

3. **What are the major pharmacokinetic differences among the NSAIDs?**
   All the NSAIDs possess similar absorption characteristics. In general, they are rapidly absorbed after oral and rectal administration. They are highly protein-bound and metabolized primarily in the liver. However, durations of action vary markedly. Some drugs, such as ibuprofen, require dosing every 4 to 6 hours, whereas piroxicam can be given once a day. The newer COX2 inhibitors also require only once or twice daily dosing.

4. **List the most common side effects associated with the traditional NSAIDs.**
   Gastrointestinal (GI) irritation, nausea, and impairment of platelet aggregation are the most common side effects associated with the traditional NSAIDs. These side effects may lead to dyspepsia, GI ulcers, and bleeding. Some of the nonacetylated salicylates (e.g., choline magnesium trisalicylate) do not inhibit platelet function. Other known side effects include peripheral edema and elevated blood pressure.

5. **Describe the clinical presentation for acute acetaminophen overdose.**
   Symptoms of acetaminophen overdose include vague abdominal pain during the first week, followed by signs of hepatic failure. At doses of 200 to 250 mg/kg, acetaminophen is hepatotoxic. Acetaminophen, at doses of 400 mg/kg, can be fatal.

6. **What are the risks of combining NSAIDs with acetaminophen?**
   The risk of analgesic nephropathy appears to increase when different NSAIDs are used together or in combination with acetaminophen. This effect is generally seen in long-term use. The primary lesion is papillary necrosis with secondary interstitial nephritis.

7. **What is the risk of nephrotoxicty with NSAIDs?**
Aspirin and NSAIDs at therapeutic doses generally do not cause renal disease in patients with normal renal function. However, problems such as nephrotic syndrome, acute interstitial nephritis, and acute renal failure have been observed when aspirin and other nonsteroidals are given to patients with abnormal renal function. This can occur as a result of the inhibition of renal prostaglandin production by NSAIDs and the coxibs. Congestive heart failure, hepatic cirrhosis, collagen vascular disease, intravascular volume depletion, and arthrosclerotic heart disease are known contributing factors that may increase the risk of renal failure.

8. **Which groups of NSAIDs are available in the United States?**
   - Traditional, or nonselective, COX1 and COX2 Inhibitors
     - Salicylate (salsalate, diflunisal, and choline magnesium trisalicylate)
     - Proprionic (ibuprofen, ketoprofen, naproxen, fenoprofen)
     - Indole (indomethacin, sulindac, tolmetin)
     - Fenamate (mefenamic, meclofenamate)
     - Mixed (piroxicam, ketorolac, diclofenac)
   - Selective COX2 Inhibitors
     - Celecoxib (Celebrex)

9. **Which agent is considered to be the drug of choice for pain control?**
There is no conclusive evidence supporting one NSAID over another for analgesia. Frequency of dosing, cost, and side-effect profile should be considered when deciding on a specific NSAID agent for pain control. Following a review of the overall efficacy of the NSAIDs and their potential risk for cardiovascular disease, the Food and Drug Administration (FDA) Arthritis Panel currently suggests Naprosyn, or Celebrex if there are risk factors that mitigate against the use of Naprosyn, as the preferred agents for the treatment of arthritis pain.

10. **Describe an adequate trial of NSAIDs for pain control.**
An analgesic should not be considered a failure unless it has been given an adequate trial. For non–cancer-related pain, 2 weeks of treatment with a maximum scheduled dose constitutes an adequate trial. For cancer-associated pain, 1-week duration of continuous dosing is considered sufficient. However, ketorolac is not recommended for more than 5 days' duration because of the risk of serious gastrointestinal and other side effects.

11. **If one NSAID fails to provide sufficient pain relief, how should a clinician proceed?**
If an adequate trial of one class of NSAID does not cause analgesia, the clinician should switch to an alternative class of NSAID. For example, if an agent from a salicylate group is considered ineffective it is recommended to change to a proprionic or indole group. On the other hand, when one group of NSAID is effective but produces intolerable side effects, the clinician should first search for another agent in the same class before switching to another group of NSAID.

12. **List the potential risk factors for the traditional NSAID-associated GI toxicity.**
   - Advancing age
   - Concomitant administration of corticosteroids
   - History of either ulcer disease or prior GI complications from NSAIDs

13. **What is the role of protective therapies in association with administration of traditional NSAIDs?**
To date, only misoprostol has been proved to reduce the risk for serious GI toxicity. Misoprostol diminishes the incidence of endoscopically detectable lesions. However, no evidence has confirmed that misoprostol diminishes the risk of complications from the lesions when they occur. Protective agents may be indicated in patients over the age of 60 years of age and patients with predisposition to GI problems.

14. **Do the selective COX2 inhibitors have a lower risk for gastrointestinal toxicity compared to the traditional NSAIDs?**
Yes. The COX2 inhibitors were associated with a lower incidence of symptomatic ulcers compared with traditional NSAIDs at standard doses. The decrease in upper GI toxicity was strongest among patients not taking aspirin concomitantly.

15. **What are the major distinctions among the mechanisms of action of aspirin, acetaminophen, NSAIDs, and the COX2 inhibitors (coxibs)?**
Aspirin is an irreversible inhibitor of the COX enzymes. The exact mechanism of action of acetaminophen is not known. However, it is a weak nonselective inhibitor of both the COX1 and the COX2 enzymes. NSAIDs inhibit the activity of both COX1 and COX2 enzymes. The coxibs selectively inhibit the COX2 enzyme.

16. **Which COX2 inhibitor(s) are currently available in the United States?**
Originally, there were three selective COX2 inhibitors in the United States. Presently, celecoxib is the only oral selective coxib available in the United States approved for osteoarthritis and rheumatoid arthritis. The FDA removed rofecoxib from the U.S. market because of increasing evidence that it increased risk for cardiovascular disease. Of note, valdecoxib was removed by the FDA primarily because of the high risk of skin lesions (i.e., Stevens-Johnson syndrome) attributed to it.

17. **What are the documented precautions with celecoxib?**
Celecoxib is contraindicated in patients who have had an allergic-type reaction to sulfonamide drugs. This agent is not recommended for patients with severe hepatic insufficiency or advanced renal disease. In postmarketing studies, patients receiving celecoxib concurrently with warfarin experienced bleeding events in association with an increase in prothrombin time. Therefore, if celecoxib therapy is initiated or changed, the International Normalized Ration (INR) should be monitored, especially in the first few days. In addition, the clinician should be aware of the potential interaction with lithium and cytochrome P450 inhibitors when patients are taking celecoxib.

18. **Discuss some cardiovascular issues associated with selective COX2 inhibitors.**
NSAIDs and coxibs do not provide the same protective effects as low-dose aspirin. Coxibs (selective COX2 inhibitors) decrease vascular prostacyclin (PGI2) production and may affect the balance between prothrombotic and antithrombotic eicosanoids. However, the available studies can suggest only that there is a potential increase in cardiovascular events compared to the traditional NSAIDs. In patients taking a coxib agent, the recommendation is to maintain low-dose daily aspirin in patients who are at significant risk of a cardiovascular event. However, the use of low-dose acetyl salicylic acid (ASA) does not consistently negate the potential cardiovascular risk of COX2 inhibitors.

19. **List the potential central nervous system side effects associated with NSAIDs.**
All NSAIDs have the potential to produce central nervous system side effects, including sedation, dizziness, and headaches. Headaches occur in about 10% of patients taking indomethacin. Usually side effects are mild and transient.

20. **What are the only parenteral NSAIDs available in the United States?**
Ketorolac and diclofenac is the only parenteral NSAID available in the United States. Doses of 10 to 30 mg parenteral ketorolac are equivalent to 10 to 12 mg of parenteral morphine. However, the risks of bleeding limit its use to no more than 5 days. Contraindications to ketorolac and diclofenac include a history or current risk of gastrointestinal bleeding, risk of renal failure, compromised homeostasis, hypersensitivity to aspirin or other NSAIDs, labor, delivery, and nursing. There are ongoing trials of parenteral forms of COX-2 inhibitors.

KEY POINTS

1. Multiple nonsteroidal antiinflammatory medications (NSAIDs), including both nonselective agents and one selective agent, are commercially available. Unlike opioid analgesics, these medications appear to have a ceiling effect.

2. The risk for nephrotoxic effects appear to be increased when different NSAIDs are used in combination with each other or with acetaminophen.

3. If an adequate trial of one type of NSAID does not result in adequate pain relief, the clinician should consider switching the patient to a different type of NSAID.

4. The clinician should prescribe these drugs cautiously, especially in view of the potential for cardiovascular, gastrointestinal, and renal adverse effects.

BIBLIOGRAPHY

1. Bombardier C, Laine L, Reicin A, et al: (The VIGOR Study Group): Comparison of upper gastrointestinal toxicity of rofecoxib and naproxyn in patients with rheumatoid arthritis, *N Engl J Med* 343:1520-1528, 2000.

2. Crofford LJ: Rational use of analgesic and anti-inflammatory drugs, *N Engl J Med* 345(25):1844-1846, 2001.

3. Giovanni G, Giovanni P: Do NSAIDs and COX 2 inhibitors have different renal effects? *J Nephrol* 15(5):480-488, 2002.

4. Macario A, Lipman AG: Ketorolac in the era of cyclo-oxygenase 2 selective nonsteroidal anti-inflammatory drugs: a systemic review of efficacy, side effects, and regulatory issues, *Pain Medicine* 2(4):336-351, 2001.

5. Mukherjee D, Nissan SE, Topol EJ: Risk of cardiovascular events associated with selective COX 2 inhibitors, *JAMA* 286:954-959, 2001.

6. Nikles CJ, Yelland M, Del Mar C, et al: The role of paracetamol in chronic pain: an evidence-based approach, *Am J Ther*, 12(1):80-91, 2005.

7. Olsen NJ: Tailoring arthritis therapy In the wake of the NSAID crisis, *N Eng J Med* 352:2578-2580, 2005.

8. Scheiman JM, Fendick AM: Practical approaches to minimizing gastrointestinal and cardiovascular safety concerns with COX 2 inhibitors, *Arthritis Res Ther* (Suppl 4):523-529, 2005.

9. Silverstein, FE, Faich G, Goldstein GL: Gastrointestinal toxicity with celecoxib vs. nonsteroidal anti-inflammatory drugs for osteoarthritis and rheumatoid arthritis, The Class Study, *JAMA* 284(10):1247-1255, 2000.

CHAPTER 34

OPIOID ANALGESICS

Ronald Kanner, MD, FAAN, FACP

1. **Tolerance to the analgesic effects of opioids is well known. Does tolerance occur to the side effects, as well as the effects?**

   Yes, tolerance occurs to the side effects, as well as the effects, but the rate of tolerance may be different. For example, pupillary constriction and constipation are chronic side effects that may continue as long as opioid dosing continues. However, tolerance to respiratory depression develops more rapidly. As opioid doses are increased to overcome analgesic tolerance, constipation and pupillary constriction persist, whereas respiratory depression may become less of a problem.

2. **What is an opioid?**

   "Opioid" is the term used to refer to a group of substances that have the analgesic and other properties of morphine. This includes the naturally occurring opiates, semisynthetic opiates, and endogenous opioids. The term "opiate" was initially used to denote any derivative of the poppy plant. As synthetic and semisynthetic products became available and endogenous peptides with morphinelike activity were identified, it became clear that the term had to be modified. It still holds some of its literary significance as any substance capable of assuaging suffering.

3. **What is the role of opioids in pain management?**

   Opioids have been the mainstay of treatment of moderate to severe pain in patients with cancer and in many acute pain syndromes. Although many patients with chronic noncancer pain have been successfully treated with opioids, their role in chronic pain of noncancer origin is still being defined. In the 1960s and 1970s, opioid treatment was considered the antithesis of good treatment for chronic pain of noncancer origin. In the 1980s and 1990s, it gained greater acceptance. For treatment of both cancer and noncancer chronic pain, there are few true long-term studies to help practitioners fully understand the potential benefits and risks of such therapy. In recent years, guidelines have been established for the safe and efficacious use of opioids in the treatment of many noncancer pain syndromes. The guidelines suggest that opioid therapy for chronic noncancer pain should be considered only after other reasonable attempts at analgesia have failed. A history of substance abuse or severe character pathology should be considered relative contraindications. One practitioner should manage the prescribed opiates, and he or she must be experienced in their use and able to recognize and deal with adverse reactions such as cognitive impairment, constipation, and aberrant use. The potential risks and benefits should be discussed with the patient and clearly documented in the patient file. New guidelines regarding the use of opioids in chronic noncancer pain are being developed as a collaborative effort among several major pain organizations and should be available soon.

4. **What is a narcotic?**

   Narcotic is now a term that has more legal implications than it does pharmacologic ones. It was initially used to denote any drug capable of producing sleep (narcosis). It was generally applied to the opiates. However, the term is now used to denote drugs of abuse that are controlled by government agencies. The old name for one of the federal agencies was the Bureau of Narcotics and Dangerous Drugs. Currently, the main regulatory agency on a national level is the Drug Enforcement Agency (DEA). The term *opioid* is now preferred instead of *narcotic* when describing opioid analgesics.

5. **What are the two main, naturally occurring opioid alkaloids used in clinical practice?**
Morphine and codeine are two of the most widely used naturally occurring opioid alkaloids. Morphine is the prototype of the opioid drug. It binds primarily to mu receptors, producing analgesia and respiratory depression.

6. **Describe the mechanism of opioid analgesia.**
Opioid analgesia is thought to be mediated through a direct interaction with an opioid receptor. Thus far, the opioid receptors responsible for analgesia have been identified in the spinal cord, the brainstem, and the cerebral cortex. It is less clear at present what analgesic role is played by the opiate receptors that have been identified in the peripheral nervous system.

7. **What is the difference between a "weak" and a "potent" analgesic?**
The weak analgesics have a ceiling effect. This implies that there is a dosing level after which side effects accrue more rapidly than analgesic effects. The potent opioids have no such ceiling. As tolerance develops or disease progresses, the doses can be increased.

8. **Name some of the "weak" opioids and the problems associated with them.**
Codeine is one of the most commonly used weak opioids. As doses escalate, nausea and constipation limit efficacy. For example, though 30 mg of codeine provides more analgesia than 15 mg, and 60 mg provides more than 30 mg, etc., higher doses are limited by side effects. Oxycodone is often listed as a weak opioid. However, this designation is mainly a function of the acetaminophen or aspirin with which it is commonly combined, and in reality, oxycodone by itself is likely more potent than morphine. When used as a single agent and not in combination with another agent, oxycodone can be given in increasing doses, without as clear a ceiling.

9. **Name some "potent" opioids.**
Morphine is the prototype of the potent group, against which other opioids have been judged despite the fact that other commonly prescribed drugs, including hydrocodone and oxycodone, are more potent than morphine. Morphine is a relatively short serum half-life drug (2 to 3 hours), as is hydromorphone. Methadone, another potent opioid, has a much longer terminal serum half-life, potentially extending to 54 hours; however, its analgesic serum half-life is often much shorter (6 to 8 hours, for example). Prescribing methadone in particular can be very challenging as a result because increasing the dose too quickly can lead to serious and potentially fatal outcomes.

10. **What subtypes of opioid receptor are important in analgesia?**
The three main opioid subtypes are the mu, kappa, and delta receptors. From the standpoint of analgesia, the mu receptor seems to be the most important. There may be subtypes of these receptors, with different drugs having different affinities for given receptor subtypes and different patients having different receptor subtypes as well. There also may be analgesic activity at the delta and kappa sites.

11. **Explain what is meant by a mixed agonist-antagonist drug.**
When a drug combines with a receptor site and produces the action of that receptor, it is considered an agonist. A drug that binds with a receptor and inhibits activity is considered an antagonist. Naloxone is an example of a pure antagonist drug. Semisynthetic and synthetic products have been produced that are both agonist and antagonist at opioid receptors. The hope in producing these drugs was that they would be agonist for analgesic effects and antagonist for the respiratory depression and sedative effects of the opioids. Examples of mixed agonist-antagonist drugs include pentazocine, butorphanol, and buprenorphine. New preparations of these drugs, specifically buprenorphine, are being or have been developed. In fact, the

administration of a mixed agonist-antagonist drug to a patient who is physically dependent on an agonist may produce a withdrawal syndrome.

12. **What are the endogenous opioids?**
The first endogenous opioids to be discovered were the endorphins and enkephalins. These are polypeptides that are synthesized in the brain and spinal cord. They bind with opioid receptors and produce analgesia. Since the discovery of endorphins and enkephalins in the early 1970s, a number of other peptide products have been described.

13. **How do mixed agonist-antagonist drugs differ from pure agonist analgesics?**
Clinically, the most important concept is that these mixed drugs have a ceiling effect. That is, with increasing doses, side effects supervene, and further analgesia cannot be achieved. When tolerance develops to pure agonist drugs, drug doses can be increased to obtain further analgesia. In patients who are opioid dependent, administration of a mixed agonist-antagonist may precipitate withdrawal.

14. **Differentiate efficacy and potency.**
Efficacy refers to the ability of the drug to produce a given response in an appropriate clinical setting. Potency refers either to the number of milligrams required to produce an effect or to the affinity with which a drug binds to a receptor. Thus a drug may be very potent (able to produce a response at a very low dose) but not have great efficacy (because of intolerable side effects).

15. **If a patient is taking a potent opioid, how can it make sense to add a nonsteroidal antiinflammatory drug to the regimen?**
Opioids and nonsteroidal antiinflammatory drugs work at different sites. As noted earlier, the opioids combine with the opioid receptor, primarily in the central nervous system. The nonsteroidal antiinflammatory drugs are cyclooxygenase inhibitors and their primary site of action is in the peripheral nervous system.

16. **What is meant by an equianalgesic dose?**
Most studies done to determine the clinical potency of the opioid analgesics were done against a standard dose of 10 mg of intramuscular (IM) morphine. Thus the number of milligrams of a given drug required to produce the same degree of analgesia as 10 mg of morphine is referred to as the "equianalgesic dose." Most opioids are far more potent when given parenterally than orally. To achieve a dose equianalgesic to 10 mg of IM morphine, 20 to 60 mg would have to be administered orally. This is because of a "first pass" effect in the liver: approximately 50% to 80% of an opioid is inactivated by hepatic metabolism after oral administration. The extent of this first pass effect varies from drug to drug. Hydromorphone, for example, is five times as potent on a milligram basis after IM injection than it is after oral administration. Methadone, on the other hand, has only a 2:1 ratio.

17. **By the intramuscular route, what are the equianalgesic doses of hydromorphone, methadone, demerol, and levorphanol that would equate with 10 mg of intramuscular morphine?**
To match the analgesic effects of a 10-mg dose of IM morphine, a patient would require 1.5 mg of hydromorphone, 10 mg of methadone, and 2 mg of levorphanol. (See Table 30-5 for equianalgesic doses of various opioids; this information is also available in most pharmacology textbooks.)

18. **Do these calculations hold for chronic dosing?**
No, the equianalgesic calculations do not necessarily hold for chronic dosing. Unfortunately, there is a paucity of data on long-term dosing, and there appears to be a very wide range of ratios that do not fit the numbers cited in Question 16, which were derived from acute dosing. Importantly, methadone appears to be much more potent than previously estimated. When switching to methadone from another opioid, the calculated dose should be decreased by about 75%! Discrepancies may also exist depending on the direction of the switch (methadone to morphine, or morphine to methadone).

19. **What are the major differences among the opioid analgesics?**
    The first major difference is between agonists and mixed agonist-antagonist drugs. The relatively pure opioid agonists include drugs such as morphine, codeine, oxycodone, oxymorphone, levorphanol, fentanyl, and methadone. The mixed agonist-antagonist drugs that are in popular use are pentazocine, butorphanol, and buprenorphine.

    The next major differentiation is between long serum half-life and short serum half-life. Methadone and levorphanol are two of the most commonly used long serum half-life drugs, having a half-life of anywhere from 12 to over 50 hours. (With prolonged use, half-life extends markedly.) Morphine and hydromorphone are prototypes of the short serum half-life drugs.

20. **What are appropriate dosing intervals for the opioid analgesics?**
    When used as immediate-release products, morphine and hydromorphone should generally be dosed every 2 to 4 hours. If a sustained-release or controlled-release product is used, morphine can be dosed every 8 to 12 hours. The long serum half-life drugs may have a greater duration of efficacy and can often be dosed every 4 to 6 hours. Despite the long serum half-life, analgesic efficacy does not directly parallel the serum half-life.

21. **What is a rescue dose?**
    Patients who are treated with a sustained-release product may have breakthrough pain (unexpected increases in pain that was previously well controlled) and require intermittent doses of an immediate-release product. It is probably best to use the same medication for the rescue as for the standing dose. It should be offered on an as needed basis every 2 to 3 hours and should be approximately 10% of the total daily dose.

22. **What routes of administration are available for the opioids?**
    Opioids can be successfully delivered by virtually any route. In general, the most convenient route is orally. However, allowances must be made for the "first pass" effect in the liver (see Question 16). When given by the parenteral route, opioids are anywhere from two to five times as potent on a milligram basis than when given orally. They are also readily absorbed after subcutaneous injection and can be administered intravenously. Rectal and sublingual preparations are also available for some opioids. Fentanyl is available as a transdermal patch. In general, the intramuscular route should be avoided. The injection itself is painful and offers little or no advantage over the subcutaneously or intravenous routes.

23. **What are the benefits and drawbacks of transdermal fentanyl?**
    Fentanyl is a relatively potent opioid analgesic. The application of a transcutaneous patch allows for relatively stable serum levels of fentanyl over 48 to 72 hours. This cuts down the need for repeated dosing and for the pain of parenteral administration. However, after application of the first patch, there is a delay of 12 to 24 hours in achieving adequate analgesia. During this time, rescue doses must be given. Furthermore, if side effects ensue, removal of the patch will not immediately eliminate them because a subcutaneous reservoir of drug has been formed. The dose of drug is directly related to the surface area of the patch. It is available as 12, 25, 50, 75, and 100 micrograms per hour. Direct equianalgesic studies with morphine have not been published, but a 100-micrograms-per-hour patch applied every 72 hours is approximately equianalgesic to 200 mg per day of morphine.

24. **What are some of the adverse reactions that are peculiar to the transdermal application of opioids?**
    Absorption varies with the state of vascular dilatation. Fever or local heat can produce vasodilatation that produces more rapid absorption and systemic distribution of the opioid preparation. Patients must be cautioned not to apply a heating pad to the area where the patch is applied. Local reactions to the adhesive have also been described.

25. **List some of the most common side effects of the opioids.**
    Constipation is the most common and bothersome clinical side effect of the opioids. It is usually defined as a reduction in the frequency of bowel movements to less than one every three days, or difficulty in passing stool. Although respiratory depression, tolerance, dependence, and addiction get the lion's share of the adverse press, constipation is the problem the clinician most often has to address. It is also a complication to which tolerance does not usually develop. All patients being started on opioid analgesics should be given a bowel regimen. In general, a combination of the senna alkaloids and a stool softener is sufficient. However, care should be taken not to allow constipation to progress too far. Once the patient has missed more than a few days of bowel movements, disimpaction may be necessary.
    Nausea and vomiting are not uncommon at the start of opioid therapy. However, tolerance usually occurs within days to weeks, and a specific therapy is not usually required. If nausea persists, opioid rotation may be tried, or the route of administration may be changed.
    Neuroendocrine side effects including hypogonadism need to be considered in patients on chronic opioid therapy.

26. **Under what circumstances is respiratory depression a serious worry in patients treated with opioids?**
    If opioids are used carefully, in gradually increasing doses, respiratory depression usually is not a problem. However, there are two circumstances in which respiratory depression may occur unexpectedly. First, when using long serum half-life drugs, remember that five serum half-lives are required to reach steady state. Thus, when using a drug such as methadone or levorphanol, it may require more than a week to achieve steady state. During this titration period, great care must be taken because serum levels may be escalating despite stable dosing.
    The second circumstance occurs in patients who undergo a pain-relieving procedure after they have been on large doses of opioids. Patients may tolerate large doses while they are in pain. However, if they undergo radiation therapy, cordotomy, or some other procedure directed at the pain syndrome itself, they may no longer be as tolerant to the opioids. Patients should be monitored carefully for a number of days following these procedures. If respiratory rate decreases or they become overly somnolent, doses should be cut back. On the rare occasion that an opioid antagonist must be administered for severe respiratory depression, it should be diluted and injected slowly to avoid the risk of a severe withdrawal syndrome.

27. **How should opioid overdose be treated?**
    Treatment depends directly on the situation in which the overdose has occurred and the severity of side effects. If there is only somnolence, without respiratory depression, simply cutting back on the dose or holding a few doses is usually enough to reverse the side effects. If there is severe respiratory depression, more urgent measures are required. In these cases, naloxone may be administered intravenously. However, if it is given as a bolus, patients who have been taking opioids chronically may experience withdrawal. Therefore, naloxone should be diluted in 10 ml of saline and administered slowly. Keep in mind that opioids primarily depress respiratory rate. Therefore, simply counting respirations as they increase is enough to judge efficacy of opioid reversal. Naloxone, however, has a much shorter serum half-life than most opioids. Repeated doses may be required.

28. **What is meant by tolerance? What are its clinical manifestations?**
    Tolerance refers to a situation in which decreased effects are noticed despite stable doses of a drug, or increasing doses of a drug are required to maintain a given effect. In experimental models, this can develop quite rapidly. Clinically, however, many patients with stable pain syndromes can be maintained on steady doses of opioids for prolonged periods of time. As pain increases (as with advancing cancer), progressively higher doses of drug may be used to control pain. In these cases, increasing analgesia may occur without significant respiratory depression or somnolence.

29. **Define physical dependence.**

   Physical dependence is a state in which rapid discontinuation of a drug or administration of an antagonist produces an abstinence syndrome. With the opioids, an abstinence syndrome is characterized by abdominal discomfort, borborygmus, goose flesh, nausea, and yawning. In addicted subjects, there is marked drug craving. In nonaddicted subjects, there is simply severe discomfort.

30. **Does physical dependence define addiction?**

   No. Physical dependence can develop entirely separate from addiction. Although "psychological dependence" has often been used interchangeably with addiction, physical dependence (as defined earlier) is a physiological phenomenon that occurs as a result of repeated administration of a drug. The mechanism of physical dependence occurs at a molecular level, not a societal one.

31. **What is meant by opioid addiction?**

   Addiction is a biopsychosocial condition in which there is psychological dependence on a drug, preoccupation with securing its supply, use despite harm, use for nonmedical purposes, and a high incidence of recidivism. This is actually quite rare in patients treated appropriately with opioids for pain. Even in patients with pain of nonmalignant origin, opioid addiction is quite uncommon. (See Chapter 35, Addiction and Pain Management, for a more thorough discussion of the subject.)

32. **What is opioid unresponsiveness? How can it be handled?**

   Opioid responsiveness is the analgesia that can be achieved from opioids as the dose is titrated to an endpoint defined either by intolerable side effects or the occurrence of acceptable analgesia. By contrast, if side effects impose a limit on dose escalation, the pain is said to be relatively opioid unresponsive. There is always a balance between effects and side effects. A number of factors can influence opioid responsiveness, including the type of pain (neuropathic pain is often relatively unresponsive), the temporal pattern of the pain (incidence of pain may be difficult to control), opioid tolerance or disease progression (may require very high doses), and idiosyncratic patient issues (may limit responsiveness).

   Strategies to overcome opioid unresponsiveness include more aggressive management of side effects (an attempt to "open the therapeutic window"), the use of adjuvant drugs that may have analgesic effects of their own, the use of drugs that may enhance opioid analgesia (calcium-channel blockers and clonidine), or "opioid rotation."

33. **Describe "opioid rotation." What is the rationale behind it?**

   Cross-tolerance among the opioids is not complete; a patient who is tolerant to a given opioid may not be completely tolerant to a different opioid. If analgesia cannot be obtained with a specific drug, it may make sense to try different opioids. This can be done sequentially, until an appropriate balance is found between analgesia and side effects.

34. **What is patient-controlled analgesia?**

   As generally used today, patient-controlled analgesia (PCA) refers to an arrangement whereby patients are able to administer their own drugs on a set basis. Usually this is by the intravenous route. Intravenous access is established, and a system is attached by which the patient may bolus small amounts of opioid every few minutes. A "lockout period" is also established to avoid overdosing. PCA can be done with or without a continuous infusion. This modality is most often used for patients in acute pain settings, such as those experiencing postoperative pain.

KEY POINTS

1. Opioid analgesics may be effective for both cancer and noncancer pain.

2. There are many different opioid analgesics currently available; the prescriber should be knowledgeable of the relative potency of the prescribed drugs and other unique characteristics of specific drugs before prescribing them.

3. Opioid analgesics are available as short acting and longer acting preparations.

4. Opioid analgesics may be administered through multiple routes depending on patient needs and, in some instances, patient preference.

5. The prescriber needs to be aware of the risks of opioids, including aberrant behaviors, as well as potential adverse effects and must screen for these and monitor for these before and during treatment with opioids.

BIBLIOGRAPHY

1. Anderson R, Saiers JH, Abram S, Schlicht C: Accuracy in equally analgesic dosing: conversion dilemmas, *J Pain Symptom Manage* 21(5):397-406, 2001.

2. Angst MS, Clark JD: Opioid-induced hyperalgesia: a qualitative systematic review, *Anesthesiology* 104(3): 570-587, 2006.

3. Arnold RM, Han PK, Seltzer D: Opioid contracts in chronic nonmalignant pain management: objectives and uncertainties, *Am J Med* 119(4):292-296, 2006.

4. Aronoff GM: Opioids in the chronic pain management: is there is significant risk of addiction? *Curr Rev Pain* 10(2):112-121, 2000.

5. Dean M: Opioids in renal failure and dialysis patients, *J Pain Symptom Manage,* 28(5):497-504, 2004.

6. Mehta V, Langford RM: Acute pain management for opioid dependent patients, *Anaesthesia* 61(3):269-276, 2006.

7. Mercandante S, Portenoy RK: Opioid poorly-unresponsive cancer pain. Part 1: Clinical considerations, *J Pain Symptom Manage* 21(2):144-150, 2001.

8. Murray A, Hagen NA: Hydromorphone, *J Pain Symptom Manage* 29(Suppl 5):57-66, 2005.

9. O'Mahony S, Coyle N, Payne R: Current management of opioid-related side effects, *Oncology* 15(1):61-82, 2001.

10. Page GG: Immunologic effects of opioids in the presence or absence of pain, *J Pain Symptom Manage* 29(Suppl 5):25-31, 2005.

11. Paice JA, Toy C, Shott S: Barriers to cancer pain relief: fear of tolerance and addiction, *J Pain Symptom Manage* 16(1):1-9, 1998.

12. Passik SD, Weinreb HJ: Managing chronic nonmalignant pain: overcoming obstacles to the use of opioids, *Adv Ther* 17(2):70-83, 2000.

13. Pasternak GW: Molecular biology of opioid analgesia, *J Pain Symptom Manage* 29(Suppl 5):2-9, 2005.

14. Pereira J, Lawlor P, Vigano A, et al: Equianalgesic dose ratios for opioids: a critical review and proposals for long-term dosing, *J Pain Symptom Manage* 22(2):672-687, 2001.

15. Portenoy RK: Opioid analgesics. In Portenoy RK, Kanner RM, editors: *Pain management: theory and practice,* Philadelphia, 1996, FA Davis, pp 248-276.

16. Portenoy RK: Opioid therapy for chronic nonmalignant pain: a review of critical issues, *J Pain Symptom Manage* 11(4):203-217, 1996.

17. Reissig JE, Rybarczyk AM: Pharmacologic treatment of opioid-induced sedation in chronic pain, *Annals of Pharmacotherapy* 39(4):727-731, 2005.

CHAPTER 35

ADDICTION AND PAIN MANAGEMENT

Ronald Kanner, MD, FAAN, FACP

1. **What is addiction?**

   Addiction is a primary, chronic, neurobiologic disease, with genetic, psychosocial, and environmental factors influencing its development and manifestations. It is characterized by behaviors that include one or more of the following: impaired control over drug use, compulsive use, continued use despite harm, and craving. This definition was accepted by the American Academy of Pain Medicine, the American Pain Society, and the American Society of Addiction Medicine in February of 2001. It implies that addiction is neither tolerance nor physical dependence, but a more complex, biopsychosocial phenomenon.

2. **Is addiction common in patients treated with opioid analgesics for chronic pain syndromes?**

   Regarding addiction in patients treated with opioid analgesics for chronic pain syndromes, prevalence figures in various studies have ranged from 1% up to 45%. The low end of the range was based on a study that looked only at patients who had received a single-dose of an opioid during a hospital stay for a non–drug-use-related problem. It is, perhaps, not a figure with great applicability, because it is far lower than the likely true prevalence of opioid addiction in the general population. The higher number was derived from a study that examined a small group of patients with a history of prior opioid addiction now treated with opioids for chronic pain. Although it is a strikingly high number, it also shows that up to 55% of patients—even with a prior history of addiction—can be treated successfully with opioids.

   The real addiction risk lies somewhere in between these two figures and is determined by a number of factors. (See Chapter 34, Opioid Analgesics, for a discussion of the issues that must be taken into account when prescribing opioids for chronic pain of noncancer origin.) When opioids are used appropriately for pain management, the risk of de novo addiction is likely acceptably low.

   As the work done by the American Academy of Pain Medicine, the American Pain Society, and the American Society of Addiction Medicine has suggested, "Addiction, unlike tolerance and physical dependence, is not a predictable drug effect, but represents an idiosyncratic and chronic adverse reaction in biologically and psychosocially vulnerable individuals. Addiction is a primary chronic disease, and exposure to drugs is only one of the etiologic factors in its development."

3. **List the five main characteristics of addiction.**

   The five C's can be used as a memory aid for recalling the five main characteristics of addiction
   - **C**hronic
   - **C**ontrol impaired
   - **C**ompulsive use
   - **C**ontinued use, despite harm
   - **C**raving

4. **What is physical dependence?**

   Physical dependence is a state of adaptation that is manifested by a drug class–specific withdrawal syndrome that can be produced by abrupt cessation, rapid dose reduction, decreasing blood level of the drug, and/or administration of antagonist. The presence of physical dependence does not, in itself, define addiction. It should be kept in mind that physical dependence is not unique to opioids.

5. **What is tolerance?**
Tolerance is a state of adaptation in which exposure to a drug induces changes that result in a diminution of one or more of the drug's effects over time. The presence of tolerance does not, in itself, define addiction.

6. **A patient is using progressively higher doses of the opioids prescribed and is requiring prescriptions sooner than anticipated. What are some of the possible causes?**
   - Worsening of the underlying disease. This is the most common cause of dose escalation in patients with pain caused by cancer. Whenever a cancer patient has a worsening pain syndrome, the underlying disease should be the primary suspect.
   - Tolerance. One of the first signs of tolerance in the patient being treated with opioid analgesics is a shortening of the duration of action. The patient may not need a higher dose, but he or she may require more frequent dosing. Care should be individualized.
   - Drug diversion. Persons other than those for whom the drug is prescribed may be taking them. This could be a family member or friend, without the knowledge of the patient, or the patient may be intentionally giving or selling the drugs to a third party.
   - Addiction.

7. **What is the utility of written medication agreements in patients suspected of opioid abuse?**
Although a written agreement may provide some security to the prescriber, it can have mixed effects. It is unclear that it prevents abuse or that it would have any legal standing. In some patients, it may create an unneeded friction between the patient and physician. However, it can be used as a means for the prescriber to outline what he or she expects from the patient with respect to appropriate medication use.

8. **What should be done if addiction is suspected?**
Addiction is an uncommon and undesirable side effect of chronic opioid treatment. Recognize it as such. Conduct a frank discussion with the patient regarding addiction. If necessary, referral to an addiction specialist can be beneficial. Although it is not illegal to prescribe opioid medications to an addicted patient for pain control, it is illegal to prescribe methadone for addiction maintenance therapy, outside of an approved addiction therapy center.

9. **What are some of the newer options for the outpatient management of opioid dependence?**
Buprenorphine (a partial opioid agonist) and the combination product of buprenorphine/naloxone have recently been approved for the outpatient treatment of opioid dependence. As a partial agonist, buprenorphine can suppress some of the withdrawal symptoms that dependent patients can feel upon a limitation of their drug. It is less likely to produce significant respiratory depression. These treatments should be used only by physicians with adequate training and sufficient support staff to supply the needed medical and psychological support for these patients.

10. **Even though methadone is a good analgesic, do patients on methadone maintenance therapy still require postoperative medications?**
Yes. Although methadone has a very long serum half-life (17 to 54 hours) and can effectively block symptoms of withdrawal during that time, its analgesic efficacy is only about 4 to 8 hours. If methadone is to be used as analgesic, it would have to be dosed at least three times per day.

11. **Can other analgesics be efficacious in patients who are on methadone maintenance therapy?**
    Yes. During the postoperative period, a reasonable program is to cover the patient's prior methadone intake and add short serum half-life analgesics for acute pain management.

12. **Is there strong evidence to suggest that hydromorphone is more likely to be abused than other opioid analgesics?**
    No. Hydromorphone is not more likely to be abused than other opioid analgesics. This is urban legend that has not been substantiated by any appropriately designed studies.

13. **Define pseudoaddiction.**
    Pseudoaddiction is a term used to describe patient behaviors that may occur when pain is undertreated. Patients may embellish their symptoms in an attempt to obtain enough medication to provide adequate pain relief or may merely express their discomfort and hoard their medications for times of severe pain. These behaviors are interpreted by the physician as signs of addiction, and medications are cut back further. This leads to a vicious cycle in which the patient is requesting more and more drug to relieve pain, and the physician is prescribing less and less, because of the fear of addiction.

14. **What is DAWN?**
    DAWN is the Drug Abuse Warning Network. It records drug-related mentions in emergency reports. Data suggest that prescription drugs account for about 25% to 30% of all drug abuse. This figure has remained stable over a number of years.

15. **True or false: "Overprescribing" and "underprescribing" are helpful terms when considering a therapy regimen.**
    False. *Overprescribing* and *underprescribing* are relatively useless terms. What is more important is "appropriate prescribing practices." If drugs are used for legitimate medical purposes, in the usual course of professional practice, and documented in medical records, it is highly unlikely that any legal action could be successfully taken against the practitioner.

16. **What types of action on the part of the practitioner typically lead to sanctions from regulating bodies?**
    Activities involving sex for drugs, money for drugs, and drugs for drugs are the types of practitioner actions that typically lead to sanctions from regulating bodies. Some physicians have actually kept records of their illicit activities, noting what they expected to receive in turn for the prescriptions.

17. **Is there any relationship between the "street value" of the drug and the likelihood of its deviation from legal, prescribed uses?**
    Yes. The "street value" of a given drug depends on a number of issues. Rapidity of onset, intensity, short duration of action, potency, the ability to create an injectable form, and brand recognition all may lead to greater desirability of a drug and therefore also lead to a greater likelihood that it will be misused.

18. **How common are severe penalties against physicians for violations of the Controlled Substances Act?**
    In the year 2000, controlled substances violations represented 7% of the total actions against physicians. Only 9% of those resulted in license revocation.

19. **What actions on the part of the patient should alert you to the possibility of "drug-seeking" behavior?**
    Any of the following may be a red flag that drug diversion or illicit use is occurring:
    - Frequent calls when another practitioner is covering
    - Calls toward the end of office hours, when a patient cannot be seen in person

- Requests for drugs without requesting evaluation
- Urgent need for drugs
- Unwillingness to provide prior medical records
- Frequent complaints of "lost prescriptions"
- Lack of follow-up on referrals

20. **How can a practitioner prevent drug diversion?**
The first rules to follow to help prevent drug diversion are the same rules of good medical practice: perform a detailed history and physical examination, and document your diagnosis and treatment plan. If you see any of the signs of drug-seeking behavior, discuss them with the patient, document it in the chart, and seek expert help, if needed. Be aware of state and federal laws and regulations. You may want to use prescription pads that are not easily copied and carry serial numbers. Prescription pads should be kept in a safe place and not made available to other practitioners. It is good practice to write numbers out fully. Designate the number of refills, even when it is "zero." Consider using risk assessment tools such as the Opioid Risk Tool (ORT) before prescribing to help you understand if the patient you are about to prescribe opioids to is at low, medium, or high risk of misusing the prescription. You can then decide if a particular patient is at an acceptable risk level for YOUR practice. If the patient's risk level is considered by you to be high, BUT you feel the patient is still an appropriate candidate for opioid treatment, consider referring the patient to a subspecialist for comanagement. Define to the patient when initially prescribing opioids what you feel is a minimally acceptable clinical response for continuing a patient on such therapy. Moniter the patient carefully while on opioid therapy for benefits and adverse effects of such treatment, and specifically consider random urine drug testing to help ensure that the patient is using the prescription appropriately.

21. **What resources are available to learn more about signs, risks, and treatments for addiction?**
The American Society of Addiction Medicine maintains a website that can be quite helpful. The American Academy of Pain Medicine and the American Pain Society also offer a number of publications regarding addiction medicine.

KEY POINTS

1. Addiction is a chronic neurobiologic disorder that needs to be distinguished from tolerance and physical dependence.

2. Even patients with known drug addiction may need to be treated with opioid analgesics and under most circumstances, with appropriate training of the prescriber and with appropriate monitoring of the patient, this is considered appropriate.

3. Prescribers should be aware of "best" practice approaches to the prescribing of opioids to patients in general, as well as to known addicts in particular, and implement these in their practice.

WEBSITES

1. U.S. Drug Enforcement Administration
   http://www.usdoj.gov/dea/agency/mission.htm

2. http://www.projectphysicianquality.org/jcaho.htm

3. University of Wisconsin: Pain & Policy Studies Group
   http://www.medsch.wisc.edu/painpolicy

4. American Pain Society
   http://www.ampainsoc.org

5. American Academy of Pain Medicine
   http://www.painmed.org

BIBLIOGRAPHY

1. Alford DP, Compton P, Samet JH: Acute pain management for patients receiving maintenance methadone or buprenorphine therapy, *Annals of Internal Medicine* 144(2):127-134, 2006.

2. American Academy of Pain Medicine, American Pain Society, American Society of Addiction Medicine: Consensus Document: Definitions related to the use of opioids for the treatment of pain. April, 2001.

3. American Society of Addiction Medicine: Public policy statement on definitions related to the use of opioids in pain treatment, *J Addict Dis* 17(2):129-133, 1998.

4. Arnold RM, Han PK, Seltzer D: Opioid contracts in chronic nonmalignant pain management: objectives and uncertainties, *Amer J Med* 119(4):292-296, 2006.

5. Compton P, Darakjian J, Miotto K: Screening for addiction in patients with chronic pain and "problematic" substance use: evaluation of a pilot assessment tool, *J Pain Symptom Manage* 16(6):355-363, 1998.

6. Fiellin DA, Kleber H, Trumble-Hejduk JG, McLellan AT, Kosten TR: Consensus statement on office-based treatment of opioid dependence using buprenorphine, *Journal of Substance Abuse Treatment* 27(2):153-159, 2004.

7. Mehta V, Langford RM: Acute pain management for opioid dependent patients, *Anaesthesia* 61(3):269-276, 2006.

8. Murray A, Hagen NA: Hydromorphone, *J Pain Symptom Manage* 29(Suppl 5):57-66, 2005.

9. Passik SD, Kirsh KL, McDonald MV, et al: A pilot survey of aberrant drug-taking attitudes and behaviors in samples of cancer and AIDS patients, *J Pain Symptom Manage* 19(4):274-286, 2000.

10. Passik SD, Portenoy RK, Ricketts PL: Substance abuse issues in cancer patients. Part 1: Prevalence and diagnosis, *Oncology* (Wiliston Park) 12(4):517-521, 524, 1998.

11. Passik SD, Weinreb HJ: Managing chronic nonmalignant pain: overcoming obstacles to the use of opioids, *Adv Ther* 17(2):70-83, 2000.

12. Portenoy RK: Opioid therapy for chronic nonmalignant pain: a review of the critical issues, *J Pain Symptom Manage* 11(4):203-217, 1996.

13. Portenoy RK, Dole V, Joseph H, et al: Pain management and chemical dependency: evolving perspectives, *JAMA* 278(7):592-593, 1997.

14. Sung S, Conry JM: Role of buprenorphine in the management of heroin addiction, *Annals of Pharmacotherapy* 40(3):501-505, 2006.

15. Weissman DE, Haddox JD: Opioid pseudoaddiction—an iatrogenic syndrome, *Pain* 36(3):363-366, 1989.

CHAPTER 36

REGULATORY ISSUES

Ellen Cooper, MS, and Charles E. Argoff, MD

1. **Do patients with painful medical conditions generally receive adequate treatment for pain?**

   No. Both acute pain and chronic pain caused by cancer are generally undertreated. This is particularly true of treatment with opioid drugs. Surveys of patients in the postoperative period demonstrate that up to 75% suffer pain of moderate or severe intensity. Because virtually all postoperative pain can be controlled with proper medication, an alarmingly high number of patients suffer from unnecessary pain. Similarly, in patients with advanced cancer, simple drug regimens can provide relief for more than 70%. However, 70% of patients with advanced cancer still report significant pain! On a global scale, the statistics are even more alarming. More than 3.5 million people suffer from cancer pain, but only a small fraction receives adequate treatment. This is particularly striking in view of the fact that pain can be controlled with appropriate drug regimens in approximately 90% of these patients.

2. **What factors stand in the way of adequate pain treatment?**

   Barriers to good analgesic therapy exist on the professional, societal, and governmental levels. From a professional point of view, physicians and nurses often have the misconception that the prescription of opioid medications will lead inexorably to tolerance, dependence, and addiction. Even physicians who understand that this is not true tend to underprescribe medications, possibly because of fear of other side effects. Furthermore, worry about regulation by outside agencies also tends to impede a physician's prescribing practices. Many physicians do not understand government regulations on opioid prescribing, and their concerns are often unjustified. Certain government regulations, however, do limit prescribing practices. For example, in states that require a triplicate prescription for opioid medications, opioid prescribing decreases by about 50%.

   Patients also have many misconceptions about opioids. Their fear that the opioids represent a "last-ditch effort" makes them reluctant to take these drugs early in their disease. They also may be afraid of addiction, other side effects, or the societal stigma that goes along with taking opioid medications.

3. **Are patients with medical illness and no history of substance abuse at significant risk of addiction if opioids are administered?**

   Studies in patients with cancer have demonstrated that the main reason for escalating drug intake is progression of disease rather than aberrant behavior. This same pattern has been demonstrated in patients with pain caused by noncancer conditions. Although tolerance and physical dependence may occur, addiction is a rather rare phenomenon in patients treated appropriately with opioid medications for their pain. (See Chapter 35, Addiction and Pain Management.)

4. **What are the differences among opiates, opioids, and narcotics?**

   "Opioid" is a generic term used to refer to codeine, morphine, and other natural and synthetic drugs whose effects are mediated by specific receptors in the central and peripheral nervous systems. The original term, "opiate," was taken to mean any derivative of *Papaver somniferum*, the poppy plant that produces opium. Opioid also includes the endogenous opioids, such as endorphins and enkephalins.

The term "narcotic" was initially used to denote a drug capable of producing sleep (narcosis). It was mainly applied to the opioids. However, narcotic is now more of a legal term, used in reference to all substances covered by the 1961 Single Convention on Narcotic Drugs, including opiates as well as synthetic substances such as meperidine and fentanyl. The term covers not only the opioids but also cocaine and many other drugs of abuse.

5. **At what governing levels do drug regulations exist? How do they pertain to individual practitioners?**
There are three tiers of drug regulations: international, federal, and state. The regulation of professional practice in medicine, nursing, pharmacy, social work, and other professions occurs at the state, and not the federal, level. There have been a number of recent changes in state laws, because of concerns about inappropriate discipline of physicians for prescribing opioid analgesics.

6. **What is the historical background that led the federal government to become involved in monitoring opioids?**
Twentieth-century governments recognized the dangers of abuse and trafficking of opioids, including opium, morphine, and heroin. Concerns, particularly about the opium trade in China and the Philippines, prompted governments throughout the world to join together and set controls on the ever-increasing diversion of illegal substances.

Studies of addicts in the 1950s and 1960s seemed to show that many addicts had their first exposure to opioids from prescriptions during a painful illness. The finding was incorrectly extrapolated to suggest that medical treatment was a common cause of addiction.

7. **What is the International Narcotics Con l Board?**
The International Narcotics Control Board (INCB) is a Vienna-based arm of the United Nations International Drug Control Program. It monitors the implementation of the Single Convention on Narcotic Drugs, an international treaty. The INCB recommends steps that governments and health professionals should take to address this problem.

8. **What do governments perceive as the major impediments to the medical use of opioids?**
In a survey of 65 governments performed by the INCB, concern about addiction was the most frequently stated impediment to the medical use of opioids; this concern appeared in 72% of statements. The next most frequently stated issue was insufficient training of health care practitioners. Sixty-five percent of the governments surveyed reported that they had national policies to improve the use of opioids.

9. **Are legal restrictions on opioid prescriptions prevalent throughout the world?**
The following is a quotation from literature produced by the World Health Organization (WHO) that addresses cancer pain:

The WHO has observed that physicians and pharmacists may become reluctant to prescribe or stock opioid analgesics due to strict requirements and fear of punishment. In the survey, many governments reported they required special government-issued prescription forms and other special permissions. The maximum sentence for a physician who fails to comply with prescriber requirements is 22 years in prison; the maximum fine afforded is up to 1 million dollars. Some governments reported having mandatory minimum penalties as high as 10 years in prison for such offenses. Forty-three percent of the governments required health professionals to report patients who receive opioid prescriptions.

None of the regulations in the United States are as stringent as this statement indicates. The majority of U.S. legislation is aimed at avoiding diversion of drugs rather than regulating appropriate prescribing practices.

10. **Which federal legislation regulates the prescribing practices of opioid analgesics?**

The Harrison Narcotic Act of 1914 is the hallmark legislation that marked the federal government's interest in the prescribing and controlling of opioids. In 1961, the INCB was established to receive reports from governments about the movement of opioids and to ensure that supply and demand for opioids were in balance, hoping to prevent undersupply for legitimate purposes. All governments involved are required to furnish the INCB with statistics on an annual basis. In 1971, the Federal Comprehensive Drug Abuse Prevention and Control Act repealed all previous laws and took over the control of prescription drugs. Opioids and drugs with potential for abuse were placed into five schedules.

Hill (see Bibliography) summarized the source of the government's authority to regulate as follows:

Government regulations on controlled substances are authorized by two legislative sources: (a) Health Care Practice Acts (HCPAs) including medical, nursing, pharmacy, dental, etc. which set standards of practice for the use of controlled substances and all other aspects of professional practice, and (b) Controlled Substances Acts (CSAs) which mandate how such substances are to be handled when used for medical purposes. States exert influence on health care practice through enactment of HCPAs and the evaluation of practitioners' practices, based on standards set forth in them. Federal influence is primarily through CSAs.

11. **What is the controlled substances act?**

The following is taken from the U.S. Drug Enforcement Administration (DEA) website (see Bibliography):

The Controlled Substances Act, Title II of the Comprehensive Drug Abuse Prevention and Control Act of 1970, is the legal foundation of the government's fight against the abuse of drugs and other substances. This law is a consolidation of numerous laws regulating the manufacture and distribution of narcotics, stimulants, depressants, hallucinogens, anabolic steroids, and chemicals used in the illicit production of controlled substances.

The CSA places all substances that are regulated under existing federal law into one of five schedules. This placement is based on the substance's medicinal value, harmfulness, and potential for abuse or addiction.

12. **What are the schedules into which all opioids and drugs with potential for abuse are classified?**

The five schedules into which all opioids and drugs are classified under the Federal Comprehensive Drug Abuse Prevention and Control Act are as follows:

Schedule I—Drugs with high abuse potential and no accepted medical use.

Schedule II—Drugs with a high potential for abuse and severe likelihood to produce psychic or physical dependence. Schedule II controlled substances consist of certain opioid drugs and drugs containing amphetamines or methamphetamines as the single active ingredient or in combination. Examples are opium, morphine, codeine, hydromorphone, methadone, cocaine, and oxycodone. Most drugs that are effective in the management of pain caused by cancer fall into this category.

Schedule III—Drugs with a potential for abuse that is less than for that of drugs in schedules I and II. Examples are drugs containing limited quantities of certain opioids and certain nonopioid drugs.

Schedule IV—Drugs with a low potential for abuse that leads only to limited physical dependence or psychological dependence relative to drugs in schedule III. Examples are chlordiazepoxide and diazepam.

Schedule V—Drugs with a potential for abuse that is less than that of drugs in schedule IV and consist of preparations containing moderate quantities of certain opioid drugs. Examples include antidiarrheal medications.

13. **How does the federal government define an addict?**
Federal law defines an addict as "any individual who habitually uses any narcotic drug so as to endanger the public morals, health, safety, or welfare, or who is so far addicted to the use of narcotic drugs as to have lost the power of self-control with reference to his or her addiction." This definition is somewhat vague, but publications by the DEA have made it clear that the agency's function is not to hinder physicians from using opioid analgesics to provide pain relief.

According to the medical definition of addiction, the patient must have a preoccupation with securing the drug, spend a great deal of time either using the drug or recovering from its effects, and continue to use the drug despite harmful effects.

14. **What is the role of the Drug Enforcement Administration (DEA)?**
The Drug Enforcement Administration (DEA) is the federal agency responsible for enforcing national drug laws. It is responsible for registering manufacturers, distributors, and practitioners who handle opioid drugs. The DEA works closely with the Food and Drug Administration and the National Institute on Drug Abuse, which determines annual quotas for amounts of the various opioids that can be manufactured and distributed.

15. **What is the mission of the DEA?**
According to the DEA website (see Bibliography):

The mission of the DEA is to enforce the controlled substances laws and regulations of the United States and bring to the criminal and civil justice system of the United States, or any other competent jurisdiction, those organizations and principal member organizations, involved in the growing, manufacture, or distribution of controlled substances appearing and/or destined for illicit traffic in the United States; and to recommend and support non-enforcement programs aimed at reducing the availability of the illicit controlled substances on the domestic and international markets.

16. **What have been the benefits, if any, of the federal drug control laws?**
Before the establishment of the international drug control system, legitimate manufacturers were the primary source of abused opioid drugs, including heroin. After 1925, legitimate production of opioids has rarely been a source of drugs in the illicit traffic. Because the federal definition of addiction is generally vague, it has not particularly limited prescribing practices. The goal of the federal laws has been to ensure that a therapeutic drug is available to patients when it is needed; laws do not restrict the size of prescriptions or set limits on refills. Many state laws, however, limit prescriptions to a 1-month supply and may even limit the number of doses.

17. **What potentially detrimental perceptions have resulted from the federal drug control system?**
By essentially waging a "war on drugs," the government may have unintentionally restricted medical access to essential medications. The drugs often necessary for managing pain in cancer and other medical illnesses are also the commonly abused drugs. This unfortunate coincidence has negatively influenced the effective treatment of pain worldwide. Regulation of drugs communicates that they are dangerous and reinforces fears. Legitimate manufacturers are concerned about production, physicians are reluctant to prescribe them, and patients are reluctant to take them for fear of being labeled addicts. Forcing physicians to register with the federal government to prescribe opioid medications has significantly curtailed their use.

18. **How have state laws affected prescribing practices?**
    Although most state controlled substance laws are patterned after the Federal Uniform Controlled Substances Act, there are many important differences. Many state laws do not recognize the essential medical uses of controlled substances or the importance of ensuring availability within the state. Many state laws do not have provisions allowing opioid treatment of intractable pain.
    There is a great deal of confusion among physicians about what the laws really say. Nearly one fourth of physicians polled in one study felt that it was probably a violation of federal or state laws to prescribe opioids for chronic nonmalignant pain. One half of the physicians surveyed thought that prescription was illegal for patients with a history of opioid abuse. In point of fact, the law considers prescription of opioids illegal *only if it is done to maintain an addiction*. Methadone maintenance can be prescribed only through a methadone maintenance program.

19. **Have state laws affected prescribing practices and availability of controlled substances?**
    In the past, multiple-copy prescription programs existed in many states and resulted in statewide reductions of more than 50% in the number of prescriptions written for opioids. Physicians must purchase registered and numbered books of prescriptions from the state. Each prescription has three copies: one goes to the pharmacist, one to the office chart, and one to the state. Many state laws limit the amount of medication that can be dispensed at one time, increasing costs and number of patient visits to a physician.

20. **What are more recent trends in state pain policies?**
    In the past decade, concerns about inappropriate discipline of physicians for use of opioid analgesics for treatment of chronic pain has led to changes in state laws, medical board regulations, and guidelines. State medical boards have begun to participate in pain management workshops and have begun to adopt new guidelines to encourage improved pain management. For further information regarding the role of state medical boards, the reader is invited to view information at www.fsmb.com.

21. **What are Electronic Data Transmission (EDT) programs?**
    As a result of pain initiatives, several states have moved to Electronic Data Transmission (EDT) programs, eliminating triplicate prescriptions. Currently, California, Idaho, Illinois, Michigan, and Texas are moving toward eliminating their triplicate programs and beginning EDT programs. Hawaii, Indiana, Massachusetts, Nevada, Oklahoma, Rhode Island, Utah, West Virginia, and New York have already moved to EDT.

22. **Is it permissible to use opioids for the treatment of chronic pain of noncancer origin?**
    Yes. Opioids are the mainstay for the treatment of pain of moderate to severe intensity in patients with cancer. Under appropriate guidelines (see Chapter 34, Opioid Analgesics), they can be used for many patients with pain of noncancer origin. Even patients with a prior history of addiction can be treated, although with great care.

23. **How can a practitioner avoid trouble with regulatory agencies over the prescription of opioid analgesics?**
    Document, document, document. The chart should contain a record of a complete history and physical examination, the diagnosis, and indications for the use of opioid analgesics. It

should be clear that the risks and benefits have been discussed with the patient and that these risks and benefits are documented in the chart. At each visit, pain relief and side effects should be noted. Very few state investigations for opioid prescribing result in actions against a physician's license. Those that do are almost invariably the result of unimaginably poor record keeping or clearly felonious activity.

24. **What are the educational issues surrounding lack of appropriate prescribing practices?**
Standard physician education falls short of appropriately preparing physicians for necessary training in pain management. Even physicians who understand the pharmacokinetics and pharmacodynamics of analgesic medications tend to underprescribe them. State cancer pain initiatives are addressing the issues of education of health care providers and interaction with regulatory agencies.

25. **What is the Oregon Death with Dignity Act? Why is the federal government trying to overturn it?**
In October 1997 Oregon became the first state in the nation to legalize physician-assisted suicide. As of this writing, the Bush administration was seeking the permission of the federal courts to overturn Oregon's Death with Dignity Act.

26. **What are the provisions of the Oregon Death with Dignity Act?**
Under the Oregon Death with Dignity Act, doctors must certify that a patient has an illness that leaves him or her with less than 6 months to live. The patient must be at least 18 and an Oregon resident. The patient must be deemed capable of making health care decisions independently.

27. **What is the doctrine of double effect?**
The doctrine states that all medications have both effects and side effects. Opioid analgesics produce pain relief, but may also suppress respirations. In patients with severe pain, it is recognized that increasing doses of opioids intended to relieve pain may hasten death. If the express intent is pain relief, but death ensues, the intervention is not considered physician-assisted suicide, or euthanasia.

28. **What is the Joint Commission on Accreditation of Healthcare Organizations (JCAHO), and what does it want from us?**
The Joint Commission on Accreditation of Healthcare Organizations (JCAHO) is an independent, not-for-profit organization that evaluates and accredits nearly 19,000 health care organizations and programs in the United States. It sets standards for patient evaluation, treatment, and education. Health care organizations are surveyed on a regular basis. Recently, with the help of nationally recognized pain management experts, standards for pain management were established. The standards state that pain must be evaluated in all patients; that an appropriate plan of action must be established; and that patients, families, and health care providers must be educated with regard to pain management.

KEY POINTS

1. Physicians' concerns regarding regulatory scrutiny remain a significant barrier for the effective treatment of patients' pain.

2. Technically the term *narcotic* refers to drugs other than opioids, including cocaine and many other nonopioid drugs that are abused; thus, *opioid* is clearly the preferred term when referring to this class of analgesic medications.

3. It is permissible for an appropriately trained practitioner to prescribe opioids for both cancer as well as noncancer moderate to severe pain; when doing so the chart should contain a record of a complete history and physical examination, the diagnosis, and indications for the use of opioid analgesics. It should be clear that the risks and benefits have been discussed with the patient and that these risks and benefits are documented in the chart. At each visit, pain relief and side effects should be noted and the rationale for continuation or discontinuation of opioid therapy clearly documented.

WEBSITES

1. http://www.usdoj.gov/dea/agency/mission.htm

2. http://www.medsch.wisc.edu/painpolicy/domestic/resource.htm

3. http://www.fsmb.com

BIBLIOGRAPHY

1. Angarola RT, Joranson DE: Recent developments in pain management and regulation, *APS Bulletin* 4(1):9-11, 1994.

2. Dahl JL: State cancer pain initiatives, *J Pain Symptom Manage* 8(6):372-375, 1993.

3. Gilson AM, Joranson DE: Controlled substances and pain management: changes in knowledge and attitudes of state medical regulators, *J Pain Symptom Manage* 21(3):227-237, 2001.

4. Hill CS: Government regulation influences on opioid prescribing and their impact on the treatment of pain of nonmalignant origin, *J Pain Symptom Manage* 11(5):287-298, 1996.

5. International Opium Convention of 1925, League of Nations Treaties Series, Vol 81, 317: *Convention of 1931 for Limiting the Manufacture and Regulating the Distribution of Narcotic Drugs*, League of Nations Treaty Series 139:301, 1931.

6. Joranson DE, Gilson AM: Pharmacists' knowledge of and attitudes toward opioid pain medications in relation to federal and state policies, *J Am Pharm Assoc* (Wash) 41(2):213-220, 2001.

7. Joranson DE, Gilson AM, Dahl JL, Haddox JD: Pain management, controlled substances, and state medical board policy: a decade of change, *J Pain Symptom* 23(2):138-147, 2002.

8. Kanner RM: How much is knowledge really worth? *J Pain Symptom Manage* 6(5):340-341, 1991.

9. Kanner RM: Opioids for severe pain: little change over 15 years (letter), *J Pain Symptom Manage* 21(2):3, 2001.

10. Max MB: Pain relief and the control of drug abuse: conflicting or complementary goals? In Hill CS Jr, Fields WS (editors): *Advances in pain research and therapy*, vol. 11, New York, 1989, Raven Press.

11. Steinbrook R: Physician-assisted suicide in Oregon—an uncertain future, *New Engl J Med* 346(6):460-464, 2002.

12. Verhovek SH: As suicide approvals rise in Oregon, half go unused, *New York Times*. Wysiwyg://9/http://www.nytimes.com/2002/02/07/national/07suic.html

CHAPTER 37

ADJUVANT ANALGESICS

Brian Thiessen, MD, Russell K. Portenoy, MD, and Charles E. Argoff, MD

1. **What are adjuvant analgesics?**

   Adjuvant analgesics (Table 37-1) are drugs that have primary indications other than pain but are analgesic in some painful conditions. This definition distinguishes a very diverse group of drugs from the traditional analgesics, which comprise the nonopioid analgesics (acetaminophen and the nonsteroidal antiinflammatory drugs) and the opioid analgesics.

   ## TABLE 37-1. ADJUVANT ANALGESICS: MAJOR CLASSES

Multipurpose Analgesics	Analgesic Agents for Neuropathic Pain Syndromes	Analgesic Agents for Musculoskeletal Pain Syndromes
Antidepressants	Antidepressants	Muscle relaxants
Alpha-2 adrenergic agonists	Anticonvulsants	Benzodiazepines
Corticosteroids	GABA agonists	Analgesic agents for bone pain
Topical anesthetics	Oral local anesthetics Topical anesthetics Sympatholytics NMDA receptor blockers Calcitonin	Corticosteroids Osteoclast inhibitors Radiopharmaceuticals

   GABA = gamma-aminobutyric acid, NMDA = N-methyl-D-aspartic acid.

2. **For whom and in which situations are adjuvant analgesics appropriate?**

   As suggested by the label "adjuvant," these analgesics are often coadministered with the traditional analgesics. In some patient populations, particularly those with cancer pain, the conventional approach involves the addition of an adjuvant analgesic drug only after the dose of a traditional analgesic (usually an opioid) has been optimized. In these populations, the adjuvant analgesics are administered for the following purposes:
   - To manage pain that is refractory to the traditional analgesics
   - To allow reduction in dose of the traditional analgesic for the purpose of lessening side effects
   - To concurrently treat a symptom other than pain

   In some clinical settings, adjuvant analgesics have become so well accepted that they are administered as the first-line drug. This is particularly true for chronic neuropathic pain syndromes unrelated to cancer, such as postherpetic neuralgia, trigeminal neuralgia, or painful polyneuropathy (see Question 25). In these situations, the term adjuvant is a misnomer.

3. **What factors should be considered prior to prescribing an adjuvant analgesic?**
The physician must be aware of the drug's clinical pharmacology and its particular use in patients with pain. Learn the following about the analgesic:
- Approved indications
- Unapproved indications widely accepted in medical practice
- Common side effects and uncommon, but potentially serious, adverse effects
- Important pharmacokinetic features, including half-life, usual time-action relationships, extent of interindividual variability, and factors that may alter disposition (e.g., age or interactions with other drugs)
- Specific dosing guidelines for pain

4. **What are the special considerations for the older person?**
In the medically frail and the older population, a cautious approach to the use of the adjuvant analgesics is warranted. It is prudent to select a drug with a good safety profile and begin therapy at a relatively low dose. Gradual escalation of the dose is the safest technique for confirming an effective regimen or determining that the drug is ineffective.

5. **Are responses to the adjuvants uniform?**
No. There is considerable interindividual and intraindividual variation in the response to adjuvant analgesics. This variation underscores the potential utility of sequential drug trials, which may be needed to identify a drug with a favorable benefit-to-risk ratio. Moreover, most trials benefit from the use of gradual dose escalation to identify the most optimal dose.

   Explain dose escalation and the potential need for multiple trials to patients who are about to begin therapy with an adjuvant analgesic. The information will help the patient maintain appropriate expectations and will reduce frustration during a period of ineffective dosing.

6. **Which classes of adjuvant analgesics may be considered multipurpose, nonspecific analgesics?**
Adjuvant analgesics that have been demonstrated to be effective in diverse pain syndromes can be designated multipurpose analgesics. The best characterized of these drugs are the tricyclic antidepressants (TCAs). Other classes that can be considered multipurpose include the alpha-2 adrenergic agonists (e.g., clonidine) and the corticosteroids. Although there is some evidence to support the labeling of local anesthetic drugs in this way, conventional practice now limits the use of this class to patients with neuropathic pain syndromes (see next question).

7. **What is the evidence that antidepressant drugs are multipurpose analgesics?**
Antidepressant drugs, especially the TCAs, have been extensively evaluated in many different pain syndromes, including neuropathic pain, low back pain, headache, fibromyalgia, arthritis, cancer pain, and others. They have been found to have multipurpose analgesic effects. A trial of an analgesic antidepressant is warranted in most patients with chronic pain.

8. **Which antidepressants are recommended for chronic pain?**
The tertiary amine compound amitriptyline has been best studied, but there is evidence supporting the analgesic efficacy of other tertiary amine tricyclic drugs as well, including imipramine, clomipramine, and doxepin. Of the secondary amine tricyclic compounds, which are generally better tolerated than the tertiary amine drugs, desipramine has been most carefully studied, and nortriptyline is also probably analgesic. Compared with the tertiary amine drugs, these secondary amine compounds are less likely to produce sedative, anticholinergic, or hypotensive side effects. (However, see Question 9.)

   Among the newer classes of antidepressants, analgesic effects have been noted for the serotonergic noradrenergic reuptake inhibitors (SNRI) agents duloxetine, venlafaxine, and milnacipran. Duloxetine is in fact approved by the Food and Drug Administration (FDA) for diabetic peripheral neuropathic pain and fibromyalgia. Milnacipran is available in Europe but not in the United States. Analgesic effects have been suggested for bupropion, trazodone, maprotiline, and paroxetine, which is a selective serotonin reuptake inhibitor (SSRI). Of these newer classes, the SSRIs and SNRIs are usually better tolerated than the TCAs.

9. **What is the relative analgesic efficacy of the various antidepressant classes?**
There have been few studies directly comparing the analgesic efficacy of the various antidepressant drugs. From the very limited data available, an analgesic response is most likely to be produced by the tertiary tricyclic drugs; amitriptyline is preferred because of the extensive data available for this drug. The secondary amine tricyclic drugs, such as desipramine, are probably less analgesic than the tertiary amine drugs, but are more likely to be effective than the SSRIs. But SSRIs have fewer side effects than either secondary or tertiary amines (Table 37-2). Based on this information, the clinician should attempt to select the drug most likely to provide benefit and be tolerated by the patient.

TABLE 37-2. COMPARISON OF ANTIDEPRESSANT SIDE EFFECTS			
	Somnolence	Cardiotoxicity	Anticholinergic
Tertiary amines Amitriptyline	+ +	+ + +	+ + +
Secondary amines Nortriptyline Desipramine	+	+ +	+
SSRIs Paroxetine	+/−	−	−

SSRI = selective serotonin reuptake inhibitors.

10. **Do the monoamine oxidase inhibitors have analgesic effects?**
The monoamine oxidase inhibitors (MAOIs), such as phenelzine and tranylcypromine, have been evaluated as analgesics in relatively few clinical settings. In a controlled trial, phenelzine was analgesic in patients with atypical facial pain, and a few uncontrolled trials suggested analgesic properties in other types of chronic pain. Despite these findings, use of MAOIs as analgesics has been limited because of the risk of hypertensive crises and the need for significant dietary restrictions.

11. **True or false: Relief of depression and analgesia are codependent.**
False. Relief of depression is not required for the analgesia produced by antidepressant drugs, although improvement in mood no doubt plays a role in some patients. The analgesia produced by the TCAs occurs at a dose significantly lower than that required to treat depression and usually appears within 1 week after this dose is reached—much sooner than the antidepressant effects typically appear.

12. **What mechanisms may be responsible for antidepressant analgesia?**
The primary pharmacologic action of the antidepressants is to block reuptake of monoaminergic neurotransmitters (e.g., serotonin and norepinephrine) in the central nervous system. Descending pain modulatory pathways that use serotonin and norepinephrine as neurotransmitters have been well characterized, and altered activity in these pathways could be the mechanism by which these drugs yield analgesic effects. The TCAs also interact with many other receptors, some of which have been implicated in other pain-modulating systems.

Interestingly, recent studies have shown that the SSRIs do not yield as much analgesia as the TCAs in patients who are not depressed. The so-called dirty drugs (those affecting multiple receptors, such as TCAs) may exert their effects through multiple systems.

13. **What are the adverse effects of the antidepressants?**

The secondary amine TCAs are less toxic than the tertiary amine compounds, and the SNRIs and SSRIs are less toxic than either tricyclic subclass (see Table 37-2). At doses commonly used for pain control, the tricyclic compounds have few serious adverse effects. Cardiovascular toxicity, including hypotension and cardiac arrhythmia, is the most serious concern. Significant heart disease, including conduction disturbances, arrhythmias, or heart failure, is a relative contraindication to treatment. Secondary amine compounds, SNRIs, and SSRIs have a lower incidence of cardiotoxicity and are preferred if cardiac disease is present.

The more common side effects of the TCAs are less serious. Anticholinergic effects include dry mouth, urinary retention, blurred vision, and constipation. Somnolence and mental clouding are often transient but are a particular problem in the older person.

Nausea is usually the most common side effect of the SSRIs. Some patients report tremulousness or insomnia, and some experience somnolence. Sexual dysfunction can be a problem for others.

14. **Do any particular characteristics among patients suggest a trial of an antidepressant analgesic?**

A trial of an antidepressant analgesic is potentially appropriate for any type of chronic pain. The presence of a psychiatric disorder that may also respond to these drugs, such as major depression or panic disorder, suggests an early trial. Insomnia may justify an early trial of an antidepressant analgesic, such as amitriptyline, which has sedating properties.

When the antidepressants are used to treat chronic neuropathic pain (see Question 26), they are often considered first-line drugs for the management of pain characterized by continuous dysesthesias. These dysesthesias are often described by patients as burning, electrical, or painful numbness. Although lancinating (stabbing) neuropathic pain can respond, antidepressants are not usually considered first-line drugs for pain of this type.

In the management of cancer pain, the usual indication for a trial of an antidepressant is chronic neuropathic pain that has not responded adequately to opioid analgesics. In this setting, these drugs are used as adjuncts to an optimized opioid regimen.

15. **A healthy 70-year-old man is beginning therapy with amitriptyline for painful neuropathy. What is an appropriate starting dose and dosing schedule?**

The starting dose of any tricyclic agent should be low, especially in the older person. For example, the recommended initial dose for amitriptyline is 10 mg/day in the older person and 25 mg/day in younger patients. The dosage can be gradually increased every 2 to 3 days until an effective dose is reached. For amitriptyline and desipramine, the effective dose is usually 50 to 150 mg/day. Blood levels can help guide therapy. The tricyclic drugs are usually administered as a single nighttime dose, thereby allowing sedative effects to occur while the patient is asleep. Some patients, however, experience a morning "hangover" and respond better to divided doses.

The inability to tolerate a trial of amitriptyline or the existence of relative contraindications to this drug (such as preexisting cognitive impairment, prostatism, constipation, or dry mouth) might be addressed by a trial of a secondary amine tricyclic, such as desipramine. If the risks associated with a TCA are too high, consider a trial of an SSRI, such as paroxetine.

16. **What role do tizanidine and clonidine have as adjuvant analgesics?**

Alpha-2 adrenergic agonists can be multipurpose, nonspecific analgesics; tizanidine and clonidine are used for this purpose in the United States. Although one study suggests that only a small proportion of patients with chronic pain respond to clonidine, responders may attain excellent analgesia. Clonidine has been shown to be analgesic in chronic headache, chronic neuropathic and nonneuropathic noncancer pain syndromes, and cancer-related neuropathic pain. Because of limited experience, clonidine is not generally considered a first-line drug, but it may be used in refractory cases. Clonidine is actually FDA-approved when epidurally administered for the treatment of cancer-associated neuropathic pain. The major side effects are dry mouth and sedation. Hypotension may occur, and these drugs must be used cautiously in patients predisposed to this effect. Tizanidine is less likely than clonidine to cause hypotension.

17. **What is the mechanism of analgesia produced by alpha-2 adrenergic agonists?**
The mechanism or mechanisms that produce analgesia are unknown. Noradrenergic pain-modulating systems exist in the central nervous system, and it is possible that the alpha-2 adrenergic receptor is involved in the functioning of this pathway. Activation of the alpha-2 receptor inhibits the release of norepinephrine. Central sympathetic inhibition may be the analgesic mechanism involved in those pain syndromes sustained, at least in part, by sympathetic efferent activity (so-called sympathetically maintained pain).

18. **What is the role of neuroleptic drugs in the treatment of pain?**
The role of neuroleptic drugs in the treatment of pain is quite limited. Methotrimeprazine is a phenothiazine neuroleptic that was demonstrated to be a multipurpose analgesic. The drug is no longer available. Although the experience with methotrimeprazine suggested that neuroleptic drugs can be nonspecific analgesics, there is actually very little evidence that other drugs in the class have analgesic effects. Anecdotal reports have suggested that drugs such as haloperidol or fluphenazine may be analgesic in neuropathic pain, and, on this basis, a therapeutic trial of one of these drugs is sometimes administered in cases of neuropathic pain and pain that has been refractory to other therapies. As yet, there is no good evidence that the newer neuroleptics, such as olanzapine, are effective analgesics.
   In migraine headache, a number of trials have shown efficacy for parenterally administered chlorpromazine and droperidol. Some of the success may have been due to antinauseant effects.

19. **Describe the extrapyramidal side effects of neuroleptics.**
The extrapyramidal effects of neuroleptics can be divided into two groups: those that occur early in the course of treatment and those that are delayed in onset. The early effects include acute dystonic reactions (such as torticollis), parkinsonism, akathisia, and neuroleptic malignant syndrome. The late effects include tardive dyskinesia and other tardive movement disorders. The ability to produce extrapyramidal syndromes is directly related to the potency of the antipsychotic, whereas the anticholinergic effects are inversely related to potency. Therefore, haloperidol is more likely to produce extrapyramidal effects and less likely to produce orthostatic hypotension than is chlorpromazine.
   Other side effects include sedation, orthostatic hypotension, and anticholinergic effects such as dry mouth, blurred vision, and urinary hesitancy. Mental clouding and confusion are relatively common in the older and medically ill patients. Rarely, neuroleptics may cause idiosyncratic side effects such as skin rashes, blood dyscrasias, and hepatic damage.

20. **List some of the common pain syndromes for which corticosteroids have shown benefit.**
In the noncancer pain population, short courses of corticosteroids are often given to provide symptomatic relief of acute herpetic neuralgia, carpal tunnel syndrome, and reflex sympathetic dystrophy. Long-term therapy is avoided because of the risk of toxicity. Epidural administration of corticosteroids may be beneficial for some patients with acute exacerbations of low back pain. Local injections of corticosteroids are also used for carpal tunnel syndrome and acute bursitis.
   In the cancer population, the use of these drugs is far more extensive. Controlled trials and clinical series have shown that corticosteroids can be beneficial in many types of cancer pain, including malignant epidural spinal cord compression, bone pain, pain caused by increased intracranial pressure, neuropathic pain from compression or infiltration of peripheral neural structures, and pain from expansion of visceral capsules or obstruction of a hollow viscus.

21. **Which corticosteroid is the agent of choice in patients with cancer?**
Dexamethasone is the preferred corticosteroid in the cancer population. Use is justified by the low mineralocorticoid effects produced by this drug.

22. **How do corticosteroids produce analgesia?**
It is likely that corticosteroids have a variety of analgesic mechanisms. Corticosteroids have direct antiinflammatory effects, reducing the tissue concentrations of inflammatory mediators that activate nociceptors. They also reduce the aberrant firing that can originate from sites of nerve injury. Pain related to malignant compression may lessen because of steroid-induced reduction of peritumoral edema and, in cases of steroid-responsive neoplasms, reduction of tumor bulk.

23. **List the common side effects associated with corticosteroid use.**
Acute treatment with corticosteroids is usually well tolerated. Potential toxicities include hyperglycemia, fluid retention (which may cause hypertension or cardiac failure in predisposed patients), dyspepsia, peptic ulcer disease, insomnia, and neuropsychological effects (ranging from frank delirium to isolated mood or cognitive or perceptual disturbances).

Chronic administration of corticosteroids can cause the following adverse effects: cushingoid habitus, weight gain, hypertension, osteoporosis, myopathy, increased risk of infection, hyperglycemia, and peptic ulcer disease. Rarely, chronic treatment results in aseptic necrosis of the femoral or humeral head.

24. **What dosing regimens are commonly used when corticosteroids are administered for pain?**
When corticosteroids are administered for pain, dosing regimens are divided into low-dose and high-dose schemes. A high-dose regimen in cancer is most commonly a 100-mg loading dose of dexamethasone followed by 24 mg every 6 hours. It is often initiated in the setting of very severe, often rapidly escalating pain ("crescendo pain") that has not responded promptly to an opioid. Severe bone pain and worsening malignant plexopathy are examples of such pain syndromes. In addition, oncologic emergencies that are steroid-responsive, such as superior vena cava syndrome and malignant epidural spinal cord compression, are commonly managed with high-dose steroid regimens.

Low-dose dexamethasone regimens vary from 4 mg every 6 hours to 1 to 2 mg twice daily. They are commonly used in the setting of advanced medical illness with pain refractory to opioids and other adjuvant agents. Given the side effects of these agents, the patient must be continually assessed for efficacy and toxicity during long-term therapy. In all cases, the lowest dose that achieves the desired analgesic benefit should be sought.

Other corticosteroids, including prednisone and methylprednisone, have also been used as analgesics. There have been no comparative trials of the various drugs, and the doses that have been administered have varied.

25. **What is neuropathic pain?**
Neuropathic pain describes a diverse set of pain syndromes in which the sustaining mechanism is believed to involve aberrant somatosensory processing in the peripheral or central nervous system. The term includes syndromes such as painful polyneuropathy, trigeminal neuralgia, central pain, postherpetic neuralgia, and phantom pain.

26. **What is the role of the adjuvant analgesics in the treatment of chronic neuropathic pain?**
Neuropathic pain syndromes are often refractory to traditional analgesics. Thus the adjuvant analgesics are extremely valuable for these diverse disorders. Although data from clinical trials are inadequate to guide the selection of specific drugs, some general guidelines can be recommended on the basis of clinical experience.

Patients with neuropathic pain characterized by continuous dysesthesias (often described as constant burning or electrical sensations) are usually offered an anticonvulsant or antidepressant analgesic early (Table 37-3). Orally administered local anesthetics are also commonly used, and other multipurpose analgesics (such as tizanidine or clonidine) may be considered in refractory cases.

TABLE 37-3. ADJUVANT ANALGESICS TYPICALLY SELECTED FOR NEUROPATHIC PAIN WITH PREDOMINATING CONTINUOUS DYSESTHESIAS

First Line	Examples
Anticonvulsants	Gabapentin, carbamazepine, valproate, clonazepam, pregabalin, others
Tricyclic antidepressants	Amitriptyline, desipramine
"Newer" antidepressants	Paroxetine, duloxetine
Oral local anesthetics	Mexiletine, tocainide, flecainide
For Refractory Cases	
Alpha-2 adrenergic agonists	Clonidine, tizanidine
Topical agents	Capsaicin, local anesthetics
NMDA receptor antagonists	Dextromethorphan, ketamine
Calcitonin	
Baclofen	

NMDA = N-methyl-D-aspartic acid.

Patients with lancinating (stabbing) pain or neuropathic pain characterized by a paroxysmal onset and longer duration are usually first offered trials of anticonvulsants or baclofen, a gamma-aminobutyric acid agonist (Table 37-4). Trials with the drugs used for continuous neuropathic pain usually follow.

Finally, patients suspected of having neuropathic pain sustained by efferent activity in the sympathetic nervous system (sympathetically maintained pain) are sometimes treated with adjuvant analgesics that may modulate sympathetic function.

TABLE 37-4. ADJUVANT ANALGESICS TYPICALLY SELECTED FOR NEUROPATHIC PAIN WITH PREDOMINATING LANCINATING OR PAROXYSMAL DYSESTHESIAS

First Line	Examples
Anticonvulsants Baclofen	Gabapentin, carbamazepine, valproate, clonazepam, pregabalin, others
For Refractory Cases	
Oral local anesthetics	Mexiletine, tocainide, flecainide
Tricyclic antidepressants	Amitriptyline, desipramine
Newer antidepressant	Paroxetine, duloxetine
Alpha-2 adrenergic agonists	Clonidine, tizanidine
Topical agents	Capsaicin, local anesthetics
NMDA receptor antagonists	Dextromethorphan, ketamine
Calcitonin	

NMDA = N-methyl-D-aspartic acid.

27. **How are anticonvulsants used in the management of neuropathic pain?**
Abundant survey data and controlled studies have established the efficacy of anticonvulsant drugs for neuropathic pain (see Table 37-4). Gabapentin and pregabalin are most widely used for this indication, but other anticonvulsants, including phenytoin, carbamazepine, valproate, and clonazepam, have been used for many years. Gabapentin and pregabalin are useful in diabetic peripheral neuropathy and postherpetic neuralgia. Each appears to have a favorable safety profile.

Other anticonvulsants that are used for neuropathic pain include lamotrigine, topiramate, tiagabine, oxcarbazepine, and zonisamide. In general, the anticonvulsants should be started at a low dose and titrated gradually.

28. **List some painful conditions with prominent lancinating or paroxysmal symptoms for which the anticonvulsant agents have shown benefit.**
Trigeminal neuralgia was the first painful condition for which the analgesic benefit of carbamazepine was described. Other anticonvulsants have also been used to treat this condition. Studies have demonstrated the efficacy of these drugs in the treatment of lancinating pain associated with postherpetic neuralgia and painful diabetic neuropathy. Other reports suggest benefit in glossopharyngeal neuralgia, tabetic lightning pains, paroxysmal symptoms of multiple sclerosis, stabbing pain following laminectomy, lancinating pain caused by cancer, and posttraumatic mononeuropathy.

29. **Can anticonvulsants be used for continuous dysesthesias?**
Although many practitioners believe that anticonvulsants are most efficacious for lancinating pain, studies have indicated that patients with continuous dysesthesias, such as the constant burning reported by many patients with painful polyneuropathy, do experience relief from anticonvulsant drugs (see Table 37-3).

30. **What are the adverse effects associated with carbamazepine?**
Of all the analgesic anticonvulsants, carbamazepine has been most widely used. Other anticonvulsants are less likely to cause side effects, however. Carbamazepine commonly causes sedation, dizziness, diplopia, unsteadiness, and nausea. These effects can be minimized by starting with low initial doses (100 mg, two or three times per day) and increasing the dose gradually (by 100 mg every other day). The effective analgesic dose is variable, and dosing should be increased until pain is relieved, side effects occur, or the plasma concentrations exceed the therapeutic range for seizure control.

Carbamazepine often lowers white blood cell counts, but clinically significant leukopenia or thrombocytopenia occurs rarely. A complete blood count should be obtained prior to therapy, several weeks later, and then 2 or 3 months after that. Therapy should be discontinued if a serious decline in blood count (e.g., a leukocyte count below 3000/ml) occurs. Hepatotoxicity is also rare with carbamazepine, but the possibility dictates periodic monitoring of liver function tests. Hyponatremia resulting from inappropriate secretion of antidiuretic hormone is an uncommon and usually asymptomatic adverse effect. Hypersensitivity reactions, usually rash, occur rarely. Cases of Stevens-Johnson syndrome have been reported.

31. **Is there much individual variation in the response to drugs used for the management of lancinating or paroxysmal dysesthesias?**
Yes. Patients with lancinating or paroxysmal dysesthesias may respond to one anticonvulsant but not to others, or they may not respond to any of the anticonvulsants but do well with one of the other drugs used to treat pain of this type (see Question 32). For this reason, it is appropriate to undertake sequential trials of anticonvulsant drugs in patients with refractory pain.

32. **What other drugs are used in the management of lancinating or paroxysmal dysesthesias?**

Baclofen, a gamma-aminobutyric acid-B receptor agonist, is generally considered the best alternative to the anticonvulsants in the treatment of lancinating or paroxysmal dysesthesias, including trigeminal neuralgia. Treatment is usually started at 5 mg three times per day and slowly increased to the range of 30 to 90 mg/day. Baclofen must not be withdrawn abruptly, as this can precipitate a withdrawal syndrome characterized by restlessness, delirium, and seizures.

Many other drugs have also been used to treat refractory lancinating neuropathic pain. Orally administered local anesthetics are often selected if an anticonvulsant and baclofen have failed. A butyrophenone neuroleptic, pimozide, has been shown to be effective for trigeminal neuralgia and has been used for similar pains. This drug has a high side-effect profile, however, and is often poorly tolerated. Other drugs, including antidepressants (e.g., amitriptyline) and agents usually selected for neuropathic pains of other types, are also used in this setting.

33. **What is the role of systemically administered local anesthetics in the treatment of neuropathic pain?**

Systemically delivered local anesthetics have been used to treat both acute and chronic pain for many years. Brief intravenous infusions of lidocaine or procaine can potentially relieve diverse types of pain, including those not categorized as neuropathic. The need for careful monitoring during this therapy and uncertainty about the optimal dosing guidelines and durability of effects have limited its utility.

Treatment with systemic local anesthetics has become commonplace with the advent of oral local anesthetic drugs, such as mexiletine, tocainide, and flecainide. The use of these drugs has focused on neuropathic pain because of evidence of efficacy from several controlled trials in painful polyneuropathy and painful traumatic mononeuropathy. A trial of an oral local anesthetic is usually recommended in patients without medical contraindications who have continuous dysesthesias that have been refractory to antidepressant treatment, and in those with lancinating neuropathic pain that has not responded to anticonvulsants or baclofen. In the United States, mexiletine is the preferred drug for this indication.

34. **What are the relative contraindications to the use of oral local anesthetic agents?**

Cardiovascular toxicity is a major concern when using oral local anesthetic agents. Toxic concentrations of systemically delivered local anesthetics can produce cardiac conduction disturbances and myocardial depression. Patients with a history of cardiac failure or arrhythmia and those at risk for these problems (e.g., patients with known coronary artery disease) should not receive these drugs without an appropriate evaluation. Referral to a cardiologist may be required.

35. **When using oral local anesthetic agents, how should you monitor the potential for cardiovascular toxicity?**

Most patients older than 50 and all those with known heart disease should be monitored with repeated electrocardiograms (ECG) during dose escalation of oral local anesthetic agents. Younger patients with no known cardiac disease should also undergo an ECG if relatively high doses are reached. The first sign of local anesthetic toxicity is prolongation of the PR interval and QRS duration. With higher concentrations, bradycardia and arrhythmias occur.

Additional toxicities include dizziness, perioral numbness, encephalopathy, and seizures. Nausea and vomiting are common with mexiletine. Liver damage and blood dyscrasias are rare complications.

36. **What is the role of topical drugs in the treatment of pain?**

Three types of topical drugs have been used in the management of chronic pain: local anesthetics, capsaicin, and nonsteroidal antiinflammatory drugs. Although these drugs are most often used in the treatment of neuropathic pains, they are sometimes used in other syndromes as well. A trial of a topical local anesthetic is often considered for neuropathic pain syndromes characterized by a predominant peripheral mechanism and continuous dysesthesias and for nonneuropathic pain syndromes attributable to a focus of cutaneous or subcutaneous tissue injury. A lidocaine-impregnated patch is approved in the United States for treatment of postherpetic neuralgia and can be tried in other conditions.

37. **Which topical local anesthetic produces cutaneous anesthesia?**

Only one commercially available formulation can produce dense cutaneous anesthesia: a 1:1 mixture of lidocaine and prilocaine known as a eutectic mixture of local anesthetics (EMLA). This drug, which is approved for the prevention of pain caused by needle punctures, was shown to be beneficial in a limited study of patients with postherpetic neuralgia and has been used to treat a variety of chronic pain syndromes. Cutaneous anesthesia is produced if the cream is applied in a thick layer and covered with an occlusive dressing for at least 1 hour.

The need for cutaneous anesthesia for pain relief has not been established in all syndromes, however, and it is possible that some patients will respond to a thin application of EMLA without a dressing, or to other commercially available topical anesthetic preparations that do not produce cutaneous anesthesia. Therefore, patients who are offered a trial with EMLA should be encouraged to try different modes of application. If an occlusive dressing is needed and a large area of skin must be covered, ordinary plastic wrap often suffices.

38. **How is topical capsaicin used in the treatment of chronic pain?**

Capsaicin, an ingredient in hot peppers, is known to deplete small peptides in primary afferent neurons, including those involved in pain transmission. For example, this compound releases and then depletes the peptide known as substance P, which mediates pain transmission at the first central synapse in the dorsal horn of the spinal cord. The evidence suggests that some patients with neuropathic pain will benefit from the topical application of this drug to the painful site. Several controlled trials indicate that patients with painful arthritic small joints can also benefit from the topical application of this drug.

39. **Discuss the method of application of capsaicin.**

Capsaicin cream is commercially available in 0.025% and 0.075% concentrations. The higher concentration has been tested most often in clinical trials and in most instances should be tried first. The cream is applied locally to the painful region three to four times per day. A minimum 4-week trial is necessary to obtain maximal benefit. The major adverse effect is local burning, which can be intense and necessitate discontinuation of the cream. Initial burning may diminish with repeated applications. Alternatively, applying a topical local anesthetic or ingesting an analgesic prior to application of the capsaicin may allow continuation of the therapy.

40. **Are topical nonsteroidal antiinflammatory drugs effective?**

There is evidence that topical nonsteroidal antiinflammatory drugs can reduce musculoskeletal pain. Such a formulation is sometimes administered for arthritis and other painful disorders.

41. **What is sympathetically maintained pain? How is it diagnosed?**

Sympathetically maintained pain is a form of neuropathic pain in which the pain is believed to be sustained through efferent sympathetic activity. The diagnosis is usually suspected when patients fulfill criteria for reflex sympathetic dystrophy or causalgia. The latter two syndromes, which have recently been renamed by the International Association for the Study of Pain as complex regional pain syndrome (CRPS) types I and II, are characterized by the association of pain and local autonomic dysregulation and/or trophic changes. This constellation of findings raises the possibility of sympathetically maintained pain, which could potentially be ameliorated by interruption of sympathetic outflow to the painful site. Sympathetic interruption is usually accomplished by sympathetic nerve blocks. This procedure can be both diagnostic and therapeutic. (See Chapter 28, Neuropathic Pain).

42. **When is drug therapy appropriate for complex regional pain syndrome? Which adjuvant agents are useful for the treatment of sympathetically maintained pain?**
Drug therapy is usually considered for patients with CRPS type I or II who are not candidates for sympathetic nerve blocks or who have had unsuccessful blocks. Anecdotal reports have described the use of virtually all of the multipurpose analgesics and the adjuvant analgesics for neuropathic pain. Although the mechanism of action is unknown, a trial of intranasal calcitonin is often administered on the basis of a successful controlled trial.

Several drugs modulate the activity of the sympathetic nervous system and have also been used anecdotally for the diagnosis or treatment of sympathetically maintained pain. Intravenous phentolamine, an alpha-1 adrenergic antagonist, has been touted as a diagnostic test for sympathetically maintained pain, and anecdotal reports have suggested the efficacy of other adrenergic drugs.

43. **Do benzodiazepine medications have a role to play as adjuvant analgesics?**
As previously mentioned, the anticonvulsant benzodiazepine clonazepam is used as an adjuvant analgesic, typically in the treatment of lancinating or paroxysmal neuropathic pain syndromes. Apart from this drug, however, the evidence for benzodiazepine analgesia is limited and often contradictory. Although a survey suggested that alprazolam, a benzodiazepine with antidepressant activity, is efficacious for chronic neuropathic pain in the cancer population, other benzodiazepines have not shown similar analgesic properties.

Despite the limited supporting data, the benzodiazepines may have a role in the management of some pain syndromes. Patients with pain associated with anxiety disorders may report less discomfort if the anxious mood can be improved. In addition, benzodiazepines such as diazepam and lorazepam have been used to lessen muscle spasm and may be helpful in patients whose pain is related to spasm or spasticity.

44. **What is the role of the so-called muscle-relaxant drugs?**
Musculoskeletal pain syndromes are among the most common ailments encountered in medical practice. Many of these conditions can be managed with nonpharmacological approaches. Muscle relaxants represent a diverse group, which includes antihistamines (e.g., orphenadrine), chemicals similar in structure to tricyclic compounds (e.g., cyclobenzaprine), and drugs of other structures (e.g., methocarbamol, carisoprodol, chlorzoxazone). Although each of these drugs has been demonstrated in controlled trials to offer analgesic effects in musculoskeletal pain, there is no evidence that they actually relax skeletal muscle. Nonetheless, these drugs are analgesic and are generally well tolerated. Sedation is the major side effect. They are usually used on a short-term basis and, like the benzodiazepines and opioids, should not be prescribed over a long period unless patients are carefully monitored by experienced clinicians.

45. **Which adjuvant analgesics are used in the management of cancer pain?**
As noted, patients with neuropathic cancer pain are offered trials of the same adjuvant analgesics used to manage nonmalignant neuropathic pain syndromes. Other adjuvant analgesics may be useful in other cancer pain syndromes. The most important of these are adjuvant analgesics for the treatment of malignant bone pain or pain caused by bowel obstruction.

46. **Discuss the analgesic potential of calcitonin.**
The effects on bone produced by calcitonin may yield analgesia in malignant bone pain and other painful conditions of bone, such as osteoporosis. This drug also has analgesic potential

beyond these indications. Clinical trials have shown efficacy in the treatment of sympathetically maintained pain and phantom limb pain, suggesting a possible role for this agent in patients with diverse types of refractory neuropathic pain syndromes. The mechanisms that account for analgesia in the latter conditions are unknown.

47. **What is the role of psychostimulants in pain management?**
The main role for psychostimulants in pain management is to "open the therapeutic window" for opioids. In those patients in whom excessive sedation is limiting the physician's ability to increase doses of opioids, small doses of psychostimulants, such as dextroamphetamine, may reverse sedation sufficiently to allow for higher doses and better analgesia. In postoperative pain and in headaches, caffeine has been shown to potentiate opioid analgesia.

48. **How are radiopharmaceuticals used in the treatment of bone pain?**
Radiopharmaceuticals are radionuclide compounds that have preferential uptake into bone and thereby deliver a concentrated dose of radiation to bony metastases. Phosphorus-32 orthophosphate was the initial compound used in treating pain from bony metastases. Although it relieved bone pain in up to 80% of patients, it had a tendency to produce significant bone-marrow suppression. Of the newly developed radiopharmaceuticals, strontium-89 and samarium-153 are commercially available in the United States.

Some degree of pain relief occurs in approximately 80% of patients receiving strontium-89; 10% achieve complete relief. Onset of action occurs 7 to 21 days postinjection, and the duration of action is typically 3 to 6 months. Bone marrow suppression is the major toxicity, occurring in 30% of patients.

KEY POINTS

1. Adjuvant analgesics are drugs that have primary indications other than pain but are analgesic in various painful conditions.

2. Antidepressants and anticonvulsants are the most widely used adjuvant analgesic medications.

3. Knowledge of the adverse effects of the various adjuvant medications used as analgesics is essential for safe prescribing.

BIBLIOGRAPHY

1. Backonja M: Anticonvulsants (antineuropathics) for neuropathic pain syndromes, *Clin J Pain* 16 (Suppl 2): 67-72, 2000.

2. Breitbart W: Psychotropic adjuvant analgesics for pain in cancer and AIDS, *Psychooncology* 7(4):333-345, 1998.

3. Cherny NI, Portenoy RK: Cancer pain: principles of assessment and syndromes. In Wall PD, Melzack R (editors): *Textbook of pain*, 3rd ed, Edinburgh, 1994, Churchill Livingstone, pp 787-823.

4. Fromm GH: Baclofen as an adjuvant analgesic, *J Pain Symptom Manage* 9:500-509, 1994.

5. Galluzzi KE: Managing neuropathic pain, *J Am Osteopath Assoc* 107(10, Suppl 6):ES39-48, 2007.

6. Goldstein DJ, Lu Y, Detke MJ, Lee TC, Iyengar S: Duloxetine vs. placebo in patients with painful diabetic neuropathy, *Pain* 116(1-2):109-118, 2005.

7. Hegarty A, Portenoy RK: Pharmacotherapy of neuropathic pain, *Semin Neurol* 14:213-224, 1994.

8. Holmes RA: Radiopharmaceuticals in clinical trials, *Semin Oncol* 20:22-26, 1993.

9. Monks R: Psychotropic drugs. In Wall PD, Melzack R (editors): *Textbook of pain*, 3rd ed, 1994, Edinburgh, Churchill Livingstone, pp 963-990.

10. Onghena P, Van Houdenhove B: Antidepressant-induced analgesia in chronic nonmalignant pain: a meta-analysis of 39 placebo-controlled studies, *Pain* 49:205-219, 1992.

11. Patt RB, Proper G, Reddy S: The neuroleptics as adjuvant analgesics, *J Pain Symptom Manage* 9:446-453, 1994.

12. Rowbotham MC: Topical analgesic agents. In Fields HL, Liebeskind JC (editors): *Pharmacological approaches to the treatment of chronic pain*, Seattle, 1994, IASP Press, pp 211-229.

13. Watanabe S, Bruera E: Corticosteroids as adjuvant analgesics, *J Pain Symptom Manage* 9:442-445, 1994.

14. Watson CP: The treatment of neuropathic pain: antidepressants and opioids, *Clin J Pain* 16(Suppl 2):49-55, 2000.

TEMPORARY NEURAL BLOCKADE

Michael M. Hanania, MD, Martin R. Boorin, DMD, and Charles E. Argoff, MD

CHAPTER 38

1. **Describe the role of temporary nerve blocks in pain management.**

   Nerve blocks can help in the diagnosis and treatment of pain. Peripheral and central nerve blocks help to localize the origin of the specific pain problem. When pain seems to cover multiple dermatomes, a selective peripheral nerve block helps to diagnose which nerve or dermatome is primarily responsible for the pain. Temporary nerve blocks are also necessary before more permanent neurolytic procedures can be attempted. When a permanent neurolytic procedure is contemplated, a temporary nerve block should produce significant pain relief before the longer-lasting block is instituted.

   For unclear reasons, a temporary nerve block sometimes results in prolonged pain relief, outlasting the duration of the local anesthetic. In cases of somatic pain, such as mechanical low back pain, temporary nerve blocks may break the pain cycle and allow increased function. This helps to facilitate physical therapy and rehabilitation, thereby preventing disuse muscle atrophy and joint dysfunction.

   In some syndromes (such as nerve injury) it is unclear whether the primary pain generator is peripheral (at the site of nerve injury) or central (within the spinal cord). If peripheral nerve block produces complete pain relief, it is inferred that the generator is peripheral.

2. **What is the mechanism of action of local anesthesia? What are the implications for differential blockade?**

   Local anesthetics are weak bases that reversibly block sodium channels and impair the propagation of an action potential along a nerve fiber. In general, thinner fibers are more sensitive to anesthetic blockade than thicker fibers. Unmyelinated fibers are more sensitive than myelinated fibers. Sympathetic fibers are very thin. Nociceptors (which are responsible for the perception of noxious stimuli) are A-delta fibers and C fibers (also quite thin, although somewhat thicker than the sympathetic nerves). Fibers subserving proprioception and light touch are relatively thick; motor fibers are the thickest. Thus, when progressively increasing concentrations of an anesthetic are used, sympathetic fibers are blocked first, followed by nociceptors, proprioceptors, and motor fibers. Function returns in the opposite order as anesthetics wear off.

3. **Which are the ester and amide local anesthetics? Discuss their fundamental differences.**

   The ester local anesthetics have an ester linkage between the aromatic moiety and amine group and are metabolized by plasma cholinesterases. Their half-lives in the circulation are short. A product of their metabolism is p-aminobenzoic acid, which is sometimes associated with hypersensitivity reactions. Procaine, cocaine, chloroprocaine, and tetracaine are ester anesthetics.

   The amide local anesthetics have an amide linkage and undergo primarily hepatic metabolism. They include lidocaine, mepivacaine, bupivacaine, levobupivacaine, ropivacaine, and etidocaine. Levobupivacaine and ropivacaine are relatively new local anesthetics that produce more sensory than motor blockade and have a lower cardiotoxicity profile bit otherwise have features that are identical to bupivacaine.

4. **What are the differences in duration of action among the commonly used local anesthetics?**

Duration of action of the local anesthetics depends on a number of factors including the agent in question, the vascularity of the tissue into which it is injected, and, with some of the local anesthetics, the coadministration of epinephrine. Therefore, lidocaine has a shorter duration of action than bupivacaine, levobupivacaine, and ropivacaine. Topical applications to mucous membrane (which has a high vascularity) are associated with shorter anesthesia than injection into, for example, muscle. Coadministration of epinephrine (a vasoconstrictor) prolongs the duration of action of lidocaine (a vasodilator), but has no effect on the duration of action of bupivacaine, levobupivacaine or ropivacaine (which have no significant effect on vascular tone). In addition to prolonging the action of lidocaine, epinephrine increases the maximum dose of lidocaine that can be used before toxic symptoms arise.

The concentration of local anesthetic used does not significantly alter the duration of action.

5. **List the toxic dose limits for peripheral nerve blockade for lidocaine and bupivacaine.**

Overdoses of lidocaine and bupivacaine usually produce symptoms indicative of central nervous system dysfunction (dizziness, tinnitus, metallic taste, slurred speech, and seizures). These are often followed by cardiovascular symptoms, such as hypotension, tachyarrhythmias or bradyarrhythmias, ventricular fibrillation, and, in extreme cases, electrical standstill. Toxic doses are dependent on the site of injection, with increasing risks of a toxic, as opposed to anaphylactic, reaction with injection into highly vascular tissue. Approximate maximum dose limits are as follows:

Lidocaine	2-3 mg Kg^{-1}
Lidocaine with epinephrine	6-7 mg Kg^{-1}
Bupivicaine	2-3 mg Kg^{-1}
Bupivicaine with epinephrine	2-3 mg Kg^{-1}

Remember that epinephrine should not be added to a local anesthetic where it is to be injected in the territory of an end artery (e.g., digital or penile nerve block).

6. **What is the role of neuraxial block in pain management?**

Epidural or spinal blocks provide temporary block of neural function at a spinal cord level. They help to differentiate a peripheral from a central origin of pain. If a peripheral nerve or root block has failed but a spinal block relieves pain, it may be inferred that the origin of the pain is more central (within the spinal cord), provided that the operator is confident that the nerve block has actually been achieved. Epidural blockade also offers the option of leaving the catheter in place for prolonged treatment. Thus, epidural analgesia or anesthesia can be provided on an ongoing basis or through intermittent boluses. This procedure may facilitate rehabilitation. The use of neuraxial block, while well established in acute pain management and anesthetic practice, is not supported by conclusive evidence in the field of chronic pain management.

7. **List the possible complications of epidural or intrathecal anesthetic blockade.**
   - Epidural blockade involves the risk of inadvertent dural puncture. When this occurs, cerebrospinal fluid (CSF) may leak, and a postlumbar puncture (low-pressure) headache may develop.
   - Rarely, the needle used for puncture may injure a nerve root.
   - Also rare are epidural abscesses, epidural hematoma, or injury to the cauda equina. With spinal injection, cord trauma is possible if spinal injection is made above the level of the conus.

- Local anesthetics may induce temporary neuritis.
- Cephalad migration of the anesthetic agent may produce an anesthetic level much higher than the level anticipated. In cervical blocks, cephalad migration may lead to respiratory arrest.
- Transient hypotension is fairly common as a result of vasodilatation (sympathetic nerve block).
- Intravascular injection could occur.

8. **What are the indications and contraindications for epidural steroid injections?**
Indications for epidural steroid injections (ESIs) are still controversial. Efficacy for chronic low back pain is uncertain. In acute exacerbations of radicular nerve pain, injections may be of some benefit. Radicular pain is more likely to respond to steroid injections than is mechanical low back pain. Recovery from an acutely herniated lumbar or cervical disc may be hastened by ESIs. With acute low back pain, most clinicians use 2 to 3 weeks of conservative management before attempting ESIs. An interlaminar approach to ESI seems to be least helpful in spinal stenosis, mechanical low back pain, and long-standing, chronic low back pain.

A recent study by Manchikanti and colleagues suggests that a caudal approach to epidural steroid injection is more effective for chronic low back pain than lumbar epidural. A transforaminal approach under fluoroscopic guidance is felt to sometimes help more with a far lateral disc herniation with nerve root inflammation than midline epidural.

Contraindications to any epidural injection include coagulopathy, local infection, or progressive weakness that may require surgical decompression.

9. **What is the appropriate timing of epidural steroid injections?**
A steroid formulation such as methylprednisolone or triamcinolone is usually injected in doses of 40 to 80 mg every 2 to 4 weeks to a maximum of three injections in 6 months. Evidence suggests that additional injections offer no added benefit and may increase the risk of side effects. Adrenal suppression with decreased cortisol levels has been shown to occur for 3 to 5 weeks after a typical ESI. Multiple injections may produce ligamentous laxity.

10. **What are the various brachial plexus blocks?**
The brachial plexus can be blocked proximally at the level of the nerve roots and trunks by the interscalene approach; at the level of the divisions and cords by the supraclavicular or infraclavicular approach; and distally at the level of the terminal branches or nerves by the axillary approach. A brachial plexus block can be performed by single injection or continuous catheter technique for repeated injections or infusion.

11. **For what pain conditions are brachial plexus blocks useful?**
Evidence for efficacy of brachial plexus blocks is anecdotal. However, some find them useful in conditions such as complex regional pain syndrome (CRPS), acute or postherpetic neuralgia involving dermatomes within vertebrae C5-T1, vascular insufficiency of Raynaud's disease, and phantom upper limb pain. Brachial plexus block also facilitates range-of-motion (ROM) exercises in cases of frozen shoulder, elbow, or wrist. Because the thoracocervical sympathetic nerves travel in close relation to the somatic nerves of the brachial plexus, brachial plexus block results in sympathetic blockade as well. It also may be used for postoperative pain management and prevention of phantom limb pain after amputation.

12. **What are the possible side effects and complications of the various brachial plexus blocks?**
Hematoma, neuropathy, and unintentional intravascular injection are possible with any of the brachial plexus blocks. Interscalene block may be associated with unintentional injection of local

anesthetic into the epidural or subarachnoid space; recurrent laryngeal nerve block, which causes hoarseness; phrenic nerve block; and ipsilateral Horner's syndrome. Pneumothorax is most often associated with the supraclavicular block.

13. **What is the sensory innervation of the lower extremities?**
The sciatic nerve divides at the level of the knee into the tibial and common peroneal nerves. The sural nerve, which forms from the tibial and common peroneal nerves, provides sensory innervation to the lateral aspect of the lower leg and foot. Anteriorly, the femoral nerve eventually becomes the saphenous nerve and provides sensory innervation to the medial aspect of the lower leg and foot. The lateral femoral cutaneous nerve and obturator nerve provide sensory innervation to the lateral and medial thigh, respectively.

14. **What are the applications of intercostal nerve blocks?**
Intercostal nerve blocks are useful in acute herpetic neuralgia involving the thoracic dermatomes. Early sympathetic or neural blockade may reduce the incidence of postherpetic neuralgia. The sympathetic fibers travel with the intercostal nerves and can be blocked easily at the posterior midclavicular line, along the inferior aspect of the rib. Intercostal nerve blocks can be used to determine pain origin (differentiating between pain originating in the chest or abdominal wall and pain with a visceral origin), because the intercostal nerves innervate only the outer structures. Intercostal neuralgia and scar neuromas after thoracotomy and some cases of postherpetic neuralgia may be treated by intercostal blocks. Neurolysis by cryoanalgesia or radiofrequency lesioning may be considered if satisfactory temporary relief is obtained after local anesthetic block.

15. **Describe the role of facet blockade in back pain.**
Facet joints may be the source of significant mechanical back and neck pain. Pain is usually deep in the paravertebral regions of the back or neck and associated with areas of referred pain. Pain resulting from facet disease increases with extension, rotation, or lateral flexion of the spine. The facet joint is innervated by the medial branch of the posterior primary ramus from the level involved and the level above. Hypertrophic arthropathy and eventually osteophytic degeneration and arthritic changes in these joints are postulated to cause the pain.

Local anesthetic block of the medial branch nerve helps to make the diagnosis, although false-positive results are possible. Intraarticular or periarticular steroid injections may provide prolonged relief. Cryofrequency or radiofrequency neurolysis of the medial branch nerve is an option if local anesthetic block gives good but temporary pain relief.

16. **What are the indications for a suprascapular nerve block?**
The suprascapular nerve not only supplies the supraspinatus muscle but also provides sensory fibers to the shoulder joint. Therefore, a suprascapular nerve block can temporarily relieve shoulder joint pain and allow the patient to perform active ROM exercises. Frozen shoulder syndrome as a result of immobilization may be prevented. When suprascapular nerve entrapment is suspected as the cause of shoulder pain, steroids also may be injected into the suprascapular notch at the superior border of the scapula.

17. **When is a lateral femoral cutaneous nerve block used in chronic pain management?**
A lateral femoral cutaneous nerve block is sometimes useful for treatment of meralgia paresthetica, a syndrome of pain and dysesthetic cutaneous sensation in the anterolateral thigh secondary to entrapment of the lateral femoral cutaneous nerve as it passes posterior to the inguinal ligament. This syndrome is commonly associated with obesity, diabetes, or tight belts.

18. **Describe the primary central nervous system center for nociceptive input from the upper cervical and craniofacial regions. Why is the diagnosis of orofacial pain often so difficult?**

Pain impulses from the orofacial region are carried by primary afferent fibers that pass through the trigeminal ganglion to the trigeminal brainstem sensory nuclear complex, where they synapse with second-order neurons. This orofacial sensory relay center, which extends from the pons into the upper cervical cord, can be divided into the main trigeminal sensory nucleus and the trigeminal spinal tract nucleus. The main relay for pain information occurs in the subnucleus caudalis, the most caudal section of the trigeminal spinal tract nucleus. Second-order neurons in the cervical spinal dorsal horn and in the nucleus caudalis cross to the contralateral side and ascend to the thalamus via spinothalamic and trigeminothalamic pathways.

The final signals sent to the thalamus by these two relay centers are influenced through the convergence of several afferent inputs from the skin, oral mucosa, dental pulp, temporomandibular joint, masticatory muscles, and cervical region into one neural path. This convergence on the second-order neuron may explain the often perplexing pain-referral patterns observed in the head, face, and neck.

Excitatory areas also may arise centrally, with pain perceived at a peripheral site. In such cases, treatment directed at the painful site rather than the central source is ineffective. Clinical examination and local anesthetic blockade may help to identify the true source of the pain.

Cranial nerves IX and X, as well as upper cervical nerves (C1-C3) carrying nociceptive input from the cervical spine, converge on the nucleus caudalis with the trigeminal afferent neurons. The convergence of impulses from both areas is the basis for referral of pain from the cervical spine to the face and head.

19. **From where is pain derived in myofascial pain syndrome and acute single muscle myofascial disorders?**

It is believed that pain derived in myofascial pain syndrome and acute single muscle myofascial disorders arises from trigger points (TPs) within the myofascial tissues. TPs are characterized by localized, deep tenderness in a taut band of skeletal muscle, tendon, or ligament that has the ability to refer pain to a specific anatomic distribution. The area of perceived pain referred by the irritable TP is known as the zone of reference and may be located in a distant location.

20. **How do you identify a zone of reference?**

Systematic palpation of the musculature may identify a zone of reference through a consistent and reproducible altered pain sensation in the area of complaint. Multiple TPs may have overlapping areas of referred pain. The symptoms of myofascial pain may outlast the initiating events and set up cyclical muscle pain. This cycle may be sustained by numerous perpetuating physical and psychosocial factors.

21. **How do you identify referral of pain to the face and teeth by the muscles of mastication?**

Referral of pain to the face and teeth by the muscles of mastication is identified with diagnostic anesthetic blocks. Patterns of pain referral from the muscles of mastication frequently involve regions of the face and mouth and complicate proper diagnosis and treatment. Injection of small volumes of local anesthetic solution directly into the muscle may be diagnostic.

22. **Describe the use of diagnostic anesthetic blocks in myofascial pain syndrome and other myofascial disorders.**

The temporalis muscle has three muscle-fiber regions that may refer pain to the maxillary teeth and/or ipsilateral midface, sometimes mimicking sinus disease. Diagnostic injection of the temporalis muscle requires caution to avoid intravascular injection into the superficial temporal artery. The masseter muscle may contain TPs in several regions and is readily accessible for diagnostic block. The superficial body of the masseter muscle commonly refers to regions involving the posterior maxillary and mandibular teeth, whereas the deep body may refer to the posterior mandible, styloid region, and ipsilateral ear. The lateral pterygoid muscle, although not readily palpated, is associated with pain deep into the temporomandibular joint and maxillary sinus region. Spasm of this muscle leads to acute interference with mandibular movement. The medial pterygoid muscle may refer pain to the back of the mouth and pharynx, temporomandibular joint, and ear. Diagnostic blockade may be approached via intraoral and transcutaneous injections. Pterygoid muscle blocks may be complicated by temporary facial paresthesia and intravascular injection into the maxillary artery.

23. **How are local anesthetic blocks used to manage headache?**
Although most types of headaches are treated with a combination of medications, some causes of headache or head pain are readily managed with nerve blocks. Head pains may arise from myofascial pain syndromes. However, other diseases and neoplasms involving the sensory distribution of cranial nerves V, IX, and X and cervical plexus nerve roots must be considered.

Myofascial pain syndromes are characterized by steady, aching muscle pain at multiple sites and are often associated with poor sleep, morning stiffness, chronic fatigue, depression, and TPs. TPs may lead to secondary central excitatory effects such as hyperalgesia, protective muscle spasm, or even autonomic responses. The superficial sternal and deep clavicular divisions of the sternocleidomastoid muscle may have referral patterns that lead to occipital and frontal headaches. The upper trapezius and occipitofrontalis muscles also may produce recurring, tension-type headache, which is often described as beginning in the occipital region and radiating over the parietal and frontal areas of the skull.

These TP sources sometimes can be inactivated by noninvasive measures (pharmacotherapy, spray-and-stretch therapy) or dry needling of the TP and injection of local anesthetic with or without steroid. Results of these interventions may include analgesia, relaxation of muscle fiber shortening, increases in local muscle blood flow, and, if a corticosteroid is used, an antiinflammatory effect. Complications are rare, but may involve local hematoma, local anesthetic toxicity, and pneumothorax when the trapezius muscle is treated.

24. **What are the indications for cervical epidural injections in pain management?**
Neck pain may result from nerve root irritation, myofascial dysfunction, arthritic cervical spine changes, trauma, or cancer of the head and neck. Cervical epidural injections of steroids are indicated primarily for neck pain secondary to cervical disc disease. Pain secondary to spinal stenosis, which leads to a narrowed intervertebral foramen, or a preexisting arthritic disorder may be treatable with cervical epidural steroid injections, but results are not as satisfactory. Complications can include spinal headache from dural puncture and, less often, epidural abscess, hematoma, and meningitis.

It is often not possible to restrict an epidural block with local anesthetic to the cervical segments, unless a transforaminal epidural approach is used. Cephalad spread may produce respiratory depression or extended blockade. Long-acting local anesthetics are best avoided to prevent respiratory compromise secondary to phrenic nerve blockade and cardiac effects, such as reduced isotropicity and total peripheral resistance secondary to unintentional sympathetic blockade.

25. **Discuss the role of superficial and deep cervical blocks in the management of acute and chronic pain and the relative risk with each block.**
Cervical plexus blocks, which may be used in numerous surgical procedures involving the neck and shoulder, are occasionally used for the diagnosis of vague neck discomfort in the superior cervical dermatomes (C2-C4). More definitive diagnostic or therapeutic procedures are usually performed on peripheral nerve extensions, such as the occipital nerve block. The superficial cervical plexus block, located in the posterior triangle of the neck at the midpoint of the posterior border of the sternocleidomastoid, leads to complete blockade of the cutaneous

nerve supply to the neck. The deep cervical plexus block is a paravertebral block that also blocks posterior primary rami for additional analgesia over the back of the neck.

The proximity of the vertebral artery leads to the potential for an intravascular injection. In even small doses, local anesthetic injected intravascularly can lead to rapid development of CNS toxicity and seizures. The risk of unintentional intrathecal or epidural injection as a result of needle placement also exists. Phrenic nerve paresis may result from blockade of the motor innervation of the diaphragm.

26. When is an occipital nerve block indicated? What complications may occur?
Occipital nerve block is indicated for the diagnosis and treatment of headaches resulting from occipital neuralgia. Occipital neuralgia often results from compression or trauma to the greater occipital nerve (sensory branch of C2) along its course through the semispinalis capitis and the occipital attachment of the upper trapezius muscle. Compression of this nerve induces paroxysmal dysesthesia or paresthesia of the occiput, radiating upward to the vertex.

Diagnostic TP blocks within adjacent muscles may be used to differentiate neuralgia from myofascial pain. Management of neuralgia, if anticonvulsants are unsuccessful, usually involves one or a series of nerve blocks with local anesthetic and long-acting corticosteroid. Complications consist of inadvertent subarachnoid administration, intravascular injection, and hematoma.

27. What is the gasserian ganglion? What are the indications for blockade?
The gasserian ganglion contains the cell bodies for the sensory neurons of the trigeminal (fifth cranial) nerve. It is located in Meckel's cave, an indentation in the petrous pyramid. It may be blocked with glycerol in cases of intractable trigeminal neuralgia.

28. How is the gasserian ganglion block performed? What side effects and complications may be experienced?
The trigeminal ganglion is partly contained within the dura mater, and the posterior two-thirds is bathed by CSF. The ganglion is bordered medially by the cavernous sinus and internal carotid artery and superiorly by the temporal lobe of the brain. The transcutaneous gasserian ganglion block is directed, often under fluoroscopic guidance, into the foramen ovale, through which the mandibular division exits the skull base. Paresthesia or dysesthesia is usually elicited along one of the trigeminal nerve divisions. When indicated, a sensory change in the specific division affected is sought by needle repositioning.

When adequate pain relief is obtained from local anesthetic placed into the ganglion, successful long-term pain reduction may be obtained with either a chemical or radiofrequency gangliolytic block. When the neurolytic block is performed, an increase in pain, masseteric weakness, and paresthesia may persist for weeks to months. Significant complications include bleeding, infection, facial dysesthesia, corneal hypesthesia, and anesthesia dolorosa. Acute complications, such as unconsciousness and paralysis, may result from injection into the CSF.

29. What are the branches and functions of the first division of the trigeminal nerve?
The first division of the trigeminal nerve—the ophthalmic division (designated cranial nerve V1)—is distributed primarily to the forehead and nose. The V1 division leaves the superior aspect of the trigeminal ganglion, lies in the lateral wall of the cavernous sinus, and enters the orbit through the superior orbital fissure, where it divides into three separate nerves: the lacrimal, frontal, and nasociliary nerves.

The V1 division provides sensory innervation to the bulb and conjunctiva of the eye, lacrimal gland (lacrimal nerve), and skin over the forehead, eyes, and nose. Intraorbital branches of the nasociliary nerve are blocked by retrobulbar block. The largest branch, the frontal nerve, divides shortly after entering the superior aspect of the orbit into the supratrochlear and supraorbital nerves, which are accessible for cutaneous blockade.

The supratrochlear nerve provides sensory innervation to the conjunctiva and skin of the medial aspect of the eye and the skin over the forehead. The supraorbital nerve, passing through the supraorbital notch, innervates the frontal sinus and then the upper lid, forehead, and scalp as far as the lambdoidal suture.

30. **What role do supraorbital and supratrochlear nerve blocks play in the management of herpes zoster?**
Repeated sympathetic nerve blocks, in combination with subcutaneous infiltration with a local anesthetic–steroid mixture for supraorbital and supratrochlear nerve blocks, have been shown to reduce the severity of pain associated with acute herpes zoster. The injections should be given during acute illness rather than delayed until postherpetic pain is experienced. Pain may be eliminated for periods greatly exceeding the length of the anesthetic block.

31. **What are the major nerve branches of the maxillary division of the trigeminal nerve? How are nerve blocks of the maxillary division used in pain management?**
The maxillary division (designated as cranial nerve V2) is purely sensory, providing innervation of the nose, cheek, eyelids, midface, maxillary sinus, and associated structures of the upper jaw. Mucosal sensory innervation includes part of the nasopharynx, tonsil, palate, and maxillary gingiva as well as maxillary teeth. The maxillary division exits the middle cranial fossa via the foramen rotundum, traverses the pterygopalatine fossa medial to the lateral pterygoid plate, and enters the orbit through the inferior orbital fissure. Major nerve branches arise in the cranial vault, pterygopalatine fossa, and orbit, as well as on the face.

Blockade of the maxillary division provides pain relief in some cases of local disease of the midface region. The major nerve trunk can be blocked via an extraoral approach under the zygomatic arch as well as by an intraoral approach.

Intravascular injection and hematoma may result from the vascular nature of the pterygopalatine fossa and presence of the maxillary artery medial to the pterygoid plates. Wide dispersal of local anesthetic may lead to temporary anesthesia of the ocular muscles or optic nerve and loss of the corneal reflex.

32. **How is the sphenopalatine ganglion block used for the management of pain conditions of the head?**
The sphenopalatine ganglion is a parasympathetic ganglion of the facial nerve. Postsynaptic fibers leave the ganglion and distribute with branches of the maxillary division of the trigeminal nerve. These fibers provide parasympathetic innervation to the lacrimal and mucosal glands of the nasal fossa, palate, and pharynx. In a similar fashion, the maxillary nerve carries sympathetic nerve efferents from the superior cervical ganglion to target structures.

The sphenopalatine ganglion block has been associated with alleviation of the frequency and intensity of headaches, specifically cluster headache and migraine, which are poorly controlled with conventional drugs such as beta-blockers. The block is carried out on a daily basis for 5 to 7 days, using topical application of local anesthetic to the nasopharynx posterior to the inferior and lower middle turbinate.

Adverse effects include bleeding, orthostatic hypotension, and local anesthetic systemic toxicity. Excessive pressure with the anesthetic applicator against the cribriform plate may increase the risk of a high spinal block with respiratory embarrassment. Further controlled trials are needed to define the indications and efficacy of this procedure.

33. **Does the addition of corticosteroids have an effect on the duration of local anesthetic block?**
No evidence exists that addition of steroids to local anesthetics has any effect on nerve blocks undertaken for acute pain management. Anecdotal evidence, however, suggests that they can significantly prolong the pain relieving effect of local anesthetic nerve block when used for

chronic pain conditions. Commonly used steroids include methylprednisolone and triamcinolone acetonide. Usually long-acting corticosteroids such as these are used.

34. How could steroids have an effect on local anesthetic nerve block?
Steroids have a number of effects on neural function that may enhance local anesthetic action. These include antiinflammatory and membrane-stabilizing effects, an action in reducing ectopic neural discharge, and an effect on dorsal horn cell function.

35. How can the certanty of achieving a good-quality nerve block be increased?
A number of strategies exist that can make it more likely that a satisfactory nerve block is achieved, including the following:
- By using a nerve stimulator to ensure that accurate placement of the injectate is achieved
- By aiming to site the nerve block at areas where landmarks are identifiable on X-ray imaging and undertaking the nerve block under radiological control
- By using a large volume injectate so that even if the needle tip is not directly beside the nerve, spread of solution will still allow satisfactory nerve blockade (remembering to avoid toxic doses)

36. List common nerve blocks with examples of potential indications.
Common nerve blocks and some of their potential indications include the following:
- Ilioinguinal nerve block—ilioinguinal neuritis
- Brachial plexus block—CRPS
- Median nerve block—carpal tunnel syndrome
- Intercostal nerve block—intercostal neuralgia
- Suprascapular nerve block—supraspinatus tendonitis, frozen shoulder
- Accessory nerve block—unilateral neck muscle spasm
- Cervical plexus block—neck pain
- Lateral femoral cutaneous nerve block—meralgia paresthetica
- Medial branch of the posterior primary ramus block—facet joint pain

KEY POINTS

1. Temporary nerve bock can help define the nerve or nerve root involved in a pain condition and is a prerequisite of a neurolytic block.

2. The evidence for the use of many nerve blocks in chronic pain management is anecdotal, but they are still widely used as a treatment.

3. Certainty of achieving a nerve block is increased by using a nerve stimulator and by choosing blockade sites where the nerve is adjacent to fixed anatomical landmarks.

4. Local anesthetic allergy is rare if amide local anesthetics are used. Toxicity is more common and is related to the dose used and the vascularity of the injection site.

BIBLIOGRAPHY

1. Manchikanti L, Boswell MV, Giordano J, Kaplan E: Assessment: use of epidural steroid injections to treat lumbar radicular lumbrosacral pain: report of the therapeutics and technology assessment subcommitte of the American Academy of Neurology, *Neurology* 69:1190, 2007.

CHAPTER 39

PERMANENT NEURAL BLOCKADE AND CHEMICAL ABLATION

Michael M. Hanania, MD, and Charles E. Argoff, MD

1. **What is neurolysis?**
   Neurolysis is the application of a chemical or physical destructive agent to a nerve to create a long-lasting or permanent interruption of neural transmission.

2. **List the types of agents commonly used in neurolysis.**
   Chemical agents commonly used in neurolysis include alcohol, phenol, glycerol, ammonium compounds, chlorocresol, and aminoglycosides. Hypotonic or hypertonic solutions may also be used. The most commonly used physical agents are cold (cryotherapy) and heat (radiofrequency lesions or laser).

3. **What are the indications for neurolysis?**
   Neurolysis is almost exclusively reserved for the treatment of intractable cancer pain. Rarely, some forms of nonmalignant pain can be treated with these neurolytic agents (for example, intractable postherpetic neuralgia and chronic pancreatitis). Neurolysis using cryoanalgesia or radiofrequency is more precise and reversible; thus these agents are often used for chronic nonmalignant pain conditions.

   Several requisites must be met before neurolysis is performed. In most cases, successful pain relief should be demonstrated with temporary blockade. The painful area must be sufficiently limited to be served by a readily accessible nerve or plexus. A thorough knowledge of the relevant anatomy and the mechanism by which the agent destroys nerve tissue are essential. Neurolysis should be regarded as an irreversible and potentially permanent procedure to be considered only when other treatment modalities have failed.

4. **What are the potential side effects or complications of neurolysis?**
   Extravasation or malplacement of the solution, resulting in injury to nerves other than the target nerve, can produce unwanted sensory and motor block. Neuritis, anesthesia dolorosa, or pain in the deafferentated area may occur. Systemic effects, such as hypotension, can be severe enough to require resuscitation.

5. **How do commonly used neurolytics, such as alcohol and phenol, work?**
   Alcohol and phenol cause protein coagulation and necrosis of the axon without disruption of the Schwann cell tube. Thus, axonal regeneration can occur. Recovery is faster with phenol than with alcohol. However, if cell bodies are destroyed along with axons, as is more likely with alcohol, regeneration is not possible, and permanent blockade results.

6. **What are the indications for celiac plexus neurolysis?**
   Celiac plexus neurolysis is a commonly performed neurolytic procedure that is useful in reducing visceral pain from structures that have sensory fibers passing through the celiac plexus. The structures innervated through the celiac plexus include the lower esophagus, stomach, small intestine, large intestine to the midtransverse colon, liver, pancreas, adrenals, and kidneys. Pancreatic cancer pain is most commonly treated with this block.

7. **Under what circumstances is celiac plexus neurolysis preferred over systemic opioids for the management of pain from pancreatic cancer?**
Most patients do well with systemic opioids and require no further intervention for controlling pain from pancreatic cancer. In fact, analgesia after celiac neurolysis may not be superior to that after treatment with systemic opioids. However, patients who develop severe side effects from systemic opioids benefit most from celiac neurolysis. Following celiac neurolysis, a decreased need for opioids is observed as well as fewer associated side effects, such as sedation, confusion, nausea, and constipation.

8. **Where is the celiac plexus? What are the approaches and techniques for celiac plexus blockade?**
The celiac plexus is the largest plexus of the sympathetic nervous system. It lies near the aorta, just anterior to the body of the first lumbar vertebra. Guidance by fluoroscopy or computed tomography (CT) scan must be used when injecting neurolytic solution to ensure correct needle placement. One technique is a posterior percutaneous approach using a needle to pass transaortic or anterior to the crura of the diaphragm at the level of L1 where the celiac plexus is situated. Variations of this approach exist, including using two needles for bilateral injection in the retrocrural region. Recently, an anterior percutaneous approach was described.

9. **What must be done prior to actual neurolysis of the celiac plexus?**
A celiac plexus block using local anesthetic must be performed first to determine if significant pain relief is likely with celiac neurolysis. The patient should therefore reduce opioid consumption the day of the procedure so that pain relief can be assessed.

10. **What is the success rate with celiac plexus neurolysis for pancreatic cancer pain?**
A success rate of 85% to 94% of good to excellent pain relief has been obtained in several large series of patients undergoing neurolytic celiac plexus block for pain from pancreatic cancer. In a series of 136 patients, analgesia was present until the time of death in 75% of cases. Repetition of the block is required in some patients. The earlier in the disease process the block is performed, the better the results. This may be due to better spread of neurolytic solution around the celiac plexus when tumor infiltration is minimal.

11. **List the potential complications of celiac neurolysis.**
Reported complications of celiac neurolysis include pneumothorax, chylothorax, pleural effusion, convulsions, and paraplegia. Postural hypotension and diarrhea occur frequently secondary to the sympathetic blockade, but they are usually self-limited.

12. **What is intrathecal neurolysis? When is it used?**
Intrathecal neurolysis is a form of chemical rhizotomy in which a neurolytic agent is introduced into the cerebrospinal fluid to block specific dermatomes. This can be performed at any spinal level up to the midcervical region. At higher levels, there is risk of spread of neurolytic agent to the medullary centers. Indications for intrathecal neurolysis include any peripheral pain within a specific dermatomal distribution.

13. **How is intrathecal neurolysis performed using phenol or alcohol?**
Studies have demonstrated that all nerve fibers are affected indiscriminately by both phenol and alcohol. The concentration and quantity of agent used determines the extent of nerve

fiber destruction and, therefore, the degree and extent of sensory loss. Phenol is hyperbaric relative to cerebrospinal fluid; therefore, the patient should be positioned so that the sensory nerve roots are aligned with gravity (i.e., semisupine). Alcohol is hypobaric, so the nerve roots involved need to be in the up position or against gravity (i.e., semiprone). Positioning of the patient and use of small incremental doses of neurolytic solution are critical for obtaining the proper block. Average duration of analgesia is 3 to 4 months, with a wide range of distribution.

14. **What are typical concentrations and volumes for intrathecal neurolysis with phenol or alcohol?**
Recent reports suggest that a higher success rate of analgesia is obtained with intrathecal phenol in preparations of 10% and 15% solution, versus a 7.5% solution, for treating pain resulting from a variety of neoplasms. Absolute alcohol may be used in increments of 0.1 ml until pain relief is obtained (usually a total of 0.7 ml is required).

15. **What are the complications associated with intrathecal neurolysis?**
If intrathecal neurolysis is performed at the lumbar level, bowel and bladder dysfunction are among the most feared complications, although the actual incidence and severity are low, regardless of the agent used. At the thoracic level, solution is introduced distant from the major limb plexuses and nerve subserving bladder and bowel function; however, intercostal muscle paresis can occur. Chemical rhizolysis at the cervical level has to be carefully performed so as not to involve the medullary centers. Acute spinal cord injury with paraplegia has also been reported.

16. **List the advantages and disadvantages of intrathecal neurolysis.**
The advantages of intrathecal neurolysis include the following: ease of performance (usually done as a one-time injection) and completeness and long duration of the block.
    The disadvantages of intrathecal neurolysis include the following: the possibility of spread to anterior motor nerve roots, thereby producing paralysis. The patient must remain in an unchanged position for at least 30 minutes after injection, and there is initial burning with injection of alcohol.

17. **List the advantages and disadvantages of epidural neurolysis.**
The advantages of epidural neurolysis include the following: positioning of the patient is not as critical; neurolysis can be carried out over a large number of dermatomes; permanent motor block is unlikely if phenol is used; and neurolysis can be carried out over a period of 2 to 4 days by repeated injections of phenol through an epidural catheter.
    The disadvantages of epidural neurolysis include the following: incompleteness and shorter duration of nerve blockade and the need for repeat injections over several days. A larger dose and volume of neurolytic solution are needed; hence, inadvertent intrathecal migration can be disastrous.
    Success rates with epidural neurolysis have not been adequately documented, although anecdotal reports of success range from 33% to 90%.

18. **What is cryoanalgesia?**
Cryoanalgesia is the application of extremely low temperatures using a cryosurgical probe; this achieves pain relief by blocking peripheral nerves or destroying the nerve endings with extreme cold. The cryoprobe works on the principle of the Joule-Thompson effect. It includes an inner tube, an outer tube, and a working tip. When high-pressure gas is allowed to expand in the probe tip, there is a rapid fall in temperature.

19. **By what mechanism does prolonged neural blockade occur after cryoprobe application?**
    Application of a cryoprobe produces a local icy lesion (cryolesion) at the nerve. After the nerve is frozen, axonal disintegration, wallerian degeneration, and disruption of the myelin sheath occur, although the integrity of the epineurium and perineurium is maintained. Thus the conduction block produced by a cryolesion is a temporary effect, and regeneration of the nerve eventually occurs.

20. **What influences the duration of the block after cryolesioning?**
    Duration of nerve blockade depends on the rate of axonal regrowth and the distance of the cryolesion from the end organ. Clinically, a peripheral cryolesion results in sensory blockade from weeks to months, typically 1 to 2 months. The closer the iceball is to the nerve and the larger the cryolesion, the better the chance for successful and prolonged blockade.

21. **What is radiofrequency neurolysis?**
    Radiofrequency neurolysis uses high-frequency waves to produce thermal coagulation of the nerves. A probe is inserted percutaneously, and correct position is confirmed by fluoroscopy and motor and/or sensory stimulation. Local anesthetic is administered and the current increased to coagulate the nerve.
    Note that lower-temperature pulsed radiofrequency appears to be a safer technique with almost similar results.

22. **List the advantages and disadvantages of radiofrequency lesioning.**
    The main advantage of radiofrequency lesioning is that a lesion is produced using a small probe, resulting in a prolonged block.
    The disadvantages of radiofrequency include the possibility of neuritis, as with chemical ablation, and the expense of the radiofrequency equipment compared with that of phenol or alcohol.

23. **List the advantages and disadvantages of cryolesioning.**
    The advantages of cryolesioning are as follows: a reversible lesion is produced, neuritis rarely occurs, and cost of equipment involved is less than that of radiofrequency neurolysis.
    The disadvantages of cryolesioning are as follows: a transient nerve block is produced that may require repeat cryolesioning; a large cryoprobe is required, so the percutaneous procedure can be uncomfortable; and success of blockade depends greatly on the proximity of the iceball to the nerve.

24. **Why do neuritis and neuroma occur occasionally after neurolysis?**
    Regeneration of peripheral nerve in particular sometimes results in neuritis or neuroma. It has been suggested that alcoholic neuritis is related to incomplete destruction of somatic nerves and that the incidence is less when a complete and prolonged block has been obtained. Nerve irritation is less common in cranial nerves than in other peripheral nerves. Some agents, such as alcohol, have more of a propensity to produce local irritation.

25. **What is deafferentation pain?**
    Deafferentation pain is usually a burning pain that can be more uncomfortable than the original pain. Central nervous system maladaptation to deafferentation, as well as a local phenomenon, may account for this complication of neurolysis. A prior local anesthetic diagnostic block can help to determine if deafferentation pain may occur.

26. **List the following neurolytic techniques in order of greatest to least incidence of neuritis: Radiofrequency, phenol, cryoanalgesia, alcohol.**
    1. Alcohol
    2. Phenol
    3. Radiofrequency
    4. Cryoanalgesia

27. **What are indications for lumbar sympathetic neurolysis?**
    Lumbar sympathetic neurolysis, also known as lumbar sympatholysis, is useful in controlling pain associated with peripheral vascular disease; specifically, patients with pedal ischemic rest pain with a cool extremity and without gangrene are the ideal candidates. It is performed in patients who are not candidates for peripheral bypass procedures because of technical or medical reasons. This procedure is sometimes used for sympathetically mediated pain that responded very well to local anesthetic blockade, but only for the duration of the local anesthetic. There are small series and case reports of good results with sympatholysis for otherwise unresponsive, prolonged ischemia of the digits in Raynaud's disease, although long-term success is minimal.

28. **What are the complications of lumbar sympathetic neurolysis?**
    Common side effects of lumbar sympathetic neurolysis are hypotension and transient diarrhea. The incidence of groin pain after lumbar sympathetic neurolysis may be as high as 20%. In the male patient there is a risk of impotence, particularly if the block is in the high lumbar region.

29. **How can lower abdominal or pelvic cancer pain be managed with neurolysis?**
    Plancarte and co-workers (1990) described a superior hypogastric plexus block at the anterolateral border of the first sacral vertebral body for alleviating pain from pelvic cancer. Intrathecal neurolysis can also be performed; however, bladder and bowel dysfunction occur in a high proportion of patients.

30. **Describe the treatment for trigeminal neuralgia that is unresponsive to conventional medical management.**
    Neurolysis with radiofrequency lesioning, glycerol, phenol, or alcohol has been successfully employed for the treatment of trigeminal neuralgia. In one series, radiofrequency retrogasserian rhizolysis was successful in 95% of patients, with a recurrence rate of 16% over 4 to 12 years. Glycerol rhizolysis is more comfortable for the patient, with good results lasting an average of 2 years. In one of the largest series using alcohol, 70% of patients had no recurrence of pain when followed for more than 3 years. Phenol was used with a similar long-term success rate. Neurosurgical microvascular decompression procedures have been successful in 80% to 90% of patients.

31. **What are the complications of trigeminal neurolysis?**
    Side effects, which are usually transient, include Horner's syndrome from block of the paratrigeminal sympathetic fibers, corneal anesthesia with consequent loss of corneal reflex and possibly paralytic keratitis, loss of sensation on the ipsilateral side of the face and half of the tongue, paresthesia, herpetic eruptions, and anesthesia dolorosa.

32. **Who should perform permanenet neural ablative procedures?**
    In the past, neuroablative procedures were more commonly undertaken because of the relatively high rate of treatment failure with pharmacological options. The range and efficacy of pain-relieving drugs is constantly improving, and therefore the need to progress to an ablative procedure is less common. One consequence of this is that practitioners, especially those more recently qualified, have less experience at carrying out these procedures.

It would be assumed that best results are usually obtained by those carrying out interventions on a regular basis, and therefore ablative procedures are probably best carried out in specialist centers where the experience in these techniques can be concentrated.

KEY POINTS

1. Neuroablative lesioning is almost entirely restricted to patients with cancer-related pain.

2. Successful celiac neurolysis can allow a reduction in opioid consumption with a consequent reduction in opioid-related side effects.

3. Neuroablative procedures should only be undertaken by experienced practitioners.

4. Neuritis and neuroma formation can complicate neuroablative procedures.

5. A comprehensive understanding of the anatomy of the region is a requirement before any neurolytic procedure is performed.

BIBLIOGRAPHY

1. Antila H, Kirvela O: Neurolytic thoracic paravertebral block in cancer pain: a clinical report, *Acta Anaesthesiol Scand* 42(5):581-585, 1998.

2. Brown DL, Bulley CK, Quiel EC: Neurolytic celiac plexus block for pancreatic cancer pain, *Anesth Analg* 66:869-873, 1987.

3. De Leon-Casasola O: Critical evaluation of chemical neurolysis of the sympathetic axis for cancer pain, *Cancer Control* 7(2):142-148, 2000.

4. Ferrer-Brechner T: Epidural and intrathecal phenol neurolysis for cancer pain, *Anesthesiol Rev* 8:14-19, 1981.

5. Ischia S, Polati E, Finco G, et al: 1998 Labat Lecture—The role of the neurolytic celiac plexus block in pancreatic cancer pain management: do we have the answers? *Reg Anesth Pain Med* 23(6):611-614, 1998.

6. Jain S, Foley K, Thomas J, et al: Factors influencing efficacy of epidural neurolysis therapy for intractable cancer pain, *Pain* (Suppl 4):T34, 1987.

7. Kline MT, Way Y: Radiofrequency techniques in clinical practice. In Waldman SD, editor: *Interventional pain management*, 2nd ed, Philadelphia, 2001, Saunders, pp 243-293.

8. Korevaar WC, Kline MT, Donnelly CC: Thoracic epidural neurolysis using alcohol, *Pain* (Suppl 4):T33, 1987.

9. Kowalewski R, Schurch B, Hodler J, Borgeat A: Persistent paraplegia after an aqueous 7.5% phenol solution to the anterior motor route for intercostal neurolysis: a case report, *Arch Phys Med Rehabil* 83(2):283-285, 2002.

10. Moorjani N, Zhao F, Tian Y, et al: Effects of cryoanalgesia on post-thoracotomy pain and on the structure of intercostal nerves: a human prospective randomized trial and a histological study, *Eur J Cardiothorac Surg* 28(3):502-507, 2001.

11. Patt RB, Cousins MJ: Techniques for neurolytic neural blockade. In Cousins MJ, Bridenbaugh PO, editors: *Neural blockade*, Philadelphia, 1998, JB Lippincott, pp 1007-1061.

12. Plancarte R, Amescua C, Patt RB, et al: Superior hypogastric plexus block for pelvic cancer pain, *Anesthesiology* 73:236, 1990.

13. Plancarte R, Velazquez R, Patt RB: Neurolytic blocks of the sympathetic axis. In Patty RB, editor: *Cancer pain*, Philadelphia, JB Lippincott, 1993, pp 384-420.

14. Polati E, Finco G, Gottin L, et al: Prospective randomized double-blinded trial of neurolytic celiac plexus block in patients with pancreatic cancer, *Br J Surg* 85(2):199-201, 1998.

15. Raj PP, Denson DD: Neurolytic agents. In Raj PP, editor: *Clinical practice of regional anesthesia*, New York, 1991, Churchill Livingstone.

16. Rykowski JJ, Hilgier M: Efficacy of neurolytic celiac plexus block in varying locations of pancreatic cancer: influence on pain relief, *Anesthesiology* 92(2):347-354, 2000.

17. Swerdlow M: Intrathecal neurolysis, *Anaesthesia* 33:733-740, 1978.

18. Waldmab SD: Avoiding complications when performing celiac plexus block, *Pain Clinic* 6:62-63, 1993.

CHAPTER 40

SYMPATHETIC NEURAL BLOCKADE

Meir Chernofsky, MD, Michael M. Hanania, MD, and Charles E. Argoff, MD

1. **What distinguishes a sympathetic block from other neural blockade procedures?**

   The goal of sympathetic blockade is to preserve motor function and touch sensation while selectively blocking the sympathetic nerves. Because sympathetic fibers travel to almost all tissues in the body to innervate the vasculature, almost all nerve blocks involve sympathetic blockade. The separation of somatic and sympathetic function (differential blockade) is sometimes incomplete.

2. **What anatomical and physiological factors differentiate sympathetic fibers from somatic fibers? How do the differences affect neural blockade?**

   Sympathetic fibers are generally thinner than most somatic fibers and are, therefore, more sensitive to anesthetic agents. The cell bodies of somatic motor fibers are located within the central nervous system (CNS), whereas those of the autonomic nervous system are located outside the CNS as postganglionic neurons. The autonomic nervous system is a disynaptic system. The autonomic motor neuron's location outside of the CNS makes it accessible for local blockade.

3. **How can a differential sympathetic blockade be achieved?**

   There are three general ways to block sympathetic nerves while preserving somatic function:
   - Sympathetic nerves are blocked with the same local anesthetic agents (in similar concentrations) used for somatic blockade, but the blocks are performed at anatomic locations where sympathetic nerves are separate and distinct from somatic nerves. Examples of such locations are the stellate ganglion and the lumbar sympathetic ganglion.
   - The block is performed at locations that combine somatic and sympathetic nerve fibers, but low concentrations of local anesthetic are used. Because postsynaptic sympathetic nerves are small and unmyelinated, they are more sensitive than some larger or myelinated somatic fibers to dilute local anesthetic. This approach is useful for spinal and epidural blockade.
   - Specific sympathetic antagonists are employed. For example, the antihypertensive agent guanethidine can be injected into the vasculature of a limb, with a tourniquet applied and inflated to a pressure greater than the systolic arterial pressure. After a short period during which the agent has had a chance to distribute into local tissues, the tourniquet is deflated, and a local selective lysis of sympathetic function has been achieved. This technique is a variation of intravenous regional anesthesia, the Bier block. It is usually a poor choice if ischemia is the primary problem.

4. **What is the general role of sympathetic blockade in pain management?**

   Sympathetic blocks can be helpful for four types of clinical problems:
   - In some body regions, afferent pain fibers travel with sympathetic nerves. For example, the fibers that conduct painful impulses from the pancreas are closely associated with the celiac plexus. Therefore neural blockade of the celiac plexus is a convenient way to provide pancreatic analgesia. The primary target of such a procedure is the afferent fibers that

travel with the sympathetic trunk, although a sympathetic role in the maintenance of such pain has not been ruled out.

- The sympathetic nervous system (SNS) is believed to play a primary role in a certain class of painful syndromes. Directed blockade of the sympathetic fibers may be both diagnostic and therapeutic in cases of sympathetically maintained pain.

- Physicians skilled in neural blockade are occasionally asked to become involved in the treatment of ischemic syndromes of the limbs. The patient may or may not have pain, and the SNS is not implicated in the pathologic process. However, by inducing sympathetic neural blockade, the tonic baseline level of arterial vasoconstriction is reduced. Depending on the vascular pathology, blood flow to the ischemic area may be improved.

- There is also a grab-bag of indications for sympathetic blockade that do not fit into one of the above categories. For example, stellate ganglion block (see Question 10) may be useful in the diagnosis and treatment of certain cardiac dysrhythmias related to prolonged QT syndrome.

5. **Without going into specific indications just yet, what are some of the common types of sympathetic blocks?**
Blocks that take advantage of isolating the sympathetic fibers at sympathetic plexi or trunks include the so-called stellate ganglion block, the lumbar sympathetic block, the celiac plexus block, and the hypogastric plexus block. Techniques that exploit the potential of differential blockade by using low concentrations of local anesthetics include differential spinal and epidural blocks. Agents used in the Bier technique in the upper or lower extremity include reserpine, guanethidine, and the ganglionic agent bretylium. Finally, almost all somatic nerve blocks also block sympathetic nerves.

6. **What is reflex sympathetic dystrophy (RSD)?**
Reflex sympathetic dystrophy (RSD) is now termed complex regional pain syndrome type 1 (CRPS-1) as opposed to CRPS type 2, which was previously labeled as causalgia. It is a syndrome of pain and disability (altered sensory, motor, and sympathetic neural function) usually, but not always in a distal extremity. It is characterized by decreased function and signs of sympathetic overactivity. CRPS-1 is usually initiated by trauma. The degree of the initial trauma may vary from a major fracture with neurovascular injury to a trauma so minor that it is not recalled by the patient. In patients with major nerve injury CRPS-2 is more usual. Various medical conditions, such as stroke and myocardial infarction, also may be inciting factors.

7. **What does CRPS-1 look like clinically?**
CRPS-1 is a chronic, progressively evolving syndrome with different signs at different stages. Pain and decreased function are present at all stages. Initially, there may be signs of sympathetic overactivity, such as increased sweating in the affected part. The area may be a dusky blue color, although color change may be intermittent. As the condition progresses, some of these signs become less obvious, and atrophy becomes more prominent. The extremity, more commonly the hand, becomes hypersensitive and tender and is guarded by the patient. In the late stages, there is radiologic evidence of bone thinning (Sudeck's atrophy), which may be contributed to by underuse of the affected part.

8. **What is the role of the sympathetic nervous system in CRPS-1?**
The clinical signs and the marked relief after sympathetic block in early cases points to sympathetic overactivity as an important factor in maintenance and perhaps initiation of CRPS-1. However, this mechanism has recently been called into question. Where the syndrome does respond to sympathetic block, the term "sympathetically maintained pain" is used to distinguish it from those cases where sympathetic block has no effect ("sympathetic independent pain").

9. **True or false: Treatment of CRPS-1 is effective at any stage of the disease.**
False. Treatment of CRPS type 1 becomes less satisfactory in the later stages of disease. When the condition is neglected, it may progress to a disability that dominates the life of the patient. Patients may become so desperate that they request amputation. Unfortunately, early surgical adventures with amputation demonstrated that a chronic pain syndrome remains even after the limb is gone. Therefore, early diagnosis, with a trial of therapy when possible, is important.

10. **What is a stellate ganglion block?**
There is a series of sympathetic ganglia on either side of the cervical vertebral column and on either side of the thoracic vertebrae. The stellate ganglion is less a consistent anatomic structure than a general area in which the inferior cervical ganglia and first thoracic ganglia are fused—or at least in close proximity.
Virtually the entire sympathetic nerve supply to the head and neck synapses in or near the stellate ganglion. A good portion of the sympathetic innervation to the ipsilateral upper extremity also synapses in the stellate ganglion, with the remainder synapsing in adjacent ganglia. A consistent blockade of the head, neck, and upper extremity sympathetic innervation may be achieved by applying a quantity of local anesthetic (5 to 12 mL) to the area of the stellate ganglion. When the proper quantity of local anesthetic is used, spread to adjacent ganglia is common, leading to reliable upper extremity sympathectomy.

11. **How is a stellate ganglion block performed?**
The most common technique for performing a stellate ganglion block is an anterior neck approach. The patient is placed in the supine position, and the neck is extended as tolerated. After antiseptic preparation, a 3-cm needle (22-23 gauge) is introduced perpendicular to the skin (and perpendicular to the floor) at the level of the cricoid cartilage between the trachea and the anterior border of the sternocleidomastoid muscle. Retracting the sternocleidomastoid muscle laterally and palpating the anterior aspect of the C6 vertebra with two fingers facilitates introduction of the needle and avoids puncture of the carotid artery. The needle is advanced until bone is encountered. If bone is not encountered at this location, the needle is withdrawn to the subcutaneous tissues and reintroduced in a slightly caudad or cephalad direction.
When bone is encountered, the needle is withdrawn about 0.5 cm. (If this step is not done, a higher incidence of somatic blockade of the upper extremity will result.) After careful aspiration testing is negative for blood or cerebrospinal fluid, 5 to 12 ml of local anesthetic is introduced in fractional doses, and the needle is withdrawn. Given the close proximity of important structures, intravenous access should be in place and appropriate cardiovascular monitoring performed.

12. **What are the contraindications to stellate ganglion block?**
Most of the contraindications to stellate ganglion block are a matter of common sense and are relative rather than absolute. Patients who are anticoagulated or taking high-dose aspirin are at increased risk for bleeding. A local infection over the proposed site of injection is a somewhat more absolute contraindication. Patients with bullous disease of the upper lobes of the lung are at greater risk for accidental pneumothorax and must be approached with more caution. Because one of the possible complications of stellate ganglion block is vocal cord paralysis, patients with contralateral vocal cord paralysis are at risk for severe airway abnormality if the ipsilateral cord becomes paralyzed. Patients who have abnormal anatomy because of prior surgery or injury present greater technical difficulty because of the differences in anatomic landmarks. Such patients are probably better approached using fluoroscopic guidance and contrast dye or with alternative techniques, such as intravenous regional sympatholysis.

13. **What are the side effects of a stellate ganglion block?**
Stellate ganglion block causes sympathetic blockade of the ipsilateral face and arm. Therefore, a successful block produces an ipsilateral Horner's syndrome (ptosis, miosis, and anhydrosis), flushing of the face, and increased temperature of the arm. These effects are normal and last for the duration of the blockade. Slightly blurred vision and a sense of fullness around the eye may result. Local trauma from the blockade or blockade of the recurrent laryngeal nerve may produce hoarseness. Neck tenderness is fairly common, but frank hematoma is less likely. In severe cases, hematoma may threaten the airway.

14. **What are the risks of a stellate ganglion block?**
Inadvertent blockade of components of the brachial plexus may lead to upper extremity numbness and weakness or paralysis, both temporary in the vast majority of cases. If pain relief occurs in the presence of somatic blockade, the pain syndrome may have been due to a peripheral lesion, but a sympathetic origin cannot be inferred. Passive ranging of the painful joints may be dangerous in the face of somatic blockade because pain, which may warn of extreme passive strain on a structure, is blocked.

   Serious complications of stellate ganglion blockade include carotid puncture with hematoma and vertebral artery puncture. Introduction of even small amounts of local anesthetic into either of these arteries may lead to seizures (usually short-lived). Introduction of small amounts of local anesthetic into the cerebrospinal fluid may lead to high (or total) subarachnoid neural blockade with respiratory arrest, coma, hypotension, and sometimes cardiac arrest. A generalized toxic reaction to the local anesthetic load also may occur if too much local agent gains access to the circulation too fast. If the needle enters too inferiorly, a pneumothorax may occur. Late complications include the remote possibility of mediastinitis after puncture of the esophagus and the possibility of late airway compromise from hematoma or trauma.

15. **How can the complications mentioned in questions 13 and 14 be prevented or managed?**
There is no foolproof way to avoid complications of a stellate ganglion block. The incidence of complications may be reduced by proper training and experience. However, the chance of permanent injury to the patient as a result of seizure, accidental spinal anesthesia, or pneumothorax can certainly be reduced to acceptable levels with proper preparation, including the following:
   1. Perform the block only on fasting patients to avoid aspiration in case of loss of consciousness.
   2. Perform the block only in a setting in which an anesthesiologist (or an emergency physician with excellent airway management skills) is immediately available to manage complications.
   3. Start an intravenous lifeline in every patient before the block is attempted so that emergency drugs can be administered without delay.
   4. Perform the block with monitoring of blood pressure, cardiac rate and rhythm, and oxygen saturation.
   5. Administer supplemental oxygen to all patients, or have it immediately available in case of signs of trouble.
   6. Have an emergency airway cart and emergency drugs available.
   7. Take all complaints from the patient seriously, and have a high index of suspicion for pneumothorax.

16. **What is the role of the stellate ganglion block in treatment of CRPS-1?**
In cases of suspected upper extremity CRPS-1, an initial block can be performed with a short-acting local anesthetic such as lidocaine 1%. This initial block is diagnostic; its purpose is to determine whether the block is technically feasible, produces sympathetic blockade of the

upper extremity, and results in (1) subjective pain relief, (2) any increase in functional ability of the hand, or (3) objective signs of improvement on examination and functional testing.

If the first block is successful either subjectively or objectively, a series of blocks may provide sufficient relief for appropriate physical therapy. After each block, a physical therapist works with the patient to achieve functional improvement. Behavioral therapy is an important adjunct to the therapy.

17. Which somatic nerve is most likely to be blocked unintentionally in attempting a stellate ganglion block?

With an anterior approach, the stellate ganglion is anterior to the trunks of the brachial plexus. The ganglion and plexus are separated by only a layer of fascia at this location. Therefore, all of the somatic nerves formed by the C5-T1 roots may inadvertently be blocked by diffusing anesthetics. If the block is performed slightly cephalad to the described location, the deep cervical plexus may be blocked, producing loss of sensation to the neck.

18. In what other ways can sympathetic block be induced at this level? Is a stellate ganglion block the best approach? If so, why?

There are other approaches to stellate or upper thoracic sympathetic chain blockade. The area, for example, may be approached posteriorly. Approaches other than the classic anterior approach do not have easy endpoints by palpation, and the use of radiographic guidance is strongly recommended.

Sympathetic blockade of the upper extremity also may be achieved by temporarily isolating the involved upper extremity with a tourniquet (inflated above venous pressure) and injecting a sympathetic blocking agent into a vein in the hand. The technique is similar to the Bier block, a popular method of achieving regional anesthesia of the hand. Problems with this approach include side effects of the sympathetic blocker, either because the tourniquet is accidentally deflated or because some shift of drug to the central compartment is inevitable, even with good technique. The side effects include hypotension, nausea, and dizziness.

Drugs that have been used for intravenous regional sympathetic blockade include reserpine, guanethidine, and bretylium.

The posterior approach to the sympathetic chain is practical if the anterior approach involves an anatomic problem. Intravenous regional sympathetic blockade can be used in patients in whom any nerve block is contraindicated—for example, in anticoagulated patients. The intravenous regional sympathetic block is also longer-lasting than a local anesthetic neural blockade. For uncomplicated patients with definite or possible CRPS-1, the stellate ganglion block is the first-line technique.

19. Other than CRPS-1, what are some commonly accepted indications for stellate ganglion block?

The pain of herpes zoster, as well as postherpetic neuralgia of the head and neck down to upper thoracic dermatomes, may respond to stellate ganglion block. Aggressive treatment of the pain associated with early herpes zoster may prevent or modify the development of postherpetic neuralgia. The so-called shoulder-hand syndrome, which is a continuum of problems including painful decreased range of the upper extremity after stroke and other vascular episodes, can be controlled with stellate ganglion block. Physical therapy may be facilitated, just as with classic RSD.

The pain of Paget's disease, phantom limb pain, and other pain associated with upper extremity denervation of benign or malignant origin may respond to this block. Severe coronary ischemic pain may improve with stellate ganglion block, and the dysrhythmias associated with prolonged QT syndrome may be temporarily managed.

For ischemic problems of the upper extremity, including atherosclerosis and microemboli, perfusion may be improved with stellate ganglion blocks. The ischemic pain associated with scleroderma, isolated Raynaud's disease, and other vasospastic conditions also may respond.

20. **What options are available if temporary pain relief is obtained after repeated stellate ganglion blockade?**

If significant but transient pain relief is obtained following stellate ganglion blocks, a more permanent radiofrequency denervation of the stellate ganglion can be performed. However, because of the close proximity to other neural structures and vessels, we have found a safer, lower-temperature pulsed radiofrequency to be just as effective. This should also be performed under fluoroscopic guidance and confirmation.

21. **How does the treatment of lower-extremity CRPS-1 differ from treatment of upper-extremity CRPS-1? What major alternative to classic sympathetic block is more practical for lower extremity CRPS-1 than for upper?**

In principle, lower-extremity CRPS-1 is approached with the same type of algorithm as upper-extremity CRPS-1. The first-line block used is the lumbar sympathetic block (see Questions 22 and 23). The requirement for a multidisciplinary approach, including behavioral medicine and physical therapy, is identical to management of upper-extremity CRPS-1.

The introduction of very dilute concentrations of local anesthetics into the epidural space may bring about sympathetic blockade and analgesia without inducing sensory and motor blockade. The cervical epidural route is a viable alternative for the induction of upper-extremity sympathetic blockade, and the lumbar epidural route is effective for lower-extremity sympathetic blockade. However, a lumbar epidural is technically easier than a cervical epidural, with fewer potential complications.

A major advantage of the lumbar epidural route for the management of lower-extremity CRPS-1 is that an epidural catheter can be inserted on an outpatient basis and left in place for several days. Therefore, repeat blockade to facilitate therapy on a more or less daily basis is easier to perform.

When the epidural route is used to achieve sympathetic blockade, pain relief is nonspecific, because the concentrations of local anesthetic may induce somatic analgesia in addition to sympathetic blockade. Diagnostically, you cannot conclude that the source of the pain is solely sympathetic if a somatic blockade is achieved.

The option of intravenous regional sympathetic blockade with a Bier technique is equally practical for the lower extremity. Considering the relatively larger volume of the venous capacitance in the lower extremity, a larger volume of medication must be used compared with the same block in the upper extremity.

22. **What landmarks are helpful when performing a lumbar sympathetic block?**

The lumbar sympathetic chain consists of presynaptic and postsynaptic sympathetic nerves and ganglia in close association with the lumbar vertebral bodies, lying anterolaterally on both sides. Therefore, the vertebral bodies themselves are the best landmark.

23. **How is a lumbar sympathetic block performed?**

In one common approach to performing a lumbar sympathetic block, the patient is positioned prone, with a pillow under the abdomen. Precautions (including an intravenous line and appropriate monitoring) are established. The spinous processes of L3 are identified and marked. The entry point of the needle is 7 to 9 cm lateral to the midline at the L3 level.

After the area is prepared, a wheel of local anesthetic is raised. Then a stiletted needle at least 12 cm in length (21-22 gauge, preferably marked in centimeters) is introduced at the above point toward the midline, making an angle of 45° with the skin. The needle is advanced while the injectionist maintains verbal contact with the patient.

There are three possible outcomes: (1) If paraesthesias are encountered, the needle has probably entered the lumbar plexus within the psoas muscle. In this case, withdraw the needle to the skin and redirect. The needle may be too far lateral and may have to be reintroduced 1 to 2 cm more medially. (2) Alternatively, you may have used too shallow an angle. If bone is encountered at 3 to 5 cm, the needle is at a transverse process. Withdraw to the skin and redirect the needle cephalad or caudal. (3) The desired endpoint is the encountering of bone at a depth of 8 to 11 cm. This bone is the vertebral body. At this point, the injectionist should note the insertion depth, withdraw to skin, and redirect at a slightly higher angle. This step is repeated until bone is not encountered at a depth of 2 cm beyond the point of the original encounter, or until you can easily "walk off" the bone and advance the needle by 1 to 2 cm. When the needle is in proper position, there should be little resistance to advancement or injection.

After careful aspiration, a 3-mL test dose of local anesthetic is injected. If after several minutes there is no evidence of spinal block or systemic symptoms, 12 to 20 mL of local anesthetic is injected in 5-mL increments with repeated aspiration and verbal contact with the patient. The same agents used for stellate block are appropriate for lumbar block. Variations to this technique include more medial entry points and multiple needle techniques.

24. **How is the lumbar sympathetic block performed fluoroscopically? What are the advantages?**
Fluoroscopic guidance is often used to facilitate lumbar sympathetic block, because needle position can be checked during the procedure and final needle position can be confirmed. It is likely that complications can be minimized with this technique in experienced hands. Once the desired needle position is obtained under fluoroscopic imaging, contrast dye is also injected to confirm spread of solution anterior to the psoas muscle in the retroperitoneal space. The contrast material should spread longitudinally (superiorly and inferiorly) along the anterolateral aspect of the vertebral bodies.

25. **Which somatic nerve is most likely to be blocked unintentionally during an attempt at lumbar sympathetic blockade?**
The most likely somatic nerve to be blocked unintentionally during an attempt at lumbar sympathetic blockade is part of the lumbar plexus in the substance of the psoas. If this occurs and pain is relieved, you cannot automatically conclude that the pain is sympathetically mediated. Accidental epidural and spinal blockades are also possible.

26. **What are the important complications of lumbar sympathetic blockade?**
The litany of problems possible with lumbar sympathetic block is somewhat similar to that for stellate ganglion block. The good news is that airway complications, mediastinal complications, and pleural trauma are out of the picture.

Common problems include discomfort from the introduction of the needle, hematoma, and persistent paresthesias (which usually resolve in days or weeks). Potentially serious complications involve the proximity of the target area to the epidural space, subarachnoid space, and either the aorta and vena cava (in the case of higher insertion or lower-lying bifurcation) or iliac vessels.

Accidental injection of 12 to 20 mL of local anesthetic into the epidural space should not be catastrophic. A normal epidural blockade results; the patient must be monitored for high block and major sympathetic blockade with hemodynamic instability.

Accidental injection of 3 mL of a test dose of local anesthetic into the subarachnoid space results in a spinal block, with implications similar to an epidural blockade. Introduction of much more than 3 mL results in a high or total spinal block with apnea, loss of consciousness, and profound hypotension with vascular collapse.

Similarly, accidental injection of 3 to 4 mL (for example, 60 to 80 mg of lidocaine or 5 to 10 mg of bupivacaine) of most local anesthetic mixtures directly into the vasculature results in mild toxic symptoms, whereas larger amounts may cause major toxic manifestations such as seizures and cardiac arrest.

27. **How can complications of lumbar sympathetic blockade be managed or prevented?**
Careful aspiration for blood or cerebrospinal fluid is mandatory for all blocks, as is incremental injection with careful observation of the patient. Unfortunately these precautions do not prevent all such complications.

28. **For what reasons may a sympathetic block not improve the signs and symptoms of CRPS-1?**
Assuming that the diagnosis of CRPS-1 is correct, a sympathetic block may fail to relieve symptoms if it was technically inadequate, if the condition is fairly advanced or centralized to the spinal cord or brain, or if there are confounding factors such as significant peripheral nerve damage. This last condition, called causalgia in the older literature, is now known as CRPS-2.

29. **How do you decide which of the factors in question 28 is operative in a particular patient?**
If a sympathetic block does not seem to be effective, objective measurement should be made to demonstrate a decrease in sympathetic activity in the involved limb. A rise in skin temperature as demonstrated with a sensitive temperature probe or thermography is useful. If a sympathectomy is not demonstrated, it is worthwhile to try again on another day, perhaps with a greater volume of local anesthetic or with a slightly different approach (more cephalad or caudad direction of the needle). If a block that produces no relief is shown to produce limb sympathectomy, encourage the patient to undergo a second attempt. Most patients who have had a successful series of blocks state that some attempts were not as effective as others.
   Sometimes the diagnosis of CRPS-1 is hard to pin down. If a series of two sympathetic blocks completely fails to relieve symptoms, and if it was demonstrated that the blocks indeed achieved sympathectomy of the involved area, the pain is probably not sympathetically mediated. However, in the absence of another diagnosis, the type of multidisciplinary program employed for CRPS-1 may still be the patient's best hope. Future sensory blocks may be used simply to facilitate analgesia and range of motion.

30. **How can the effect of limb sympathetic blockade be clinically measured?**
Early in the course of CRPS-1, the vasculature innervated by the overactive sympathetic nerves should remain reactive, i.e., able to dilate if the sympathetic input is reversed. This is the rationale of sympathetic blockade. The most obvious measurements to confirm the efficacy of a block relate to temperature and blood flow.
   Extracting useful information from a diagnostic sympathetic block is far more complex than a single objective measurement. The full range of peripheral neuroanatomic and psychological considerations in chronic pain may influence what happens after a block.

31. **Specifically, which objective measurements of limb sympathetic blockade can be used in the clinical setting?**
The simplest and most widely used measurement of limb sympathetic blockade is to place thermometer probes on the distal part of the involved extremity and on the contralateral healthy extremity. The most reassuring response is a lower baseline temperature on the involved side (compared with the healthy side), which rises 28 Kelvin within 20 minutes of neural blockade. The problem with this measurement is that it is neither specific nor sensitive. There may be no baseline difference between the two sides, and surface temperature may poorly reflect tissue temperature for many reasons.
   If you are lucky, the veins of the distal extremity will become more prominent after blockade. This observation, however, is hardly quantitative or even objective. In classic CRPS-1, increased sympathetic activity leads to increased sweat production. A number of tests, some based on

serial measurement with indicator papers, quantify a decrease in sweat production after a successful sympathetic block. Quantitative sudomotor axon reflex testing (QSART) is more specific, but more difficult.

The psychogalvanic reflex is a change in the conductivity of skin secondary to sudden stimulation of the special sensory organs. It is thought to be mediated by vasomotor changes and is diminished after sympathetic blockade. This reflex can be measured by a simple oscilloscope, such as an electrocardiograph monitor.

Plethysmographic measurements of pulsatile blood flow should increase after a successful block. Thermography, an elegant way to demonstrate changes in sympathetic activity, is used by some pain clinics.

32. **What is the celiac plexus?**

The celiac plexus is a series of ganglia surrounding the celiac artery just anterior to the aorta. The sympathetic innervation of the abdominal viscera originates with other sympathetic nerves but does not synapse in the sympathetic chain. The sympathetic nerves exit the sympathetic chain as splanchnic nerves to synapse in a number of ganglia. Most of these are loosely associated in the celiac plexus. Most of the afferent nociceptive innervation of the visceral structures of the abdomen travel in close association with the celiac plexus. Therefore by blocking the celiac plexus, you can interrupt nociception from the viscera and also affect any sympathetically mediated pain in this area.

33. **What organs does the celiac plexus inervate?**

The celiac plexus innervates the lower esophagus, stomach, small intestines and large intestines up to the splenic flexure, omentum, liver, biliary tract, pancreas, spleen, adrenal glands, and kidneys. The capsule of the liver is not covered by the celiac plexus, and therefore pain resulting from metastatic disease causing stretching of the liver capsule will not be interrupted following a celiac plexus block.

34. **How is celiac plexus block performed? What are the risks?**

As with other sympathetic blocks, a number of approaches are possible when performing a celiac plexus block. The most common is a posterior approach, which is similar in principle to the lumbar plexus block. The patient is placed prone with a pillow beneath the abdomen. Intravenous access is secured, and appropriate monitoring is established.

The needle used is a 21-gauge or 22-gauge stiletted needle at least 12 to 15 cm in length, preferably with distances marked in centimeters. The entry point is 7 or 8 cm lateral to the midline. The exact starting point is just inferior to the end of the twelfth rib and lateral to the T12 spinous process. After local infiltration at the entry point, the needle is advanced toward the midline, making an angle of 45 degrees with the horizontal in the cross-sectional plane. The vertebral body is sought at a depth of 10 to 12 cm. Bone encountered within 5 to 6 cm is probably the transverse process. In this case, the needle is withdrawn to subcutaneous tissue and directed superiorly or inferiorly. In view of the anatomy, superior direction is a better choice. If no bone is encountered by 13 cm or so, the needle is withdrawn to subcutaneous tissue and the angle with the horizontal is decreased slightly.

Ideally, bone should be encountered as described. When it is, attempt to redirect the needle anteriorly (higher angle) and "walk off" the vertebral body. A pop is then felt as the needle is advanced by 2 cm. At this point, aspiration tests are carried out and the block is activated.

With a smaller-gauge (e.g., more malleable) needle, there is less ability to walk off the vertebra, and it is more likely you will need to withdraw and redirect. However, smaller needles may do less damage if they penetrate vital structures.

When you believe that the needle is correctly placed, perform a test dose, as described in Question 23 for the lumbar sympathetic block. If the test appears to be negative, inject the local anesthetic mixture. Large volumes may be necessary because of the extent of the loosely defined anatomic structure; 15 ml is the minimum. The local agent may be bupivacaine 0.25% to 0.5%, with or without epinephrine 2 to 5 mg/ml. For follow-up blocks, a neurolytic mixture is often used.

35. **What type of guidance can be used for celiac plexus block? When is guidance necessary?**
The celiac plexus block may be performed with fluoroscopic or computed tomographic (CT) guidance. Guidance is necessary when the anatomy is distorted by disease or body habitus. Proper placement of the needle is suggested by a characteristic pattern of spread of a contrast bolus.

36. **What are the risks of celiac plexus block?**
The risks and complications of celiac plexus block are similar to those of lumbar sympathetic blockade. The aorta, of course, is in close proximity to the celiac plexus. Aortic penetration should not be catastrophic, barring coagulopathy or severe atherosclerosis. However, you certainly do not want to inject therapeutic substances into the aorta. Frequent aspiration tests are the key.

37. **What is the clinical problem in treating the pain of pancreatic carcinoma? What is the role of local anesthetic celiac plexus blockade? What other approaches may be helpful?**
The pain from pancreatic carcinoma may arise from a number of sources: invasion and destruction of the pancreatic duct system; mass effect; invasion of neighboring structures, including nerves; and various degrees of intestinal obstruction. Although systemic narcotics are usually the first modality used, they may become ineffective or cause intolerable side effects.

Many nerve blocks target the pain of pancreatic carcinoma, including epidural blockade, subarachnoid blockade, and celiac plexus block.

The celiac block is particularly attractive because it is effective and because neurolytic agents can be delivered to the celiac plexus with relatively low risk of somatic neurolysis. Subarachnoid and epidural block, when indicated for this type of pain, are used to deliver opioids, with or without very low doses of local anesthetic. Such therapy may not be completely effective for visceral pain, which is mediated by pathways quite different from somatic pain. Subarachnoid or epidural neurolytic block is less practical for this indication.

The other advantage of celiac plexus neurolytic block is that its usual duration of effect (weeks to months) coincides with the unfortunately short life span of the patient. If necessary, a second block can be made weeks or months after the first block. Although patients often have an expected life span of weeks to months after diagnosis, they are alert until the end. To free the patient of significant pain and to preserve the alert state are real services.

The role of local anesthetic celiac plexus blockade for this indication is diagnostic. If a block with bupivacaine 0.25% to 0.5% relieves the pain, a neurolytic block is likely to provide prolonged relief.

38. **For what other painful conditions may celiac plexus blockade have a role?**
Celiac plexus blockade is potentially useful for any painful condition of the abdominal viscera, including malignancies and benign pain such as that associated with chronic pancreatitis. Local anesthetic celiac plexus blockade may be used as a diagnostic maneuver for painful abdominal conditions. A condition that arises from the viscera or involves sympathetically mediated pain may be relieved with a celiac block. Pain arising from musculoskeletal or neural structures should not be relieved.

Celiac plexus blockade with local anesthetic has a potential but limited role in the management of surgical anesthesia and pain. The block may supplement neuraxial block and permit various procedures in the upper abdomen to be performed without general anesthesia. Celiac plexus blockade was used in some centers for cholecystectomy when open cholecystectomy was common.

39. **What are potential problems with the use of the celiac plexus block to treat benign pain?**

As with many chronic pain syndromes, one must consider the presence of significant associated behavioral dysfunction. As with almost all chronic pain syndromes, there is likely to be significant associated behavioral dysfunction. If a local anesthetic celiac plexus block is effective, celiac neurolytic block can be considered. The problems are twofold. First, the analgesic effect is often temporary, and it is not known how many times such a procedure can be safely repeated. Even so, a few weeks to months of relief can help to break the chronic pain cycle and allow other modalities to take effect.

The second problem is loss of a potential signal that something is wrong. Patients with benign chronic abdominal pain may be subject to intraabdominal catastrophes such as perforations and obstructions of the gastrointestinal tract. Obviously, time is of the essence in diagnosing and treating such problems. If the potential to feel visceral pain is lost, such conditions may progress until the patient's chances of survival are diminished. This is a particular problem if the cause of the pain is alcoholic pancreatitis. An alcoholic patient may be less reliable in noting and reporting other signs of a surgical emergency, such as vomiting and abdominal pain.

40. **When using a celiac plexus block, how do you decide which side to block?**

The celiac plexus is not a lateralized structure, but it is a diffuse structure. For a diagnostic block, it is acceptable to block from one side. If the result is poor, a repeat block with bilateral needle placement may be attempted. For neurolytic block, bilateral needle placement is sometimes done to get the best spread without excessive volume of neurolytic agent. However, when the block is performed with radiographic assistance, even neurolytic block can be performed with one needle.

41. **What is the clinical challenge in treating severe malignant pelvic pain? What is the role of sympathetic blockade?**

Various cancers of the reproductive organs and lower gastrointestinal tract can cause severe pelvic pain. When oral analgesics fail to control the pain and you must resort to nerve blocks, the options are continuous spinal or epidural opioids, with or without local anesthetics, and various neuroablative procedures. All of these options yield excellent results for well-selected patients; however, they are quite invasive. In addition, neurodestructive procedures are not ideal; they occasionally result in somatic blockade, which can be distressing to a terminally ill patient who wants to maintain as much function as possible for as long as possible. The other side of the coin is that neurodestructive procedures are not as permanent as they sound. The life expectancy of some patients with malignant infiltration of the pelvis may be months and even years.

Of the many possible pathologies of pelvic pain, nerve invasion and destruction are prominent. When the pain is sympathetically mediated, a simple series of blocks can forestall the need for more invasive procedures.

42. **How is a hypogastric plexus block performed?**

The hypogastric plexus is a series of nerves that lie anterior to the lower lumbar vertebrae and then branch out to a number of minor plexi in the pelvis. This plexus system contains mainly sympathetic postganglionic nerves and afferent fibers.

Although the details of this block are beyond the scope of this chapter, the various components of the hypogastric plexus can be blocked with the patient in the prone position. Fluoroscopic assistance is usually required because hypogastric plexus block does not have a palpable endpoint. The basic approach is not unlike that used for the lumbar sympathetic block; hypogastric plexus block is performed lateral to L5 vertebra. The needle is directed caudad, and the goal is placement anterior to the lumbosacral junction. Proper needle placement yields a consistent picture on fluoroscopy and can be confirmed by injection of contrast, which shows a characteristic pattern of spread.

43. **Almost all of the indications for sympathetic blockade are chronic problems. why, then, do we perform local anesthetic sympathetic blocks, which wear off within several hours of the procedure?**
Local anesthetic sympathetic neural blockade is performed to make a diagnosis, to interrupt a cycle of pain, or to facilitate other interventions. When you are planning the management of a poorly defined, nonspecific chronic pain problem, the management plan may be altered based on response to a sympathetic block.

   For example, if atypical foot pain of relatively recent onset responds to a lumbar sympathetic local anesthetic blockade, and if you can demonstrate that no incidental somatic blockade resulted, it is acceptable to proceed with an accepted protocol for CRPS-1. Again, this is most often a multidisciplinary protocol involving a series of blocks, physical therapy, behavioral therapy, and perhaps intravenous sympatholytic injections. If, in the same patient, a lumbar sympathetic block produces good evidence of sympatholytic effect but no relief, further management is planned in other directions.

44. **When are repeated blocks beneficial?**
The most common use of repeated blocks is to facilitate physical therapy. This is the classic way of managing CRPS-1, but it is also appropriate for many other painful conditions. During the effective period of the block, stretching and range-of-motion exercises can be accomplished with less discomfort. Teamwork is essential in coordinating the block with therapy. Beyond the obvious challenge of making sure that the therapy appointment is scheduled within the effective period of the block, a mutual understanding of the diagnosis is essential. Furthermore, we insist that a fully certified physical or occupational therapist be involved in the exercise. Depending on the diagnosis, therapy carried out by an inexperienced individual may push the patient too hard and do more harm than good.

45. **How might a patient's expectations regarding a blockade affect the physician-patient relationship?**
Neural blockade with local anesthetics almost never cures a pain problem by itself. If the block is to serve its purpose as an adjunct to the multidisciplinary care plan, the patient's expectations for the block must be realistic. If patients expect a block to be curative and then feel that they are referred for behavioral therapy when it is not curative, a certain loss of hope and trust is inevitable.

KEY POINTS

1. Sympathetic block can be used to differentiate between "sympathetically maintained pain" and "sympathetic independent pain."

2. If temporary pain relief is obtained with local anesthetic stellate ganglion block, more prolonged relief can be obtained by using radiofrequency techniques.

3. Celiac plexus block can be used to treat pancreatic cancer pain.

4. Neurolytic celiac plexus block should only be used to treat noncancer pain in exceptional circumstances because the neural block produced may mask other gastrointestinal catastrophes.

5. Sympathetic nerve blocks should be used as part of a multimodal treatment of pain.

BIBLIOGRAPHY

1. Bell S, Cole R, Robert-Thomason IC: Coeliac plexus block for control of pain in chronic pancreatitis, *BMJ* 281:1604, 1980.

2. Bonica JJ: Causalgia and other reflex sympathetic dystrophies. In Bonica JJ, editor: *The management of pain*, 2nd ed, Philadelphia, 1990, Lea & Febiger, pp 220-243.

3. Brown DL, Bulley TK, Uiel EL: Neurolytic celiac plexus block for pancreatic cancer pain, *Anesth Analg* 66:869-873, 1987.

4. Ebert TJ, Kettler RE: Autonomic nervous system and sympathetic blockade. In Kirby RR, Gravenstein N, Lobato E, Gravenstein JS, editors: *Clinical anesthesia of practice*, 2nd ed, Philadelphia, 2002, WB Saunders, pp 512-526.

5. Glynn CJ, Basedow RW, Walsh JA: Pain relief following postganglionic sympathetic blockade with IV guanethidine, *Br J Anaesth* 53:1297-1302, 1981.

6. Moore DC, Bush WH, Burnett LL: Celiac plexus blockade: a roentgenographic, anatomic study of technique and spread of solution in patients and corpses, *Anesth Analg* 60:369-379, 1981.

7. Patt RB, Cousins MJ: Techniques for neurolytic neural blockade. In Cousins MJ, Bridenbaugh PO, editors: *Neural blockade*, Philadelphia, 1998, JB Lippincott, pp 1007-1061.

8. Plancarte R, et al: Hypogastric plexus block: retroperitoneal approach, *Anesthesiology* 71:A739, 1989.

9. Plancarte R, Velazquez R, Patt RB: Neurolytic blocks of the sympathetic axis. In Patty RB, editor: *Cancer pain*, Philadelphia, 1993, JB Lippincott, pp 384-420.

10. Roberts WJ: A hypothesis on the physiological basis for causalgia and related pains, *Pain* 24:297-311, 1986.

11. Rocco AG, Palomgi D, Raeke D: Anatomy of the lumbar sympathetic chain, *Reg Anesth* 20:13-19, 1995.

12. Waldmab SD: Avoiding complications when performing celiac plexus block, *Pain Clinic* 6:62-63, 1993.

13. Wenger C, Christopher C: Radiofrequency lesions for the treatment of spinal pain, *Pain Digest* 8:1-16, 1998.

CHAPTER 41

INTRASPINAL OPIOIDS

Zahid H. Bajwa, MD, Stephen A. Cohen, MD, MBA, Carol A. Warfield, MD, and Gary McCleane, MD

1. **What is meant by intraspinal opioid?**

   This term *intraspinal opioid* refers to the application of opioid medications in close proximity to the spinal cord in contrast to systemic (oral, intramuscular, intravenous) administration. Whereas intraspinal opioids act primarily on the spinal cord, the primary site of action for systemic opioids has been shown to be supraspinal receptors in the brain.

2. **How are intraspinal opioids given?**

   Intraspinal opioids may be injected into the epidural space (outside the dura mater) or into the intrathecal space (subarachnoid or spinal). Either method may be single-shot or continuous. With single-shot administration, the spinal or epidural needle is withdrawn following injection. For continuous administration, a small catheter is placed, and the drug is given via the catheter. Drugs may then be administered by intermittent bolus or via a continuous infusion device.

3. **How long have intraspinal opioids been in use?**

   In 1855, the Wood needle allowed for the first parenteral administration of morphine. However, it was not until 1979 that Wang, Nauss, and Thomas reported the first human study demonstrating the safe, effective intrathecal application of morphine. Behar and associates reported epidural applications soon after.

4. **What is the rationale for using intraspinal opioids?**

   Nociceptive input (i.e., a painful stimulus) travels to the spinal cord via primary afferents, A-delta fibers, and C fibers. These fibers synapse with second-order neurons located in the dorsal horn of the spinal cord. From there, nociceptive input is transmitted to supraspinal centers in the brain via ascending tracts.

   Melzack and Wall's gate control theory proposed that interneurons in the dorsal horn act to modulate nociceptive input. They postulated that gates could be opened and closed by stimulation and inhibition via interneurons in the spinal cord. These interneurons were later determined to be located in the substantia gelatinosa. Spinal opioids exert their inhibitory primary effects in the substantia gelatinosa (lamina II) of the dorsal horn.

5. **What evidence is there for opioid action in the substantia gelatinosa?**

   Iontophoretic, microinjection, and patch-clamp data have demonstrated that the substantia gelatinosa is the primary site of action for intraspinal opioids. Radioautographic studies have confirmed the presence of specific opioid binding in the substantia gelatinosa. The mechanism in the substantia gelatinosa is presynaptic inhibition of neurotransmitter release, although postsynaptic effects probably play a role.

6. **How do opioids reach the substantia gelatinosa?**
Once administered, subarachnoid opioids reach the spinal cord via two mechanisms: (1) direct spread from the cerebrospinal fluid (CSF), and (2) vascular absorption from the CSF, which is then delivered to the spinal cord. For epidural routes, opioid enters the CSF via direct spread through the dural cuff and then reaches the cord by the two mechanisms described above. Vascular absorption from the epidural space with subsequent delivery to the spinal cord also occurs.

7. **Which specific properties of the opioid molecule play a role in reaching the dorsal horn?**
Several pharmacokinetic properties determine the degree to which intraspinal opioids reach the dorsal horn: lipid solubility, molecular weight and shape, surface area exposed (i.e., "spread") (Fig. 41-1), and route of administration (epidural vs. subarachnoid). The most important of these appears to be molecular weight.

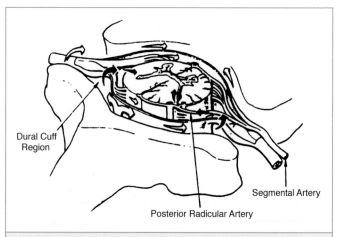

Dural Cuff
Region

Segmental Artery

Posterior Radicular Artery

Figure 41-1. Cross-section depicting opioid spread in epidural space *(white arrows)* and in spinal cord and cerebrospinal fluid *(black arrows)*. (From Cousins M, Bridenbaugh P, editors: *Neural blockade in clinical anesthesia and management of pain*, Philadelphia, 1998, JB Lippincott, with permission.)

8. **Are all opioids created equal?**
No. The most useful property for classifying intraspinal opioids is lipid solubility. Opioids can be divided into two classes: lipophilic (lipid-soluble) versus hydrophilic (lipid-insoluble). Examples of lipophilic opioids include fentanyl, sufentanil, and meperidine. Morphine and hydromorphone are hydrophilic. The octanol water coefficient is the standard for grading and comparing lipophilicity (Table 41-1).

TABLE 41-1. RELATIVE OCTANOL: WATER COEFFICIENTS (COMPARED TO MORPHINE)

Opioid	O:W
Morphine	1
Hydromorphone	4
Meperidine	40
Fentanyl	400
Sufentanil	1600

9. **What pharmacodynamic role does lipophilicity play?**
Increased lipid solubility decreases the time required for transfer of drug across lipid barriers (blood vessels, cell membranes). Clinically, this translates to more-rapid onset, shorter duration of action after spinal administration, higher equianalgesic doses, and higher incidence of systemic side effects.

10. **Why are higher equianalgesic doses required for lipophilic drugs?**
Because of the highly vascular and adipose-filled nature of the epidural space, a significant amount of lipophilic drug is absorbed by both blood and fat. This serves to reduce the amount of drug "available" to reach the dorsal horn.

11. **What factors determine duration of action of spinal opioids?**
Termination of action is accomplished after the opioid diffuses away from the receptor and returns to the CSF or is carried away from the spinal cord by venous return. Affinity for the receptor and lipophilicity determine the duration of action. To date, the role for intraspinal metabolism is unclear.

12. **What are the common side effects of intraspinal opioids?**
Classically, intraspinal opioid side effects are similar to those observed with systemic administration: respiratory depression, urinary retention, pruritus, and nausea and vomiting. Tolerance and physical dependence may also occur.

13. **Which is the most common side effect?**
Pruritus has been shown to occur quite commonly with intraspinal opioids; however, according to studies by Reiz and Westburg and by Bromage, Camporesi, and Chestnut, the incidence is highly variable: 15% to 100%. The exact mechanism is unknown, but probably does not involve histamine release. Pruritus responds to low-dose intravenous naloxone (5 mg/kg/hr) without decreasing analgesic effectiveness.

14. **How common is urinary retention when using intraspinal opioids?**
The incidence of urinary retention when using intraspinal opioids varies between 10% and 50% and does not differ from that of systemically administered narcotics, although the onset and severity may differ (see Stenseth and Breirik). Reducing the administered dose does not decrease the incidence. The mechanism of action involves inhibition of the volume-evoked micturition reflex. Urinary retention responds to low-dose naloxone.

15. **Is nausea more likely with the spinal route than with systemic administration?**
    The incidence for intraspinal-related nausea is probably 17% to 34% and may be reduced
    with lipophilic drugs, epidural (vs. intrathecal) administration, and continuous therapy
    (vs. single shot). The mechanism involves opioid receptor stimulation at the chemoreceptor
    trigger zone. Antiemetics are the first-line therapy for nausea.

16. **Is opioid withdrawal a potential problem?**
    Patients physically dependent on systemic narcotics may achieve pain relief from
    intraspinal opioids or local anesthetics. If systemic opioids are stopped abruptly, there is
    risk of withdrawal because the amount of intraspinal opioid reaching supraspinal centers
    may not be enough to prevent withdrawal signs and symptoms.

17. **What is the incidence of respiratory depression?**
    Respiratory depression is most commonly associated with intrathecal morphine and the
    narcotic-naive patient. The incidence is less than 1% with the epidural route and slightly
    higher for intrathecal opioids. Intraspinal opioids have not been shown to have a higher
    incidence of respiratory depression than systemic opioids.

18. **What is the time course of respiratory depression?**
    Respiratory depression is commonly classified as early or late. Early respiratory depression
    after spinal administration generally occurs within 1 to 2 hours postinjection. Late respiratory
    depression peaks at 6 hours, but can occur up to 12 hours postinjection. Each type has a
    different mechanism and thus different time of onset.

19. **What are the causes of respiratory depression?**
    Early respiratory depression occurs as a result of vascular absorption and is primarily
    seen after epidural administration. Overdoses of opioid (e.g., accidental spinal injection,
    dosage error) in the subarachnoid space can result in early respiratory depression via
    a nonvascular mechanism, but this is rare. Because lipophilic drugs (fentanyl, meperidine)
    are readily absorbed in the highly vascular epidural space and because higher doses are
    administered, they are much more likely to produce early respiratory depression.
      Late respiratory depression occurs as a result of rostral migration of drug in the CSF.
    Ultimately, the opioid reaches the floor of the fourth ventricle. The drug can then be
    absorbed into the medulla and affect the respiratory center. Clearly, hydrophilic drugs
    (hydromorphone, morphine) are at highest risk for this type of migration because of
    greater "spread" and relatively higher CSF concentrations. Lipophilic drugs generally do not
    develop great enough CSF concentrations or significant rostral spread because they are
    rapidly absorbed.

20. **How does vascular absorption occur?**
    Two mechanisms of vascular absorption exist when using intraspinal opioids. The most
    significant amount of absorption occurs via the epidural veins. Delivery to the systemic
    circulation transpires via the azygous vein. Once the drug reaches the systemic circulation,
    its effects, side effects, and metabolism resemble a systemically administered opioid.
      Absorption via the basivertebral venous plexus provides an alternative route of
    blood-borne redistribution. However, the basivertebral route bypasses the azygous return and
    delivers the drug to the brain. Hence, even small concentrations of drug carried by this
    system might have more profound effects, either alone or in combination, with systemically
    redistributed drug.

21. **Is bolus administration superior to continuous infusion?**

The bolus administration and continuous infusion methods each have advantages and disadvantages (Table 41-2). Bolus administration of opioid is advantageous in that a sophisticated infusion device is not required. Practically, only hydrophilic agents can be used because of their longer duration of action. However, increased side effects, including respiratory depression, can result. In addition, local anesthetic cannot be combined with the regimen; the dose-sparing, synergistic combination of local anesthetic and opioid is used commonly in both acute and cancer pain management.

Continuous infusion offers the advantage of use with local anesthetic and decreased risk of side effects. Ideally, the infusion also offers steady levels of opioid (and analgesia). Finally, the likelihood for contamination (resulting from the closed system) is also reduced when compared with the bolus technique.

TABLE 41-2. CONTINUOUS VS. BOLUS: RELATIVE ADVANTAGES OF EPIDURAL ADMINISTRATION TECHNIQUES

	Advantages	Disadvantages
Continuous Infusions	Can use shorter-acting opioids, which are more titratable Consistent analgesia (fewer peaks and troughs) Decreased risk for contamination Device eliminates need for physician to periodically inject catheter May be combined with local anesthetic solutions Reduced incidence of side effects	Requires sophisticated infusion device Higher cost
Intermittent Bolus	Does not require sophisticated infusion device Simplicity of periodic injection Inexpensive	Cannot be combined with local anesthetic Difficult to titrate dose Higher incidence of rostral spread and side effects Increased risk for contamination Requires staff to periodically inject catheter

22. **Which route is preferred: Intrathecal or epidural?**

Epidural is the preferred route for opioid administration in postoperative pain management therapies, primarily because the risk of a spinal headache is greatly reduced. In chronic and cancer pain therapies, the increased risks associated with intrathecal administration (including respiratory depression and chronic CSF leak) and the greater likelihood of meningitis should the catheter become infected lead many clinicians to opt for the epidural route.

However, the following two important considerations argue for the use of an intrathecal catheter in the chronic/cancer pain setting:

- A high opioid requirement is more easily met by the intrathecal route, because spinal dosing is generally one-tenth that of equianalgesic epidural dosing.
- Catheter-tip fibrosis, which leads to ineffective analgesia and is a common epidural catheter complication, is probably less likely to occur when the intrathecal route is chosen.

23. **When are intraspinal techniques contraindicated?**
Allergy to intraspinal opioids and systemic infection are absolute contraindications. Coagulation disorders are only relative contraindications to intrathecal and epidural techniques; however, the risk of an expanding hematoma causing spinal cord compression is a real risk. Most centers have established guidelines for acceptable aberrant coagulation parameters.

24. **In terms of pain relief, what advantages do intraspinal opioids have?**
In the acute situation, intraspinal administration presents a high concentration of opioids directly to the dorsal horn and modulates nociceptive input there. Somatic input is largely reduced when adequate doses are given. Visceral input, however, is only partially blocked; for this reason, intraspinal opioids are often combined with local anesthetics. This combination serves to block all nociceptive input, both visceral and somatic.

25. **Do these advantages apply to the chronic pain patient?**
In addition to the advantages noted in Question 24, intraspinal opioids allow for pain control in patients tolerant to systemic opioids and those unable to take these medications systemically (e.g., because of nausea and vomiting secondary to oral morphine).

26. **When are intraspinal opioids used for acute pain?**
The most common indications for intraspinal opioids include perioperative pain management, peripartum pain management, and acute pain secondary to trauma.

27. **Are intraspinal opioids alone effective for acute pain?**
Intraspinal opioids are effective in relieving somatic pain but not completely effective in relieving visceral pain. Many medical centers use morphine alone for acute pain relief; however, the majority use combinations of opioids and local anesthetics. Yaksh has demonstrated the synergistic effect of using local anesthetics with lower doses of opioids.

28. **Are intraspinal opioids useful for labor and delivery?**
Intrathecal and epidural opioids have been used for both labor and delivery. Epidural opioid administration has become the method of choice for laboring parturients. When combined with local anesthetic, excellent analgesia results. Formerly, the risk of spinal headache in young patients steered many away from the use of intrathecal opioids, but with smaller, well-designed needles, this is no longer a common complication.

29. **Are there other acute settings where intraspinal opioids may be of use?**
Trauma patients in whom systemic opioids may be detrimental (e.g., ventilatory depression with severe obstructive lung disease or multiple rib fractures) may benefit from neuraxial blockade of nociceptive stimuli.

30. **Are intraspinal opioids useful for chronic pain?**
When conventional pain therapies fail or reduce the quality of life, intraspinal opioids may be indicated. In general, this occurs when patients have pain responsive to oral or parenteral opioids, but suffer from intolerable side effects with systemic opioids. Cancer pain is the most common indication. Noncancer pain syndromes, such as complex regional pain syndromes, ischemic extremity pain, or postherpetic neuralgia, are more likely to respond to the intraspinal administration of local anesthetic than an opioid alone.

Continuous administration of opioid via an indwelling catheter can provide long-lasting pain relief with little systemic effects. Choices for administration include patient-controlled, bolus, or other infusion techniques. Catheters may be injected via an externalized port, percutaneous reservoir, or implanted pump.

31. **What other agents may be added to opioids or opioid/local anesthetic mixtures to produce intraspinal analgesia?**
    Many other classes of drugs have been studied for use in intraspinal analgesia. Two examples are: (1) The alpha-adrenergic agonist clonidine, which serves as a prototype for drugs that display analgesic activity both alone and synergistically with opioids and local anesthetics. Since its Food and Drug Administration approval in 1997, clonidine has held promise, particularly in treating cancer pain and complex regional pain syndromes. (2) NMDA receptor antagonists such as ketamine also show analgesic activity when administered intraspinally. They have not gained widespread use, however, because of their central nervous system side effects.

32. **What are the most common side effects of intraspinal clonidine?**
    Sedation, hypotension, and bradycardia are the most common side effects of intraspinal clonidine. Development of analogues to diminish these side effects progresses.

KEY POINTS

1. Intraspinal opioids may be administered either epidurally or intrathecally.

2. Intraspinal opioids may be administered through a single injection, through a catheter that is partly external to the patient or through a catheter that is part of an internal drug delivery system.

3. Many practitioners choose to use intraspinal opioids in combination with nonopioid analgesics such as clonidine and local anesthetics.

BIBLIOGRAPHY

1. Behar M, Magora F, Olshwang D, et al: Epidural morphine in treatment of pain, *Lancet* 1:527, 1979.

2. Borgeat A, Stirnenmann HR: Odansteron is effective to treat spinal or epidural morphine-induced pruritus, *Anesthesiology* 90(2):432-436, 1999.

3. Bromage PR, Camporesi E, Chesnut D: Epidural narcotics for postoperative analgesia, *Anesth Analg* 59:473-480, 1986.

4. Brownridge P: Epidural and intrathecal opiates for postoperative pain relief, *Anesthesiology* 38:74, 1983.

5. Chaney MA: Side effects of intrathecal and epidural opioids, *Can J Anaesth* 42:893, 1995.

6. Chia YY, Liu K, Liu YC, et al: Adding ketamine in a multimodal patient-controlled epidural regimen reduces postoperative pain and analgesic consumption, *Anesth Analg* 86:1245-1249, 1998.

7. Cole P, Craske DA, Wheatley RG: Efficacy and respiratory effects of low dose spinal morphine for postoperative analgesia following knee arthroplasty, *Br J Anaesth* 85(2):233-237, 2000.

8. Cousins M, Cherry D, Gourlay G: Acute and chronic pain: use of spinal opioids. In Cousins M, Bridenbaugh P, editors: *Neural blockade in clinical anesthesia and management of pain*, Philadelphia, 1988, JB Lippincott.

9. Eisenach J, De Kock M, Klimscha W: Alpha-2 adrenergic agonists for regional anesthesia: a clinical review of clonidine (1984-1995), *Anesthesiology* 85:288-296, 1996.

10. McMahon S, Koltzenburg M, editors: *Wall and Melzack's textbook of pain*, New York, 2005, Churchill Livingstone.

11. Nehme A: Intraspinal opioid analgesia. In Warfield C, editor: *Principles and practice of pain management*, New York, 1993, McGraw-Hill.

12. Ohno T, Kumamoto E, et al: Actions of opioids on excitatory and inhibitory transmission in substantia gelatinosa of adult rat spinal cord, *J Physiol* 518(Pt 3): 803-813, 1999.

13. Ozalp G, Guner F, Kuru N, et al: Postoperative patient-controlled epidural analgesia with opioid-bupivacaine mixtures, *Can J Anaesth* 45:938-942, 1998.

14. Reiz S, Westberg M: Side-effects of epidural morphine, *Lancet* 2:203-204, 1980.

15. Siddall PJ, Mollowy AR, Walker S, et al: The efficacy of intrathecal morphine and clonidine in the treatment of pain after spinal cord injury, *Anesth Analg* 91(6):1493-1498, 2000.

16. Stenseth O, Breirik H: Epidural morphine for postoperative pain: experience with 1085 patients, *Acta Anaesth Scand* 29:148, 1985.

17. Ummenhofer WC, Arends RH, Shen DD, Bernards CM: Comparative spinal distribution and clearance kinetics of intrathecally administered morphine, fentanyl, alfentanil, and sufentanil, *Anesthesiology* 92(3):739-753, 2000.

18. Wang JK, Nauss LA, Thomas JE: Pain relief by intrathecally applied morphine in man, *Anesthesiology* 50:149-151, 1979.

19. Yaksh TL: The spinal pharmacology of acutely and chronically administered opioids, *J Pain Symptom Manage* 7:356-361, 1992.

CHAPTER 42

NEUROSTIMULATORY AND NEUROABLATIVE PROCEDURES

Jason E. Silvers, BS, James N. Campbell, MD, and Charles E. Argoff, MD

1. **What is spinal cord stimulation?**

   Spinal cord stimulation (SCS) provides electrical stimulation over the dorsal columns of the spinal cord through the placement of epidural electrodes. Although the mechanism by which SCS relieves pain remains unclear, SCS results in significant pain relief for an appropriately selected group of patients.

2. **List the criteria for choosing patients who may benefit from spinal cord stimulation for treatment of pain.**
   - The patient should have a clear diagnosis for which the procedure is indicated.
   - Standard therapies to treat pain have been exhausted or are unacceptable to the patient.
   - When feasible, temporary relief of the patient's pain symptoms should be demonstrated by a trial of stimulation.
   - The pain should be distributed such that spinal stimulation can stimulate the sensory fibers that serve the painful area and create paresthesias. It is difficult to stimulate the sensory fibers that serve the spinal column, and thus spinal axis pain usually does not respond to SCS. In spinal cord injury, the sensory fibers that would ordinarily serve the painful area may be severed. The underlying substrate for stimulation (the dorsal columns) is thus missing. Not surprisingly, SCS does not relieve pain in such patients.
   - The patient must have a clear understanding of what to expect from treatment.

3. **Give examples of conditions that may respond and of those that usually do not respond to spinal cord stimulation.**

   The following conditions may respond to spinal cord stimulation:
   - Radicular pain from failed back surgery
   - Ischemic pain from peripheral vascular disease
   - Pain from peripheral nerve injury
   - Phantom limb pain or stump pain
   - Complex regional pain syndrome (reflex sympathetic dystrophy, causalgia)
   - Angina pectoris

   The following conditions usually do not respond to spinal cord stimulation:
   - Postherpetic neuralgia
   - Pain from spinal cord injury
   - Axial pain in failed back syndrome

4. **What are the theoretical bases for stimulation-produced analgesia?**

   Although there is no clear unifying theory for stimulation-produced analgesia (SPA), the most frequently employed is the "gate control theory." In its simplest form, this theory holds that stimulation of nonnociceptive fibers can inhibit the perception of activity in nociceptive fibers, and that there are central, descending pathways that also modulate the perception of pain. Electrical stimulation of certain central areas (most commonly the periventricular gray matter and thalamic nuclei) may produce analgesia through endogenous opioid mechanisms (see Chapter 1, Definitions).

5. **Why is spinal cord stimulation for failed back surgery syndrome more applicable to radicular neuropathic pain than to axial low back pain?**

It is easier to generate paresthesias in radicular distributions than in the midline of the lower back. Radicular paresthesias are elicited at almost all electrode positions, whereas achieving stimulation overlap of the lower back is technically difficult and may require complex electrode placement and extensive psychophysical testing.

6. **What are some of the complications of spinal cord stimulation for treatment of chronic pain?**

The most common complication of spinal cord stimulation for treatment of chronic pain is failure to achieve long-term pain control. Some of this may be the result of faulty patient selection. Occasionally, electrodes break or migrate from their initial site and analgesia wanes.

Other complications include infection at the site of the stimulus generator or a seroma collection.

7. **What are implantable pumps for intrathecal drug delivery?**

Implantable pumps consist of reservoirs, placed subcutaneously, which connect via a catheter into the intrathecal space. Implantable pumps allow physicians to administer opiate analgesics directly into the cerebrospinal fluid (CSF). The pumps are programmable so that the treating physicians can adjust dosages and delivery rates. The reservoir will have to be refilled on an intermittent basis: this is achieved by a percutaneous injection into the reservoir. Because the reservoir pump is driven by electricity, intermittent replacement is needed as the battery expires. More information on this technique is given in Chapter 41, Intraspinal Opioids.

8. **What are the dose advantages of spinal epidural and subarachnoid opiate delivery versus systemic administration?**

Spinal epidural opiate delivery has a dose advantage over systemic administration of one order of magnitude. On a milligram basis, epidural opioids are 10 times more potent than systemically administered opioids. Subarachnoid delivery has a two order of magnitude (100-fold) dose advantage. Of note, visceral pain responds best to intraspinal opiate delivery, whereas head and neck pain respond best to intracerebroventricular delivery. Therefore, analgesia may be obtained at dose levels significantly below those needed if oral therapy is used. This may be accompanied by a reduction in opioid-related side effects.

9. **How can externalized catheters be used to treat pain symptoms?**

Externalized catheters are placed percutaneously and connect directly into the intrathecal space. Treating physicians can administer medications directly from the outside into the CSF. However, externalized catheters are associated with high infection rates and therefore must be changed frequently. Opioids are the most frequently administered drugs, although muscle relaxants can be given in this fashion for the treatment of spasticity.

10. **What is the most common indication for opiate delivery via implantable pumps?**

The ability to administer opiates directly into the CSF has been one of the most important advances for the treatment of regional and widespread cancer pain. Opiate receptors are present on the central terminals of the sensory fibers that innervate the painful area and thus can be directly activated in this way. Direct delivery to the spinal cord also has the advantage over systemic administration in that there may be fewer associated symptomatic side effects because of the smaller doses necessary for adequate pain relief.

Note that implantable pumps should be used only in patients in whom oral delivery of opiates has failed, whether because of unacceptable side effects or lack of efficacy.

11. **What are neuroablative techniques and what are some examples?**
    Neuroablative procedures are aimed at the interruption of pathways in the peripheral and central nervous system concerned with transmission of nociceptive information. Examples include peripheral neurectomy, ganglionectomy, rhizotomy, the dorsal root entry zone operation (see Question 13), and cordotomy. It is probably true to say that these techniques are used less frequently nowadays with the advent of an increasing number of pharmacological options available for pain treatment. Therefore, the number of physicians with extensive experience in performing these techniques is declining.

12. **Can nerves be cut as a way to treat pain?**
    Severing or otherwise destroying a nerve that innervates a structure that generates pain is sometimes useful to treat pain. This is the basic idea behind procedures such as facet denervation. Unfortunately, severing a major nerve may generate a separate neuropathic condition (deafferentation pain). Small cutaneous nerves are often severed with operations or trauma. The resulting neuromas may be a source of pain. The location of the neuroma may play a critical role in the generation of pain. Relocation of the neuroma by proximal neurectomy is a relatively common and simple procedure and may relieve pain. Because transected nerves form new neuromas, another way of dealing with these problems is to perform a dorsal root ganglionectomy or rhizotomy operation. Most peripheral nerves are served by two or more ganglia (dorsal roots), however.

13. **What is the dorsal root entry zone operation?**
    In cases of traumatic avulsion of the brachial, lumbar, or sacral plexus, pain arises from abnormal signaling in the dorsal horn. This can be addressed by making microlesions in the dorsal horn, a procedure that has been termed the dorsal root entry zone (DREZ) operation. It can be used to treat certain aspects of pain from spinal cord injury.

14. **What is a cordotomy? What are the desired results?**
    A cordotomy surgically destroys the spinothalamic tract. The spinothalamic tract, located in the anterolateral part of the spinal cord, carries nociceptive information from the contralateral side of the body to the brain. Pain relief occurs a few spinal segments below the level of the lesion, but on the side of the body opposite the side of the cordotomy.

15. **How does an open cordotomy compare with a percutaneous cordotomy?**
    Open cordotomy requires a small laminectomy and incision in the spinothalamic tract, whereas percutaneous cordotomy uses radiofrequency lesions to destroy this portion of the cord. A percutaneous cordotomy is done with local anesthesia, and, prior to producing the destructive lesion, stimulation can be done to assure that the painful area will be covered by the cordotomy. Percutaneous cordotomy is usually performed at the C1-C2 vertebrae level, allowing for a high body level of pain relief. Although results from open cordotomy are favorable, percutaneous cordotomy is less invasive and results are comparable.

16. **What are the potential risks of a bilateral cordotomy performed at upper cervical levels?**
    - Respiratory depression—this may take the form of "Ondine's curse" or sleep apnea
    - Neurogenic bladder
    - Horner's syndrome—usually transient, from injury to the sympathetic fibers in the cervical cord
    - Transient hypotension
    - Sexual dysfunction
    - Bowel and bladder incontinence—usually transient

17. **How do rhizotomy and cordotomy differ in treating specific cancer lesions?**
    Rhizotomies affect only the areas served by the specific root that is cut (dermatomes), whereas cordotomies affect the entire side of the body from the level of the lesion down. Therefore, rhizotomies are considered only in very localized pain syndromes, and cordotomies can be used for more widespread pain.

18. **What is thought to be the anatomic basis for trigeminal neuralgia?**
    One proposed structural basis for trigeminal neuralgia is vascular compromise of the trigeminal nerve. Trigeminal neuralgia may also result from multiple sclerosis, collagen vascular disease, and other structural diseases that compress the trigeminal nerve near the brainstem. (See Chapter 18, Trigeminal Neuralgia, for a broader discussion and information on medical management.)

19. **Name three percutaneous ablative techniques used to treat trigeminal neuralgia and the side effects associated with these procedures.**
    - Radiofrequency retrogasserian rhizolysis attempts to produce graded anesthesia in the affected division of the trigeminal nerve. The procedure is based on the thermocoagulation of specific roots.
    - Retrogasserian glycerol rhizolysis involves glycerol injection into the trigeminal cistern. The osmotic agent produces a "chemical neurolysis."
    - Balloon microcompression involves inflation of a Fogarty-type of balloon near the gasserian ganglion.

    Regarding side effects of these techniques, loss of sensation is usually mild or not noticeable, particularly with glycerol injection. In severe cases, corneal anesthesia may lead to loss of vision. A different type of pain may emerge in the area rendered anesthetic; this pain is sometimes referred to as anesthesia dolorosa. (See Chapter 28, Neuropathic Pain, for a discussion of the mechanisms of pain production in injured nerves.)

20. **What open procedure can be used to treat trigeminal neuralgia?**
    Microvascular decompression can be used to treat trigeminal neuralgia; this procedure requires a craniotomy. The surgeon dissects vessels away from the trigeminal nerve.

21. **What is sympathetically maintained pain?**
    In some patients with neuropathic pain, abnormal activity in the sympathetic nervous system is presumed to maintain the pain. Sympathetically maintained pain (SMP) most likely results from the emergence of abnormal sensitivity of peripheral nerve pain fibers (nociceptors) to norepinephrine. The release of norepinephrine from the sympathetic nervous system activates nociceptors and thus produces pain.

22. **How can sympathetically maintained pain be diagnosed and treated?**
    One of the major stumbling blocks in treating SMP has been diagnosis. SMP must be considered in any patient suffering with severe facial or extremity pain. Also, almost all patients with SMP have cooling hyperalgesia (pain to a mild, cooling stimulus). A sympathetic block will relieve pain in every patient suffering from SMP. However, there are false-positives associated with sympathetic blocks, and placebo effects may be difficult to detect. If a technically well-done sympathetic block fails to relieve the patient's pain symptoms, the patient does not have SMP.

    Phentolamine infusion and possibly topical clonidine may also be used to test for SMP. In properly selected patients, surgical sympathectomy can be used to treat well-documented cases of SMP.

KEY POINTS

1. There should be a clear diagnosis of the condition causing the pain.

2. Where possible, pain relief with temporary stimulation should be demonstrated before more long-term spinal cord stimulation is instituted.

3. Radicular pain is more likely to respond to spinal cord stimulation than nonradicular pain.

4. Nerve sectioning may lead to deafferentation pain, which is pain arising in a numb area.

5. Invasive neurodestructive lesioning should only be carried out when simpler pain-relieving techniques have failed and then only by experienced practitioners.

BIBLIOGRAPHY

1. Bell GK, Kidd, D, North RB: Cost-effectiveness of spinal cord stimulation in treatment of failed back surgery syndrome, *J Pain Symptom Manage* 13(5):286-295, 1997.

2. Bendok B, Levy RB: Brain stimulation for persistent pain management. In Gildenberg PL, Tasker RR, editors: *Textbook of stereotactic and functional neurosurgery*, New York, 1998, McGraw-Hill.

3. Campbell JN: Diagnosis and treatment of pain associated with nerve injury. In Benzel EC, editor: *Practical approaches to peripheral nerve surgery*, Park Ridge, IL, 1992, AANS Publications Committee.

4. Coffey RF: Neurosurgical management of intractable pain. In Youmans JR, editor: *Neurological surgery*, 4th ed, Philadelphia, 1996, W.B. Saunders.

5. Gildenberg PL: Spinal cord surgery for pain management. In Gildenberg PL, Tasker RR, editors: *Textbook of stereotactic and functional neurosurgery*, New York, 1998, McGraw-Hill.

6. Loesser JD: Dorsal rhizotomy for the relief of chronic pain, *J Neurosurg* 36:745-754, 1972.

7. Nashold BS, Nashold JRB: The DREZ operation. In Tindall GT, Cooper PR, Barrow DL, editors: *The practice of neurosurgery*, Baltimore, 1996, Williams & Wilkins.

8. North RB: Spinal cord stimulation for chronic intractable pain. In Devinsky O, Beric A, Dogali M, editors: *Electrical and magnetic stimulation of the brain and spinal cord*, New York, 1993, Raven Press.

9. North RB, Kidd DH, Campbell JN, et al: Dorsal root ganglionectomy for failed back syndrome: a five-year follow-up study, *J Neurosurg* 74:236-242, 1991.

10. Onofrio BM, Yakash TL: Long-term pain relief produced by intrathecal morphine infusion in 53 patients, *J Neurosurg* 72:200-209, 1990.

11. Raja SN, Treede RD, Davis KD, Campbell JN: Systemic alpha-adrenergic blockade with phentolamine: a diagnostic test for sympathetically maintained pain, *Anesthesiology* 74:691-698, 1991.

CHAPTER 43

PSYCHOLOGICAL CONSTRUCTS AND TREATMENT INTERVENTIONS

Dennis R. Thornton, PhD, and Charles E. Argoff, MD

1. **List three possible psychological mechanisms for pain.**
   The first purely psychological mechanism that worsens pain is somatization. Psychic distress and conflict are converted into somatic complaints in an unconscious attempt to reduce intrapsychic tension. A second mechanism is psychosomatic: underlying muscle tension results in regional discomfort. Although this may be difficult to prove by examination, the fact that relaxation techniques and the use of anxiolytic drugs provide relief lends credence to the theory. The third psychological mechanism for pain represents the rare occurrence of somatic delusions or hallucinatory pain. These phenomena may occur in schizophrenia or in cases of severe depressive illness.

2. **Why is it important to recognize the manifestations and processes of somatization?**
   Expression of psychic distress via physical symptoms is universal. Up to two thirds of patients visiting a primary care service report at least one unexplained somatic symptom. In our society the prevailing belief is that more attention will be given to medically based problems over psychologically based ones. This then contributes to a preference to convey concerns with organically referenced language.

3. **What are some pointers to keep in mind when evaluating the patient with nonspecific complaints?**
   It is important to appreciate how the patient's decision to seek help and the manner in which symptoms are described are shaped by social context. Potential factors include position in the life cycle, marriage satisfaction, job status and satisfaction, level of affective distress, and the presence of any personal crisis.

4. **Name three contemporary conceptual models to help understand the process of somatization.**
   The transduction model can be seen as an extension of the concept of conversion, where emotional distress is unconsciously "transduced" into bodily sensations for which there is no physiological basis. The illness behavior model places emphasis on cognitive and appraisal factors, and sees environmental pressures and rewards as shaping health care decisions. The choice model postulates that cultural factors sanction the presentation of symptoms in somatic terms as a means of avoiding the stigma of mental illness.

5. **Identify the salient tenets of the biopsychosocial model.**
   Instead of assuming the hierarchical perspective that ruling out organic disease precedes exploration of psychosocial issues, the biopsychosocial model attempts to incorporate all aspects of the human condition and place the presenting symptoms in a broader whole life context.

6. **What are some points from the biopsychosocial model to try to incorporate into the patient evaluation?**
Avoid using blaming language if the patient presents with symptoms that do not make sense medically or do not improve with initial treatment. Attempt to reframe the symptoms in terms that reduce the need to classify the problem exclusively as either organic or psychological. Touch the symptom site during the physical exam. Suggest consideration of appropriate noninvasive, complementary treatments. Place emphasis on improved functioning rather than curing the disease as the outcome criterion. Educate the patient regarding body mechanics, adherence to treatment recommendations, and limitations and potential disadvantages of additional tests and/or procedures that you believe to be unnecessary. Open the discussion to touch upon psychosocial factors early on, rather than waiting until treatments have failed.

7. **Are the same psychosocial factors present in all pain patients?**
No. There are a variety of pathways by which individuals can come to display pain behaviors. Histories of being raised in dysfunctional homes with abuse, alcoholism, or mental illness are common in chronic pain patients. The resulting harsh superego is reflected in alcohol and drug abuse, self-sabotaging behaviors, marital discord, suicide attempts, and workaholism. An injured worker may experience not only the loss of employment but also an absence of personal gratification and a diminished sense of self, leaving him vulnerable to reemergence of anger, depression, and other negative emotions repressed from childhood. Such dynamic factors then negatively influence the patient's ability to invest in, and benefit from, psychological interventions.

8. **What is the relevance of psychoanalytic theory to understanding the experience of pain?**
Psychoanalytic theory divides the psyche into three functions: the id—unconscious source of primitive sexual, dependency, and aggressive impulses; the superego—subconsciously interjects societal mores, setting standards to live by; and the ego—represents a sense of self and mediates between realities of the moment and psychic needs and conflicts. Psychoanalytic writings discuss how pain frustrates the satisfaction of dependency and sexual needs as well as appropriate dissipation of aggressive feelings. The blocked expression of these needs leads to inner turmoil. However, when sanctioned as a bona fide physical problem, pain allows for unconscious gratification of ambivalent dependency needs. Underlying anger may be expressed indirectly, in the form of passive-aggressive behaviors, whereby the patient holds family members and treating practitioner alike as hostages to endless complaints and demands for attention. The experiences of pain satisfy the superego's need to suffer and atone.

9. **From a psychoanalytic perspective, how can the experience of pain be employed as a defense mechanism?**
Pain can be viewed as an ego defense mechanism in that the focus on somatic sensations deflects attention from intrapsychic conflicts and anxieties. The experience of physical pain is unconsciously perceived as more acceptable than the emotional pain. The patient represses his fears of loss and rejection, and the tension from these conflicts is displaced onto the body. The ensuing chronic pain behavior then serves as a form of interpersonal communication. Individuals frustrated and angry over their inability to alter their life situation in turn baffle health care professionals who attempt to treat the physical complaints, which are symbols of the underlying emotional pain.

10. **What is meant when pain patients are described as experiencing some form of "gain" from their pain experience?**
The construct of gain is described in three basic forms—primary, secondary, and tertiary—all of which are means by which pain behaviors are reinforced.

11. **What is primary gain?**
    Avoidance of a psychic conflict by converting it to a physical ailment is a primary gain the patient experiences from his or her pain. This conversion process is usually interpreted as a defense against anxiety or as a compromise solution of unconscious conflicts. While the underlying conflict is kept out of consciousness, the conflict remains unresolved and there is a continued buildup of psychic tension always ready for discharge. The anxious individual then discharges the pent-up energy by responding to ordinary or mildly painful stimuli in an exaggerated way.

12. **How is the term secondary gain applied?**
    Secondary gain applies to factors that reinforce the display of pain-related behaviors. The reinforcing factors alluded to are most commonly litigation and disability payments. However, demonstration of caring and concern is also a factor. Under these circumstances, there is a perceived incentive for the patient to persist in the complaint of pain. If the pain is resolved, the plaintiff's case will be weakened, or the love may be lost. Similarly, the injured worker who is partially improved may be pressured to return to work. Feeling in a weakened state, not ready to resume full responsibilities, the patient finds it easier to retreat into pain rather than face the threat of attempting to return to functioning and failing.

13. **How is tertiary gain different from primary and secondary gain?**
    Where constructs of primary and secondary gain apply to the individual, tertiary gain is external to the patient and involves family members or significant others who benefit from directly or indirectly reinforcing pain behaviors. The gain may be that interpersonal or family problems are suppressed as long as the patient remains ill; for example, a parent who feels inadequate successfully avoids having to work and interact with the world by caring for an ill child. By continuing to report that the child is symptomatic, the parent has a face-saving excuse for remaining dysfunctional. Similarly, the angry spouse may undermine the patient's efforts toward regaining independence because a new balance has been achieved with the advent of chronic pain and disability.

14. **Name some characteristics often associated with chronic pain syndromes.**
    - Preoccupation with pain
    - Strong and ambivalent dependency needs
    - Characterologic masochism (meeting other people's needs at one's own expense)
    - Inability to take care of self-needs
    - Passivity
    - Lack of insight to deal appropriately with anger and hostility
    - Use of pain as a symbolic means of communication

15. **What is meant by the term pain-prone disorder?**
    The concept of a pain-prone personality evolved from psychodynamic theory. The dynamic was created to codify the process by which intrapsychic conflicts predisposed the individual to seek expression for repressed feelings in the form of somatic, particularly painful, complaints. Chronic pain was viewed as a variant of depression, even though patients might see themselves as not depressed but suffering from physical ailments. In this light the depressive symptoms were "masked."

16. **Is the concept of "masked depression" still accepted as a relevant theory?**
    Proponents of psychodynamic theory believe that individuals with repressed conflicts are less distressed expressing their dependency needs through physical rather than emotional symptoms, because the former are more socially acceptable. However, it is extremely difficult to conduct research to confirm this theory. As investigators inquire more into this issue, there is mounting evidence that the experience of chronic pain and the negative lifestyle changes

imposed by it constitute a major life stressor and that dysphoria is a frequent consequence. Of course, a multitude of factors, including a premorbid vulnerability for depression, can make some individuals more vulnerable to the development of a major depressive disorder in response to the advent of chronic pain.

17. **How has learning theory been applied to the field of chronic pain?**
Learning theory proposes that there are two classes of responses that can be displayed by an organism: respondents and operants. Respondents are essentially reflexive in nature and are under the control of the antecedent stimulus, like Pavlov's dog being trained to salivate at the sound of the tone preceding the presentation of food. In contrast, operants involve actions potentially subject to voluntary control. Here the magnitude of the response depends on the nature and duration of the antecedent stimulus. In this sense, the behavior is under the control of the environmental consequences (reinforcements) and is, therefore, time-limited.

In terms of chronic pain, the theory suggests that if the behavior (e.g., moaning) is positively reinforced (by attention from others), it will increase in relation to the amount of reinforcement received and the meaning of that consequence (attention) to the person. Conversely, if the behavior is not reinforced (others ignore the moaning), the behavior will gradually extinguish. This learning theory model has been presented as an alternative to the medical model to explain how individuals evolve into chronic pain patients: their pain-related behaviors are reinforced by those around them.

18. **According to learning theory, what are the three principal pathways by which chronic pain syndromes develop?**
Operantly acquired pain behaviors are maintained through the following three basic pathways, which are not mutually exclusive:
- Direct and positive reinforcement of pain behavior
- Indirect but positive reinforcement of pain behavior by avoidance of adverse consequences
- Failure of well behavior to receive positive reinforcement

19. **Give two examples of direct and positive reinforcement of pain behaviors.**
Continued rest can become a major positive reinforcer of pain behavior. If certain movements result in pain, the person is less likely to perform such behaviors and will instead rest in bed. Initially, this may decrease the level of discomfort (direct positive reinforcement). However, as the overall activity level decreases, so does the pain tolerance, resulting in longer and longer rest periods and a downward spiraling in general functioning. Rest, as a pain contingent reinforcer, becomes self-perpetuating.

Analgesic medications provided on an as-needed basis can also foster pain behaviors. In both acute and chronic pain circumstances, patients may feel forced to take the attitude: "If the doctors will not keep me comfortable, I will have to complain and exaggerate my pain to get relief." In many inpatient programs, the cycle of drug-related pain behaviors is disrupted through detoxification.

20. **Can others, aside from health professionals, reinforce pain behaviors?**
Monetary rewards play a significant role in the maintenance of pain behaviors in a substantial proportion of chronic pain patients. Another example of how others impact the display of pain behaviors was demonstrated in a study that examined how chronic pain patients, participating in an inpatient pain program, acted in the presence of their spouses in comparison to how they acted in the presence of the staff. The spouses were classified as either solicitous or nonsolicitous, with the former group described as responding to patients' pain behaviors in a manner that would reinforce the display of such behavior. As expected, patients with solicitous spouses displayed pain-related behaviors more frequently in the presence of their spouses than when interacting with neutral staff, who did not reinforce these behaviors. Patients with nonsolicitous spouses did not show an increase in frequency of pain-related behaviors in the presence of their mates.

21. **Provide an example of indirect reinforcement (avoidance learning) of pain behaviors.**

    Much of our everyday behavior results from avoidance learning. We act to minimize or avoid behaviors and/or circumstances that may lead to adverse or punishing consequences. Pain may allow a person to avoid the unpleasant job, the test for which he was unprepared, or the argument with his spouse. Behaviors that are successful in avoiding the undesired circumstances are reinforced. Once established, these behavior patterns are extremely resistant to change. This pattern is offered as a major explanation for why so many injured employees fail to return to work once they are out of work for any prolonged period of time.

22. **Comment on the way in which failure to reinforce well behaviors can continue the pain cycle.**

    There is a clear overlap between the failure to reinforce well behaviors and the direct and indirect reinforcement of pain behaviors. The wife who actively encourages her husband to spend another day in bed resting his back before considering returning to work is both discouraging well behavior (return to work) and directly reinforcing a pain behavior (resting), which may or may not be coupled with the husband's own desire to avoid work. Similarly, the husband who rushes in to assist his wife with physical chores because of her sore hand is discouraging her attempts to resume normal responsibilities. A more appropriate response would be to offer assistance and respond only upon the spouse's cueing that help is needed.

23. **What is social learning theory?**

    Social learning theory is a psychological construct that proposes that behavior is not merely a result of inherited or acquired psychological conditions and environmental forces. Rather, individuals develop in a more complex manner by interacting in a meaningful way with their environment, with both actions and environment impacting each other. New experiences reshape views of the past and vice versa.

24. **How does social learning therapy apply to the understanding of chronic pain?**

    It is accepted that family members and other culturally important figures serve as models for both desirable and undesirable behaviors. Children are particularly open to the effects of modeling adults. Studies of children with recurrent abdominal pain were shown to be over five times as likely to have relatives (parents or siblings) who had similar symptoms in the study period than children who did not report recurrent abdominal pain. Fear of dental procedures has been demonstrated to be transmitted from fearful parents to their young offspring. Adults who scored high on a scale for hypochondriasis, dependency, and use of health services recounted that when they were ill as children, their own parents were very likely to call the doctor. There is a relatively high incidence of relatives with similar or other chronic illness reported by adults with chronic pain syndromes.

25. **What is cognitive-behavioral therapy?**

    Cognitive-behavioral therapy is a theoretical approach that acknowledges the importance of both cognitions and behaviors in the acquisition and maintenance of behavioral patterns. Cognitive behavior treatments have been applied to a wide range of psychological disorders, including depression and anxiety, as well as pain.

26. **What is implied by a cognitive-behavioral treatment approach to pain management?**

    A cognitive-behavioral treatment approach to pain management focuses on and promotes adaptive changes in the thoughts, feelings, beliefs, and behaviors of pain patients. Emphasis is placed on enlisting the patient as an active participant in the treatment program. This is often a unique experience, because many patients are maintained in a passive role when receiving unidimensional, medically oriented treatments such as surgery and/or medications. Being offered the opportunity to become a collaborator in their treatment helps pain patients attain a greater perception of self-control as well as coping skills that can mitigate suffering.

A cognitive-behavioral approach is generally active, structured, and time-limited, in contrast to more psychoanalytically oriented psychotherapy where the patient talks and the therapist listens. The patient is engaged in a dialogue regarding the personal effects of pain, learns concrete coping strategies, and works to establish steps to achieve mutually identified goals. Treatment also calls for the patient to assume personal responsibility in the form of self-monitoring, practicing relaxation and other techniques, and eventually conducting "personal experiments" to challenge and modify maladaptive beliefs, cognitions, and behaviors identified as promoting continued pain behaviors.

27. **What are the basic tenets of a cognitive-behavioral perspective?**
The following five general statements can be made concerning the basic tenets of a cognitive-behavioral perspective:
- Individuals are active processors of information and not just passive reactors.
- Thoughts (e.g., appraisals, expectancies, beliefs) can elicit and influence mood, affect psychological processes, have social consequences, and serve as an impetus for behavior; conversely, mood, physiology, environmental factors, and behavior can influence the nature and content of thought processes.
- Behavior is reciprocally determined by both the individual and environmental factors.
- Individuals can learn more adaptive ways of thinking, feeling, and behaving.
- Individuals should be active, collaborative agents in changing their maladaptive thoughts, feelings, and behavior.

28. **What are the primary objectives of cognitive-behavioral treatment programs as applied to the rehabilitation of patients with chronic pain?**
The main emphasis in cognitive-behavioral treatment programs is on functioning, as opposed to simple reduction of pain. Other goals involve reduction in the patient's reliance on analgesic medication, decreased use of the health care system, and eventual resumption of responsibilities, e.g., functioning at home and/or return to employment.

With these goals also used as central objectives for pain management, cognitive-behavioral principles are applied as an integral component of the interdisciplinary treatment approach. Cognitive-behavioral strategies are designed to assist the patient to achieve the following goals:
- Reduce the patient's sense of suffering and being overwhelmed by pain.
- Instruct the patient in the acquisition and implementation of effective coping strategies to promote more adaptive adjustment to pain.
- Promote a fundamental shift in self-perception from a stance of passive helplessness to being proactive toward rehabilitation, fostering a sense of self-efficacy.
- Assist the patient in recognizing the interplay between psychosocial factors, especially thoughts, feelings, and the experience of pain.
- Provide instruction for and model the use of cognitive-behavioral techniques to reduce distress.
- Enhance patient skill level to help anticipate setbacks, and devise plans to reduce their probability and successfully deal with those that occur.
- Promote an active role in daily activities, enhancing the patient's self-confidence and willingness to let go of pain-related behaviors.

29. **What is meant by "coping style"?**
Cognitive behavioral theory postulates that the patient's beliefs and cognitions play a significant role in the appraisal and response to pain. Beliefs serve as a perceptual lens through which the individual appraises the situation—in the case of pain, the threat—and influences the selection of coping strategies to be employed. The Coping Styles Questionnaire

(CSQ) is one of the commonly used instruments in the field of pain research. The original version identified five cognitive and two behavioral scales. Of these, the Pain Catastrophizing Scale has been shown to be the most predictive and most studied.

30. **Describe the catastrophizing coping style and give an example.**

Catastrophizing is simultaneously an appraisal, a coping strategy, and an exaggerated negative distortion. Dispositional negativism, passivity, and a sense of helplessness are cardinal traits. Individuals exhibiting this style are likely to endorse CSQ items such as the following: "It's awful and I feel that it overwhelms me"; "I worry all the time about whether it will end"; or "I feel like I can't go on."

31. **What has been the significance of the CSQ and the pain catastrophizing scale in particular?**

The CSQ has been replicated by many and recently has undergone a revision. It has also spawned additional indices assessing beliefs, attitudes, and catastrophizing—specifically, the Pain Catastrophizing Scale (PCS). The catastrophizing scale has been the most robust and has statistically linked pain with intensity, disability, and depression when other variables have been controlled for. With the PCS a ruminating factor has been found to be central to the concept of catastrophizing and shown to be predictive by itself (see Question 32).

32. **How does a patient's ruminating over his or her pain problem impact functioning?**

The "rumination factor" is a component of the PCS. This 13-item questionnaire assesses cognitions and feelings associated with the experience of pain. For example; "I can't stop thinking about how much it hurts!" In a sample of chronic pain patients, individuals scoring high on this rumination factor were more likely to present themselves as disabled. This result occurred after controlling for pain intensity and affective distress.

33. **What is "kinesiophobia"? How is it measured?**

The term *kinesiophobia* (kinesis = movement) was coined to describe the condition in which an individual is significantly encumbered by excessive and irrational fears of reinjury. Feeling perpetually vulnerable to exacerbations of pain, physical activity is minimized and avoided, leading to deconditioning and greater disability. The Tampa Scale for Kinesiophobia (TSK) is a 17-item questionnaire that estimates the degree to which the individual fears that physical activity might lead to reinjury.

34. **What is the transtheoretical model of change?**

The transtheoretical model for change proposes that people transition through defined stages in the process of altering problematic behavior patterns. The stages are defined as: "precontemplation" where no problem is acknowledged and there is no consideration given toward change; "contemplation" where a problem is acknowledged and serious thought is given to change in the future; "preparation" where some behavioral change is initiated; "action" where substantive behavioral efforts lead to alteration of the previous pattern; and, "maintenance" where change is sustained through continued effort.

35. **Illustrate how the transtheoretical model has relevance in the assessment and treatment of chronic pain patients.**

A patient in the precontemplative stage is less likely to acknowledge that any change needs to be made in his or her approach in dealing with pain. This patient would be prone to negative cognitions and coping strategies related to self-management of his or her pain. Therefore, he or she would not be a good (active) candidate for a multidisciplinary program because there is no motivation to exert effort toward making any change. Prior to becoming an active participant in a rehabilitative program such a patient would benefit more from a psychoeducational approach for assistance transitioning through the contemplation stage and into the action stage. In the action stage the patient displays greater motivation and effort toward actively altering problematic behaviors.

36. **What is meant by the concept "locus of control"?**
Patients experiencing protracted pain come to feel that their condition and suffering is out of their personal control. This mind-set contributes to a sense of helplessness and hopelessness. Principles of cognitive-behavioral therapy (CBT) are applied to assist the patient in successfully shifting his or her perception of control from externally based ("The pain controls me.") or exerted by powerful others ("I need to rely on the doctors and medication to control my pain.") to a more internally oriented stance ("I can take actions to modulate my pain.").

37. **How can this shift in perception of control be promoted and maintained?**
Instructing the patient in pain-coping strategies, promoting behavioral changes such as planning and pacing, and learning and applying relaxation techniques are among the interventions that can assist the patient in affecting a decrease in pain frequency and intensity. These interventions modify activities that contribute to flare-ups by promoting muscle relaxation and employing cognitive strategies that view the pain experience in realistic terms as opposed to fearing the worst. As more control is gained, self-efficacy is enhanced. Self-efficacy is the belief that the individual can succeed at a task, manage pain, and function at a higher level. The application of such CBT interventions for migraine is 50% efficacious, roughly equivalent to propranolol. Successful promotion of self-efficacy reduces pain behaviors and avoidance behaviors in patients with various pain states.

38. **What is the role of pacing in the rehabilitation of chronic pain patients?**
Pacing is a construct that has been receiving more attention in the field of rehabilitation. Learning how to conduct oneself in a slow and steady manner is essential to gradually increasing level of functioning. Patients with fibromyalgia are noted for their difficulties in sustaining activities at home or within the context of a rehabilitative setting. As with many patients with chronic pain, these individuals spend untold hours resting, then out of frustration try to push themselves to the point of exhaustion. This is a vicious cycle of nonfunctioning, overfunctioning, and collapse. Learning how to create more realistic expectations, plan ahead by breaking tasks into more discrete and manageable components, engaging in activities at a modulated pace, and interjecting rest periods results in improved functioning and self-efficacy.

39. **What role does anger management play in the treatment of patients with chronic pain?**
Anger is a salient emotion for many patients with chronic pain, and anger management is critical to treatment. Clinical experience links suppressed anger and expressed hostility with poor treatment outcome. In research studies, about 70% of patients report angry feelings: 74% were angry at themselves and 62% were angry at professionals. Self-directed anger was associated with greater pain intensity and depression. Generalized anger was linked with perceived disability. Anger suppression has been correlated with depression among women with recurrent headaches. In a group of men with low back pain, anger expression was a negative influence on progress in rehabilitation measures. Anger suppression, in this cohort, was positively associated with depression and negatively with general activities.

TREATMENT APPROACHES

40. **How can physicians reduce their level of frustration when working with patients who have chronic nonspecific symptoms?**
It is essential to cultivate a sense of trust with a patient who feels misunderstood and rejected by previous physicians. Reassure the patient that all appropriate medical assessments will be

conducted and results and implications discussed. Limit unnecessary tests and specialist referrals. Establish regularly scheduled nonsymptomatic follow-up visits. This will allow the patient to feel that there is a forum to discuss his or her concerns, which will in turn help reduce emergency phone calls and\or visits. Convey that the objective of treatment is not to seek a cure for the identified chronic condition but rather to assist the patient in being reasonably comfortable and as functional as may be possible without doing additional harm.

41. **How effective have psychoanalysis and psychodynamic psychotherapy been in the treatment of individuals with chronic pain syndromes?**
Although psychodynamic principles have contributed significantly to understanding the psychological problems that can foster pain behaviors, insight-oriented psychotherapy alone is not a very effective treatment approach. Many pain patients are so focused on somatic symptoms, believing them to be evidence of underlying organic disease, that there is little motivation to attain insights into the psychological underpinnings of their problem. In instances where individuals have been motivated and treatment has been successful, it has been time-consuming and costly. Thus, intensive traditional psychotherapy generally is not the treatment of choice for this patient population. However, when employed in conjunction with CBT or other treatments designed to alter maladaptive behaviors, insight can promote positive change.

42. **Name four principal behavior therapy techniques used in treating chronic pain patients.**
    - Graded activation program: Patients are taught to gradually increase their level of physical activity.
    - Social reinforcement: Significant others are enlisted as participants in the treatment program and alter their responses to the patient's behaviors to discourage the display of pain-related behaviors and reward the display of well behaviors.
    - Time-contingent use of medications: Analgesic medications are provided on the basis of time rather than the report of pain or display of pain behaviors.
    - Self-control techniques: The patient is taught self-regulatory skills to diminish the experience of pain and focus on well behaviors.

43. **When should a graded activation program be started?**
A graded activation program can be started as soon as clinically safe. Diaries are helpful in monitoring increased physical activity, and can be tailored to specific needs. Information includes "up time" (time spent in active endeavors) and "down time" (when the patient is resting, sitting, sleeping, etc.); pain intensity rating; use of medication; socialization (time spent alone or with others); as well as mood, thoughts, feelings, or self-cognitions. Diaries are best used when they are maintained for at least 7 consecutive days and are reviewed with the clinician while still current.

44. **What are some of the potential benefits derived from the use of a diary?**
    - Diaries are a reasonable reflection of the patient's experience of pain and help the clinician gauge perceived pain intensity.
    - Pain normally fluctuates over time, and patterns can be surmised and influential factors identified.
    - Effectiveness of medications and specific interventions can be readily assessed.
    - Monitoring their own behavior increases patients' awareness of factors influencing their pain.
    - Because the maintenance of a diary requires some effort and must be completed by the patient, it serves as an excellent means of assessing a patient's cognitive organization and his or her level of motivation.
    - The use of electronic diaries in research settings has confirmed moderate correlations with post-hoc questionnaire assessment.

45. **Describe how the concept of time-contingent use of medications is employed.**
The primary objective of a strategy involving time-contingent use of medications is to break the association between the display of pain behavior and the reduction of pain by analgesic medication. By providing medications on a fixed schedule, the pain behaviors are no longer reinforced, but appropriate relief can be provided. Time-contingent dosing can also be used to eliminate analgesic medication in an inpatient program.

First, a diary is employed to assess the baseline consumption of medication. Second, the total intake is divided into even doses and then provided at set intervals in the form of a "pain cocktail." The medication is combined with a liquid, e.g., orange juice, to mask the exact amount of drug provided. Over time, the amount of medication is reduced to zero, but the pain cocktail is still provided. Data have shown that patients receiving medication on a time-contingent basis reported less pain both during and after detoxification compared to those receiving medication on an as-needed basis.

46. **What are some of the formalized relaxation techniques?**
Relaxation techniques can be grouped according to the basic approach employed. The specifics of each technique can be altered to suit the needs of the individual and are not mutually exclusive, i.e., elements of one technique can be combined with other techniques.

Breathing relaxation: Adapts principles and exercises of classic yoga. Breathing is usually an automatic function, without conscious control. When conscious attention is focused on breathing, attention is removed from areas of tension. The focus is on the promotion of altered breathing, primarily abdominal or diaphragmatic breathing. This approach is extremely flexible and adaptive and often serves as the base technique to be learned.

Progressive relaxation: Created to assist individuals in becoming more aware of muscle tension and relaxation through a process of tensing, then relaxing specific muscle groups in sequence. The structured procedure requires about 20 minutes to complete.

Autogenic relaxation: Uses a series of self-statements to promote a state of inner calm and muscle relaxation. For example, "My mind is quiet," "My arms and legs feel quiet, heavy, comfortable, and relaxed," etc. These self-statements are generally pleasant and soothing, making this approach quite popular.

Guided imagery: This approach encourages the use of imagination to create pleasant scenes and experiences to promote a sense of well-being. Popular themes are the creation of a private place where the individual can go to contemplate, reflect on issues, and experience a decrease in pain. Taking an imaginary trip to the beach is commonly employed. The more sensory modalities engaged, the more profound the effect.

Meditation: Borrowed from Eastern teachings, the process of meditation is founded on the principle of uncritically focusing on one thing at a time. This may be a word, such as a mantra or a short phrase, meaningful to the meditator. Focusing on a flame, flower, or other object can also act as a mental anchor. It is important to note that the act of meditation is not simply focusing on one object to the exclusion of everything else. The mind is always drifting, and the meditator accepts this and strives toward maintaining an inner harmonious focus. Awareness, in the form of "mindfulness," produces measurable health benefits.

47. **What is the role of self-help groups for treating chronic pain patients?**
Self-help organizations have grown in popularity, and organizations exist locally and nationally for a wide variety of medical conditions, including chronic pain. Participation can be beneficial for pain sufferers. First and foremost, it provides a sense that "I am not alone." This is significant because many patients with chronic pain report that their suffering is unseen by others and may be questioned, and they experience a profound sense of isolation. Discovering that others have the same condition, have comparable experiences with the health care system, and harbor similar emotions can provide a sense of relief and belonging. Some of the groups are oriented toward teaching one another a variety of self-management techniques and reinforcing their use.

48. **Are there potential drawbacks to patients participating in self-help pain organizations?**

On the whole, the experience of patients in self-help pain organizations is positive. However, the quality of any local group is determined more by the individual leaders and members than by the sponsoring organization. This is true for all self-help groups. Group leaders are almost exclusively chronic pain sufferers themselves. Although this level of responsibility may assist some in their rehabilitation, a few may unconsciously seek to cloak themselves in pseudoprofessional, caretaker roles as a means of diverting their energies from their own recovery. Others may use self-help groups as an alternative to the traditional health care system and then chastise workers in the traditional system for failing to help them. Encourage patients to inquire about self-help organizations and use them as an adjunct to mainstream interventions.

49. **Is group therapy also applicable to treating chronic pain patients?**

Group therapy has been applied successfully in treating patients with chronic pain. Cognitive-behavioral techniques often are the mainstay of skills training. Groups tend to be psychoeducationally oriented, teaching patients about pain, the use of medication, and self-management techniques, and providing instructions for relaxation procedures, appropriate exercise, and methods to enhance self-esteem. Follow-up data indicate that patients frequently report a decrease in depressive symptoms and a reduction in pain, and they use fewer drugs. They also are more active.

50. **Should all chronic pain patients receive marital or family therapies as an adjunct to medical and physical interventions?**

Marital and/or family therapies, like all interventions, do not work for everyone. Couples therapy employed with headache sufferers revealed that those couples who completed therapy did benefit from treatment as opposed to those who dropped out, as assessed by the applied outcome measures. Of note is that dropout couples reported marital discord of greater severity and duration than the completers. Therefore, recommendations for marital therapy should be made on a selective basis.

51. **How is psychologically oriented technology being used in the area of pain control?**

Cutting-edge technology is employing virtual reality (VR) to assist patients in acute pain situations. Donning a VR headset, burn patients played Nintendo or other games while under going debridement and physical therapy. This distraction strategy deflected attention away from the painful procedures, leading to greater tolerance and less reliance on medication.

52. **What information about self-help is available to patients?**

There are two national self-help organizations for patients with chronic benign pain syndromes. The primary focus of these groups is to provide patients and concerned family members with relevant information related to chronic pain conditions. The American Chronic Pain Association (ACPA) is specifically geared to the lay public and self-help. A fundamental premise is that further medical interventions are not likely to provide additional relief. Therefore, it is incumbent upon the individual to learn new ways of dealing with pain to lead a productive life. Guidelines are provided for conducting self-help groups.

The National Chronic Pain Outreach Association (NCPOA) presents itself as a clearing house for both patients and professionals. It publishes a quarterly magazine about new treatments, maintains a listing of self-help groups and pain specialists, and offers self-help kits for those who want to initiate a self-help group of their own.

Contact information for these chronic pain organizations is as follows:

ACPA
P.O. Box 850
Rocklin, California 95677
916-632-0922
www.theacpa.org
www.chronicpain.org

NCPOA
P.O. Box 274
Millboro, VA 24460
540-862-9437
www.ncpoa@cfw.com

There are additional self-help organizations for headache sufferers. The American Council for Headache Education (ACHE) is directly affiliated with the professional organization, the American Association for the Study of Headache. The National Headache Foundation is an independent charitable organization that provides patient-related information. There are also self-help groups around the country for specific pain syndromes. Local directories can provide information about self-help clearinghouses where information about support groups of all sorts can be obtained.

Contact information for these headache organizations is as follows:

ACHE
875 King's Highway, Suite 200
West Deptford, NJ 08096
www.achenet.org

National Headache Foundation
52525 North Western Avenue
Chicago, IL 60625
888-NHF-5552
www.headaches.org

53. **Are there professional organizations from which information about pain syndromes as well as services can be obtained?**
In the United States, there are three organizations that deal specifically with pain syndromes: (1) the American Pain Society (APS), which is the national affiliate of the International Association for the Study of Pain. These organizations are interdisciplinary and academically oriented. The APS holds annual scientific meetings to keep professionals abreast of both clinical and research advances; (2) the American Academy of Pain Management, which is a smaller organization with a multidisciplinary orientation; (3) the American Academy of Pain Medicine, which is an organization for physicians specializing in pain management. All organizations hold annual meetings dedicated to the furthering of understanding in the field and sharing of treatment approaches.

American Pain Society
4700 W. Lake Avenue
Glenview, IL 60025-1485
847-375-4715
www.ampainsoc.org

American Academy of Pain Medicine
4700 W. Lake
Glenview, IL 60025
847-375-4731
www.painmed.org

American Academy of Pain Management
13947 Mono Way #A
Sonora, CA 95370
203-533-9744
www.aapainmanage.org

54. **What other organizations are available to both professionals and the public to obtain information about the quality of services provided?**
The Commission on Accreditation of Rehabilitation Facilities (CARF) is an independent organization that accredits various rehabilitation facilities (e.g., those for spinal cord injury,

head trauma, and general rehabilitation) and pain centers. CARF emphasizes a multidisciplinary, rehabilitation orientation, and patients play an active role in their rehabilitation. Stringent criteria are applied to those facilities applying for accreditation. Those facilities that have achieved CARF accreditation have demonstrated themselves to be centers of excellence.

CARF
4891 E. Grant Road
Tucson, AZ 85712
520-325-1044
www.carf.org

KEY POINTS

1. Psychological mechanisms of pain do exist and include somatization, psychosomatic, and the rare occurrence of somatic delusions or hallucinatory pain.

2. Primary objectives of cognitive-behavioral treatment programs for chronic pain include the following: a main emphasis on functioning, as opposed to the reduction of pain; reduction in the patient's reliance on analgesic medication; decreased use of the health care system; and eventual resumption of responsibilities such as functioning at home and/or return to employment.

3. Numerous patient-focused and professional pain organizations exist as resources for chronic pain and headache management.

BIBLIOGRAPHY

1. Asghari A, Nicholas MK: Pain self-efficacy beliefs and pain behaviour: a prospective study, *Pain* 94(1):85-100, 2001.

2. Arena, J, Blanchard EB: Biofeedback and relaxation therapy for chronic pain disorders. In Gatchel R, Turk DC, editors: *Psychological approaches to pain management: a practitioner's handbook*, New York, 1996, The Guilford Press.

3. Bebbington P, Delemos I: Pain in the family, *J Psychosom Res* 40(5):451-456, 1996.

4. Burns JW, Johnson BJ, Devine J, Mahoney N, Pawl R: Anger management style and the prediction of treatment outcome among male and female chronic pain patients, *Behav Res Ther* 36(11):1051-1062, 1998.

5. Davis M, Eshelman ER, McKay M: *The relaxation and stress reduction workbook*, 4th ed, Oakland, California, 1995, New Harbinger Publications.

6. Eccleston C: Role of psychology in pain management, *Br J Anaesth* 87(1):144-152, 2001.

7. Epstein RM, Quill TE, McWhinney IR: Somatization reconsidered: incorporating the patient's experience of illness, *Arch Int Med* 159(3):215-222, 1999.

8. Haythornthwaite JA, Benrud-Larson LM: Psychological assessment and treatment of patients with neuropathic pain, *Curr Pain Headache Reports* 5(2):124-129, 2001.

9. Hoffman HG, Patterson DR, Carrougher GJ: Use of virtual reality for adjunctive treatment of adult burn pain during physical therapy: a controlled study, *Clin J Pain* 16(3):244-250, 2000.

10. Jenson MP, Nielson WR, Romano JM, et al: Further evaluation of the pain stages of change questionnaire: is the transtheoretical model of change useful for patients with chronic pain? *Pain* 86: 255-264, 2000.

11. Kabat-Zinn, J: *Full catastrophe living*, New York, 1990, Dell.

12. Keefe FJ, Beaupre PM, Gil KM: Group therapy for patients with chronic pain. In Gatchel R, Turk DC, editors: *Psychological approaches to pain management: a practitioner's handbook*, New York, 1996, The Guilford Press.

13. Kole-Snijders AM, Vlaeyen JW, Goossens ME, et al: Chronic low-back pain: what does cognitive coping skills training add to operant behavioral treatment. Results of a randomized clinical trial, *J Consult Clin Psychol* 67(6): 931-944, 1999.

14. Lake AE: Behavioral and nonpharmacologic treatments of headache, *Med Clin North Am* 85(4): 1055-1077, 2001.

15. Morley S, Eccleston C, Williams A: Systematic review and meta-analysis of randomized controlled trials of cognitive behaviour therapy and behaviour therapy for chronic pain in adults, excluding headache, *Pain* 80(1-2):1-13, 1999.

16. Nielson WR, Jensen MP, Hill ML: An activity pacing scale for the chronic pain coping inventory: development in a sample of patients with fibromyalgia syndrome, *Pain* 89(2-3):111-115, 2001.

17. Okifuji A, Turk DC, Curran SL: Anger in chronic pain: investigations of anger targets and intensity, *J Psychosom Res* 47(1):1-12, 1999.

18. Patrick L, D'Eon J: Social support and functional status in chronic pain patients, *Can J Rehabil* 9(4):195-201, 1996.

19. Peters ML, Sorbi MJ, Kruise DA, et al: Electronic diary assessment of pain, disability and psychological adaptation in patients differing in duration of pain, *Pain* 84(2-3):181-192, 2000.

20. Romano JM, Schmaling KB: Assessment of couples and families with chronic pain. In Turk DC, Melzack R, editors: *Handbook of pain assessment*, 2nd ed, New York, 2001, The Guilford Press.

21. Romano JM, Turner JA, Jensen MP, Friedman LS: Chronic pain patient-spouse behavioral interactions predict patient disability, *Pain* 63(3):353-360, 1995.

22. Rosen G, Kvale A, Husebo S: Group therapy of patients with chronic pain, *Tidskr-Nor-laegeforen* 110:3602-3604, 1990.

23. Severeijns R, Vlaeyen JW, van den Hout MA, Weber WE: Pain catastrophizing predicts pain intensity, disability, and psychological distress independent of the level of physical impairment, *Clin J Pain* 17(2):165-172, 2001.

24. Sholevar GP, Perkel R: Family systems intervention and physical illness, *Gen Hosp Psychiatry* 12(6): 363-372, 1990.

25. Sullivan MJL, Stanish W, Waite H, et al: Catastrophizing, pain, and disability in patients with soft-tissue injuries, *Pain* 77(3):253-260, 1998.

26. Tunlin TR: Treating chronic-pain patients in psychotherapy, *J Clin Psychol* 57(11):1277-1288, 2001.

27. Turner JA, Jensen MP, Romano JM: Do beliefs, coping, and catastrophizing independently predict functioning in patients with chronic pain? *Pain* 85(1-2):115-125, 2000.

28. Vlaeyen JWS, Seelen HAM, Peters M, et al: Fear of movement/(re)injury and muscular reactivity in chronic low back pain patients: an experimental investigation, *Pain* 82(3):297-304, 1999.

29. Venable VL, Carlson CR, Wilson J: The role of anger and depression in recurrent headache, *Headache* 41(1): 21-30, 2001.

30. Williamson D, Robinson ME, Melamed B: Pain behavior, spouse responsiveness, and marital satisfaction in patients with rheumatoid arthritis, *Behav Mod* 21(1):97-118, 1997.

CHAPTER 44

PHYSICAL MODALITIES: ADJUNCTIVE TREATMENTS TO REDUCE PAIN AND MAXIMIZE FUNCTION

Bryan J. O'Young, MD, Mark A. Young, MD, Jeffrey S. Meyers, MD, LAc and Steven A. Stiens, MD, MS

1. **What is the role of physical modalities in pain management?**
   Physical modalities for the relief of pain are an important aspect of pain management and a time-honored adjunct of medical and interventional pain management. These modalities often serve to supplement and enhance interventional and pharmacological interventions. Physical modalities refer to any therapeutic medium that uses the transmission of energy to or through the patient. Physical forces such as heat, cold, pressure, water, light, sound, or electricity can be used as adjunctive treatment for the purpose of decreasing pain. In general, physical modalities are not meant to replace medical or other interventions; rather, they are intended to enhance overall outcomes.

2. **Give specific examples of physical modalities employed in the clinical setting.**
   Physical modalities that are employed in the clinical setting include hot packs (hydrocollator packs), cold packs, laser, therapeutic ultrasound, whirlpool, paraffin, electrical stimulation, traction/compression, massage and iontophoresis. These modalities produce effects including heating, cooling, movement, and analgesia. Heating and cooling agents are the most commonly used modalities.

   ## HEAT

3. **List the common indications for prescribing and administering mild to moderate heat therapy.**
   - Muscle spasm, tension myalgia: Heat therapy allows muscle relaxation by reducing muscle tension.
   - Pain: Heat therapy relieves pain by decreasing pain receptor sensitivity.
   - Contracture: Heat therapy increases range of motion by increasing collagen extensibility.
   - Hematoma, superficial abscess, thrombophlebitis: Heat therapy improves blood flow and circulation.

4. **What are the precautions for therapeutic heat?**
   The following precautions should be addressed when considering therapeutic heat:
   - Pregnancy: Avoid applying heat to the abdomen or low back; avoid immersing patient into a warm/hot whirlpool.
   - Impaired circulation: Use milder superficial heat in areas with poor circulation, particularly in older and younger patients. Patient may have poor vasodilatory responses and therefore may get burned.
   - Edema: Application to an edematous extremity in a dependent position has been shown to increase edema. Heat may be applied with caution with the area elevated if edema is present and is thought to be secondary to poor venous circulation.
   - Cardiac insufficiency: Monitor the patient carefully because heat can cause both localized and generalized vasodilatation.

- Metal in area: Metal has a higher thermal conductivity and higher specific heat and can become very hot with the application of heat.
- Open wound: Avoid paraffin over an open wound as it may contaminate the wound. The loss of epidermis reduces the insulation of subcutaneous tissues and therefore the application of heat should be provided with caution and at a lower temperature. Check frequently for signs of burning.
- Over areas where topical counterirritants have been recently applied: Topical counterirritants can cause local superficial vasodilatation. If a thermal agent is further applied, the vessels in the area may not be able to further vasodilate to dissipate the heat and a burn can result.

5. **Are there specific contraindications for therapeutic heat? (can I get "burned"?)**
   - Acute trauma, or inflammation: Heat can increase tissue temperature leading to increased vasodilation, which in turn may lead to increased blood flow that can aggravate the injury, increase pain, and delay recovery.
   - Hemorrhage, bleeding disorders: Heat can increase blood flow, which can restart or exacerbate the bleed.
   - Thrombophlebitis: Increase in temperature can increase risk of a thrombus becoming dislodged and moving to a vital organ.
   - Decreased sensation: Reduced ability to sense the heat increases the chance of the patient being burned.
   - Communication, alertness or judgment limitations that limit the patient's response to pain: Inability to communicate the pain increases the risk of being burned.
   - Malignancy: Avoid thermotherapy over or near malignant tissue; it may increase the growth rate or rate of metastasis.

6. **What is the therapeutic range and duration of heat?**
   The therapeutic temperature range is 40-45° C and the duration is 5 to 30 minutes. Sustained temperatures of 45° or more can cause tissue damage and burns.

7. **Are heating modalities only "skin deep"?**
   Some heating modalities, such as heat lamps, hot packs, hot-water soaks, and paraffin baths, are superficial and heat just the skin and the underlying subcutaneous tissue. Superficial heat is considered to be 1 to 2 cm. Other heating modalities are deep heating (diathermies) and are able to transmit energy through tissue and heat at depths of 3.5 to 8 cm, allowing treatment of joints like the hip.

8. **How is dosing and intensity of heat determined in the treatment of patients with physical modalities?**
   All energy applications must be applied in a given dose with a particular rate of transmission and a given therapeutic goal. A patient's sensory function at the site is the primary mechanism to judge safe application. The maximal therapeutic effect of heat in well perfused body tissues such as muscle, tendon, or ligaments is 42° C. This is normally expected to be uncomfortable for the patient with normal sensation. Sustained temperatures of 45° or more can cause tissue damage and burns. Cooling temperatures to 13° are uncomfortable but tolerated at the skin surface.

9. **Name four primary modes of heat transfer and provide some examples of each.**
   - Conduction: Heat transfer by direct contact (e.g., hot packs, paraffin baths)
   - Convection: Heat transfer by circulation of a medium of a different temperature (e.g., fluidotherapy, whirlpool)
   - Conversion: Nonthermal energy converts to heat (e.g., ultrasound, shortwave diathermy)
   - Radiation: Exchange of energy directly without an intervening medium (e.g., infrared lamp)

CONDUCTION

10. **What are hot packs, and what role do hot packs play in pain management?**
Hot packs consist of canvas bags filled with a hydrophilic silicon gel that can absorb many times its weight in water. The packs are hung in racks inside a thermostatically controlled water cabinet that stays on at all times and ensures that the packs are kept at approximately 70-75° C. During use, the packs are removed from the water baths and excess water is drained. The packs are then wrapped in six to eight layers of dry towels. Hot pack covers come in various sizes to match the hot packs and each cover can substitute for two to three layers of the towels. Packs can maintain therapeutically useful temperatures for 20 to 30 minutes.

11. **What are paraffin baths and what is their role in pain management?**
Paraffin baths are a form of thermotherapy commonly used for treating conditions including contractures, scleroderma, and rheumatoid arthritis. A mixture of paraffin and mineral oil in a 7-to-1 ratio is placed in a container and is kept at 45-50° C. Paraffin baths are effective for treating distal extremities, which benefit from a medium that can easily shape to the contour of an area. This is done by dipping the area in the bath and then removing it so the wax can harden between each dipping. Alternatively, the area can be submerged in the bath for 20 minutes for more intense heating. Paraffin can also be used to treat the knees, back, and other areas by "painting" it over the areas.

CONVECTION

12. **What is hydrotherapy?**
Hydrotherapy involves the application of water either externally or internally for treatment of dysfunction. Local immersion techniques include whirlpool, and contrast baths. Full-body immersion techniques include Hubbard tank whirlpool and water exercise in pools. Nonimmersion techniques include local irrigation devices.

13. **What are general indications for hydrotherapy?**
Hydrotherapy is used for pain control, wound care, superficial heating and cooling, control of edema, and water exercise.

14. **How is hydrotherapy used in pain control?**
Although data is lacking, it is believed that the sensory stimulation from water to the peripheral mechanoreceptors gates the transmission of pain sensations at the spinal cord level. The decreased weight bearing in water immersion techniques and the reduction of inflammation from cold submersion may also play a role.

CONVERSION

15. **What is therapeutic ultrasound?**
Therapeutic ultrasound uses sound waves of alternating compression and rarefaction at frequencies well above the human audible range (0.8 to 3 MHz) that are transmitted through a coupling gel medium into the body.

16. **What are the therapeutic effects of ultrasound? How are they used clinically?**
Heat production occurs at interfaces when tissue densities change, producing hyperemia and increasing connective tissue extensibility. Nonthermal effects of ultrasound include

mechanical deformation, forced streaming of liquid, cavitation (bubbles in fluid media), standing waves and shock waves. Collectively, these effects can disrupt tissue adhesions and scarring and clear infection. Ultrasound is effective in heating deep tissues to loosen deposits in calcific tendonitis and stretch contractures. Ultrasound should be used cautiously with continuous movement of the probe to avoid overheating at tissue interfaces.

17. How does shortwave diathermy work?
Shortwave diathermy transmits energy through tissue by inducing small microcurrents that heat tissue because of natural resistance and vibration of molecules. Maximal temperatures occur in tissues with less interstitial fluid, such as connective tissue. Radio waves are transmitted through treatment areas and tuned for maximal coupling. The advantage of shortwave diathermy over ultrasound is the capacity to treat a larger area over a sustained duration.

RADIATION

18. Describe the use of infrared lamps.
Infrared (IR) lamps using IR-A wavelengths 780 to 1500 nm increase tissue temperature directly proportional to the amount of radiation penetration of the tissue. Penetration is influenced by a number of factors including wavelength, power of radiation, distance of source to the tissue, angle of incidence of radiation to tissue, and tissue absorption coefficient. IR radiation at these wavelengths is absorbed 1 to 3 mm deep. The further the source of radiation from the tissue surface, the less the effectiveness of heating. Benefits of IR lamps include (1) the area being treated is visible throughout the treatment, and (2) the treatment does not require contact of the medium with the patient.

COLD

19. How does cold therapy work?
Cold therapy or cryotherapy works through the removal or absorption of thermal energy (heat) through agents applied superficially/topically. Both sweat and vapocoolant sprays absorb heat from the body surface and evaporate, thereby reducing the temperature over the area. Cooling agents rely on conduction and convection to achieve their effect.

20. What are the common physiological effects of cryotherapy?
Cryotherapy is known to decrease nerve conduction velocity, decrease spasticity, decrease metabolic rate, have a variable effect on muscle strength, increase pain threshold, and facilitate muscle contraction. It also initially decreases blood flow but later increases it. Decreased spasticity is believed to be related to decreased discharge in the afferent spindle fibers and Golgi tendon organs. Decreased metabolic rate is believed to be due to inhibited enzymatic activity. Facilitation of muscle contraction is temporary and is believed to be related to facilitation of alpha motor neuron activity. Nerve conduction velocity decreases in both sensory and motor nerves in proportion to the degree and length of temperature change. Myelinated and small fibers are affected the most.

21. What are the common indications for cryotherapy?
Although cold therapy in the form of ice packs is commonly used to treat acute musculoskeletal injuries, other common indications include controlling inflammation, stabilizing edema, providing analgesia, promoting vasoconstriction, and modifying spasticity.

22. **What are the contraindications for cold therapy?**
Cryotherapy should generally be avoided in situations involving decreased skin sensation, ischemia, severe hypertension, cryoglobulinemia, and cold hypersensitivity such as Raynaud's syndrome.

23. **What is the difference between cold packs and ice packs?**
Cold packs contain a gelatinous mixture covered with vinyl that is kept at 0-5° C. The gelatinous quality allows the pack to conform to the treated area. Cold packs can be made at home using frozen vegetables or a water and rubbing alcohol mixture. Ice packs are used in a similar manner but are made using crushed ice in a plastic bag and allow greater cooling than cold packs at similar temperatures because of the higher specific heat of ice.

24. **What is "cold laser"?**
"Cold" or low-intensity laser uses monochromatic (all one color), coherent (all waves in phase), and directional (with minimal beam divergence) light for biostimulation and to enhance healing. In the laboratory, cold laser has been found to alter nerve conduction and regeneration, increase adenosine triphosphate (ATP) and nucleic acid production, stimulate macrophages, stimulate fibroblasts to increase collagen production, and cause vasodilatation. The mechanism of action for these effects is still unknown.

25. **What are the indications for cold laser?**
Cold laser is frequently used for musculoskeletal disorders including arthritis and soft tissue problems. It has been shown to reduce pain and dysfunction for a variety of specific problems including chronic pain, trigger points, neck pain, low back pain, and lateral epicondylitis. Cold laser is also used to promote healing of wounds and fractures.

26. **How does one choose between cryotherapy and thermotherapy since some of the indications and effects overlap?**
A summary of the effects of cryotherapy and thermotherapy is outlined in Table 44-1.

TABLE 44-1. SUMMARY OF THE EFFECTS OF CRYOTHERAPY AND THERMOTHERAPY		
Effect	Cryotherapy	Thermotherapy
Pain	↓	↓
Muscle	↓	↓
Blood flow	↓	↑
Edema formation	↓	↑
Nerve conduction velocity	↓	↑
Metabolic rate	↓	↑
Collagen extensibility	↓	↑
Joint stiffness	↑	↓
Spasticity	↓	0

↓ = decreases, ↑ = increases, 0 = no effect.

TRACTION AND COMPRESSION

27. **What are the effects of spinal traction?**
    - Joint distraction—the separation of articular surfaces possibly decreasing load.
    - Muscle relaxation—by breaking the pain-spasm-pain cycle
    - Stretching of soft tissues—thereby increasing their length.
    - Reducing disc protrusion—through realignment, suction, or tensing of the posterior longitudinal ligament.
    - Joint mobilization—to increase mobility or decrease pain.
    - Patient immobilization—to limit mobility for prolonged periods thus decreasing symptoms related to motion. (Note: This has fallen out of favor for a number of reasons including the recognition that prolonged immobilization may result in increased pain long term.)

28. **When is traction indicated?**
    Traction is indicated for neck or back pain with or without radiation caused by disc bulge/herniation, nerve root impingement, joint hypomobility, subacute joint inflammation, or paraspinal spasm.

29. **What should be included in a prescription for traction?**
    - Positioning: Supine or seated for cervical, supine for lumbar.
    - Static or intermittent force: Static or continuous traction may be most beneficial for muscle relaxation, whereas intermittent traction may be best for reducing disc protrusion or distracting joints.
    - Amount of force: Traction force should be increased gradually but, in general, cervical traction is recommended at 25 to 30 pounds of force (including 10 pounds to overcome gravity). For lumbar traction 25% of body weight is needed to achieve vertebral separation with another 25% body weight needed to overcome the friction effects of a regular traction table.
    - Duration: Recommended parameters for both cervical and lumbar traction range from 5 to 10 minutes in the acute phase to 20 to 30 minutes in general.

30. **When is traction contraindicated?**
    General contraindications for traction include ligament-joint instability, acute injury or inflammation, local tumor or infection, history of previous trauma, pregnancy, osteopenia, osteomyelitis, achondroplastic dwarfism, significant hypertension, and in situations where there is peripheralization of symptoms with traction. Specific restrictions for cervical traction include vertebrobasilar artery insufficiency, rheumatoid arthritis, acute torticollis, and midline disc herniation. Specific restrictions for lumbar traction include pregnancy, restrictive lung disease, aortic aneurysm, active peptic ulcer, cauda equina syndrome, and gross hemorrhoids.

31. **How is compression used in pain rehabilitation?**
    Compression devices include pneumatic pumping devices and compressive garments. These devices can be used to improve venous and lymphatic circulation, limit the shape and size of tissue, and increase tissue temperature, thus preventing or alleviating pain.

Clinical indications include treatment of edema and lymphedema, prevention and treatment of deep venous thrombosis, treatment of venous stasis ulcers, residual limb shaping postamputation, and hypertrophic scar control.

TRANSCUTANEOUS ELECTRICAL STIMULATION (TENS)

32. **What is TENS and what is its role in pain management?**
TENS is an electronic device that delivers a depolarizing current through the skin to primarily sensory subcutaneous nerves and is considered a method for pain relief. Muscle contraction is a side effect of higher amperage and is not an intended effect. Pain perception is reduced by replacing one sensory stimulus for another. Electrodes are placed on or around the painful area. Type I afferents are activated and carry sensory messages to the substantia gelatinosa layer to the dorsal root entry zone likely blocking nociceptive messages (via the gate control theory). When first applied with optimized settings and placement, pain reduction is consistently observed. Unfortunately, habituation to the response often occurs after 3 to 4 months. Newer devices vary the stimulation to avoid habituation.

MASSAGE

33. **Under what circumstances is massage useful?**
   - To release and stretch areas of myofascial tension
   - To prevent and loosen adhesions and reduce contractures
   - To deactivate trigger points, and to increase circulation to an area

34. **What are the absolute contraindications to massage?**
   - Malignancy
   - Open wounds
   - Deep venous thrombosis
   - Infection

IONTOPHORESIS/PHONOPHORESIS

35. **What is iontophoresis?**
Iontophoresis uses an electrical stimulation device with low-voltage electrical currents to drive medications across the dermis over symptomatic areas. Theoretically, any charged substance can be used. Medications typically include lidocaine and salicylate.

36. **What is phonophoresis?**
In phonophoresis, ultrasound is applied with a topical medication mixed with an acoustic coupling medium. The purpose is to enhance delivery of the medication through the skin. Typical medications used with this technique include corticosteroids and topical anesthetics, but other agents including ibuprofen have been studied and show promise.

KEY POINTS

1. Physical modalities can only be integrated into a pain management program after an appropriate physical diagnosis process has been completed.

2. Physical modalities may be a part of an integrated pain management program combining these with medical and interventional approaches as needed.

3. When using therapeutic heat or cold as a physical modality, the practitioner must be certain that specific precautions and contraindications for the use of therapeutic heat or cold have been screened for and addressed appropriately.

4. When using traction as a pain-reducing physical modality, the practitioner must be aware of the specific contraindications for this technique.

5. Iontophoresis and phonophoresis are physical modalities designed to drive medications across the dermis into localized symptomatic areas.

WEBSITES

1. http://physicaltherapy.about.com/od/abbreviationsand terms/p/Modalities.htm

2. http://www.emedicine.com/pmr/TOPIC200.HTM

3. http://www.emedicine.com/pmr/TOPIC201.HTM

4. http://www.emedicine.com/pmr/TOPIC203.HTM

5. http://www.emedicine.com/pmr/TOPIC206.HTM

6. http://www.spineuniverse.com/displayarticle.php/article1853.html

BIBLIOGRAPHY

1. Atchinson JW, Stoll ST, Cotter AC: Traction, manipulation, and massage. In Braddom RL, editor: *Physical medicine and rehabilitation*, 2nd ed, Philadelphia, 2000, W.B. Saunders, pp. 413-439.

2. Basford JR, Sheffield CG, Harmsen WS: Laser therapy: a randomized, controlled trial of the effects of low-intensity ND:YAG laser irradiation on musculoskeletal back pain, *Arch Phys Med Rehabil* 80(6):647-652, 1999.

3. Basmajian JV: *Manipulation, traction, and massage*, 3rd ed, Baltimore, 1985, Williams and Wilkins.

4. Baxter D: Low intensity laser therapy. In Kitchen S, Bazin S, editors: *Clayton's electrotherapy*, 10th ed, London, 1996, W.B. Saunders.

5. Brucks R, Nanavaty M, Jung D, et al: The effect of ultrasound on the in vitro penetration of ibuprofen through the human epidermis, *Pharm Res* 6(8):679-701, 1989.

6. Byl NN: The use of ultrasound as an enhancer for transcutaneous drug delivery: phonophoresis, *Phys Ther* 75(6):539-553, 1995.

7. Cameron, MH: *Physical agents in rehabilitation: from research to practice*, 2nd ed, St. Louis, 2003, Saunders.

8. Caroll D, Moore RA, et al: Transcutaneous electrical nerve stimulation (TENS) for chronic pain (Cochrane Review). *Cochrane Database Syst Rev* 3:CD003222, 2001.

9. Choi H, Sugar R, Fish DE, Shatzer M, et al: Modalities. In *Physical medicine and rehabilitation pocketpedia*, Philadelphia, 2003, Lippincott, Williams, and Wilkins.

10. Cyriax J: *Textbook of orthopedic medicine, Vol I: Diagnosis of soft tissue lesions*, London, 1982, Bailliere Tindall.

11. Douglas WW, Malcolm JL: The effect of localized cooling on cat nerves, *J Physiol* 130:53-54, 1955.

12. Gallagher RM: Rational integration of pharmacological, behavioral and rehabilitation strategies in the treatment of chronic pain, *Am J Phys Med Rehabil* 84(Suppl):64-76, 2005.

13. Gorman PH, Alon G, Kornhauser SH: Electrotherapy: medical treatment using electrical currents. In O'Young BJ, Young MA, Stiens SS, editors: *Physical medicine and rehabilitation secrets*, 3rd ed, Philadelphia, 2008, Elsevier, pp 226-232.

14. Hinderer SR, Biglin PE. Manipulation, massage, and traction: an overview. In O'Young BJ, Young MA, Stiens SS, editors: *Physical medicine and rehabilitation secrets*, 3rd ed, Philadelphia, 2008, Elsevier, pp 216-220.

15. Judovich B: Lumbar traction therapy, *JAMA* 159:549, 1955.

16. Karu TI: Molecular mechanisms of the therapeutic effects of low intensity laser radiation, *Lasers Life Sci* 2:53-74, 1989.

17. Knight KL: *Cryotherapy: theory, technique, and physiology*, Chattanooga, TN, 1985, Chattanooga Corp.

18. Knuttsson E: Topical cryotherapy in spasticity, *Scand J Rehabil Med* 2:159-162, 1970.

19. Lentall G, Hetherington T, Eagan J, et al: The use of thermal agents to influence the effectiveness of a low-load prolonged stretch, *J Orthop Sport Phys Ther* 16(5):200-207, 1992.

20. Maitland GD: *Vertebral Manipulation*, 5th ed, London, 1986, Butterworth.

21. Matthews JA: The effects of spinal traction, *Physiotherapy* 58:64-66, 1972.

22. Miglietta O: Action of cold on spasticity, *Am J Phys Med* 52:198-205, 1973.

23. Mysiw WJ, Jackson RD: Electrical Stimulation. In Braddom RL, editor: *Physical medicine and rehabilitation*, 2nd ed, Philadelphia, 2000, W.B. Saunders, pp. 459-487.

24. Onel D, Tuzlaci M, Sari H, et al: Computed tomographic investigation of the effect of traction on lumbar disc herniations, *Spine*, 14:82-90, 1989.

25. Pal B, Mangion P, Hossain MA, et al: A controlled trial of continuous lumbar traction in the treatment of back pain and sciatica, *Br J Rheumatol* 25:181-183, 1986.

26. Price R, Lehman JF, Boswell-Bassette S, et al: Influence of cryotherapy on spasticity at the human ankle, *Arch Phys Med Rehabil* 74:300-304, 1993.

27. Saunders HD: Use of spinal traction in the treatment of neck and back conditions, *Clin Orthp* 179:31-38, 1983.

28. Seliger V, Dolejs L, Karas V: A dynamometric comparison of maximum eccentric, concentric, and isometric contractions using EMG and energy expenditure measurements, *Eur J Apply Physiol* 45:235-244, 1980.

29. Shankar K, Randall KD: *Therapeutic physical modalities*, Philadelphia, 2002, Elsevier.

30. Snyder-Mackler L, Barry AJ, Perkins AI, et al: Effect of helium-neon laser irradiation on skin resistance and pain in patients with trigger points in the neck or back, *Phys Ther* 69(5):336-341, 1989.

31. Swezey RL: The modern thrust of manipulation and traction therapy, *Semin Arthritis Rheum* 12:322-331, 1983.

32. Van der Heijden GJMC, Beurskens AJHM, Assendelft WJ, et al: The efficacy of traction for back and neck pain: a systematic, blinded review of randomized clinical trial methods, *Phys Ther* 75(2):93-104, 1995.

33. Weber DC, Brown AW: Physical agent modalities. In Braddom RL, editor: *Physical medicine and rehabilitation*, 2nd ed, Philadelphia, 2000, W.B. Saunders, pp 440-458.

34. Wieting JL, Andary MT, Holmes TG, et al: Manipulation, massage, and traction. In DeLisa JA, Gans BM, editors: *Physical medicine and rehabilitation: principles and practice*, 4th ed, Philadelphia, 2005, Lippincott-Raven, pp 285-310.

35. Worden RE, Jumphrey TL: Effect of spinal traction on the length of the body, *Arch Phys Med Rehabil* 45:318-320, 1964.

CHAPTER 45

PAIN CLINICS

Nelson Hendler, MD, MS, and Charles E. Argoff, MD

1. **What is a multidisciplinary pain treatment center?**
   A multidisciplinary pain treatment center is made up of various medical disciplines and ancillary personnel to assist with the diagnosis and management of patients with chronic and persistent pain. Centers can be organized as an outpatient, inpatient, or combined setting, and they may be freestanding or hospital-based. They are usually characterized as multidisciplinary chronic pain treatment centers (those using numerous clinicians and a broad spectrum of modalities to treat any number of syndromes), monomodality centers (using only a single type of treatment, such as nerve blocks, biofeedback, or hypnosis), and syndrome-specific clinics (treating only one disorder). In a truly multidisciplinary center, both the diagnostic component and the treatment component are multidisciplinary.

2. **How should a multidisciplinary pain treatment center be organized?**
   The central element of a multidisciplinary pain treatment center's organization is the establishment of a common philosophy among the various physicians and other health care personnel involved. This philosophy addresses (1) the use of pharmacologic agents, (2) the interpretation of various diagnostic studies, (3) attitudes toward the role of psychiatry, physical therapy, and adjunctive treatments, and (4) the goal of the chronic pain treatment center—i.e., rehabilitation, reduction of pain, and restoration of function.

3. **What are the essential elements of a multidisciplinary pain treatment center?**
   A well-run multidisciplinary pain treatment center requires that a single health care provider function as the leader of the team. This person assumes responsibility for coordinating all of the medical efforts, laboratory studies, ancillary therapies, and medications and should be available during all hours that the center is open, to provide continuity of care. Any health care provider with expertise in pain management can be the team leader for a specific patient, though it is usually more practical for the leader to be a physician.
   Members of the team may be from any and all disciplines. The most common cadre is an admixture of anesthesiologists, neurologists, psychiatrists, psychologists, physiatrists, neurosurgeons, orthopedic surgeons, and nurses. In centers treating orofacial pain, dentists are indispensable. Social workers and nonmedical personnel round out the team. The exact composition of the team is less important than the philosophy of working as a team toward the functional rehabilitation of patients in pain.

4. **Is there evidence that multidisciplinary treatment plans are better than general good care?**
   Yes. Although the data are hard to analyze, a number of studies have shown that multidisciplinary pain centers can be cost-effective for patients with low back pain, chronic abdominal pain, and a number of musculoskeletal pain disorders.

5. **What is the role of a psychiatrist in a multidisciplinary chronic pain treatment center?**

The multidisciplinary chronic pain treatment center's psychiatrist(s) can assist in the identification of psychiatric conditions that may initiate or perpetuate pain conditions. The psychiatrist should have a good working knowledge of psychopharmacology; he or she should be knowledgeable about drug interactions and dependence or addiction. A psychiatrist should either run or supervise group psychotherapy sessions and biofeedback, as well as family counseling sessions. Appropriately directed psychiatric treatment can help in withdrawal of potentially harmful medications, development of appropriate coping skills, and identification of factors that tend to perpetuate a chronic pain syndrome.

6. **What is the role of an interventional pain specialist in a multidisciplinary pain treatment center?**

An interventional pain specialist can be an invaluable member of the multidisciplinary team. He or she can provide both diagnostic and therapeutic blocks. An interventional pain specialist also can provide greater insight into drug interactions and novel means of drug delivery. Additionally, an interventional pain specialist working in conjunction with the neurosurgeon and the orthopedic surgeon of the team can provide a continuity of care, ranging from diagnostics through the anesthesia needed for surgery. The interventional pain specialist typically also has a background in anesthesiology, physical medicine and rehabilitation, or neurology.

7. **What is the role of the neurosurgeon?**

The neurosurgeon can provide diagnostic and surgical skills not available from other specialties at the multidisciplinary pain treatment center. He or she can provide both stimulatory and ablative procedures for pain relief.

8. **What is the role of the psychologist?**

The psychologist at the multidisciplinary center can provide skills usually not offered by a psychiatrist in the area of administration and interpretation of psychological testing and neuropsychological testing, and assessment of cognitive functioning. Working alone or in conjunction with the psychiatrist, the psychologist provides group therapy, supportive psychotherapy, family counseling, and individual counseling. Additionally, he or she can coordinate the activities of the social workers and help to deal with the multiple social issues usually associated with chronic pain. Many psychologists have special training in cognitive-behavioral techniques and biofeedback.

9. **What is the role of a rehabilitation specialist?**

A physiatrist can provide valuable input in the area of rehabilitation, both occupational and vocational, at the pain treatment center. He or she may supervise the occupational therapist and vocational rehabilitation specialist. The physiatrist can manage the physical therapist and select appropriate physical testing and rehabilitation efforts, such as muscle strengthening and muscle retraining. A physiatrist is also of great assistance in postoperative care and rehabilitation.

10. **Who should lead a multidisciplinary pain treatment center?**

The answer to this question is rather complex. The experience of many chronic pain treatment centers indicates that care is facilitated by a physician as leader. A physician can prescribe and regulate medications, coordinate medical testing, and serve as a medical coordinator among the various consultants. This role would be very difficult for a Ph.D., who may be knowledgeable in these areas, but unfortunately would not have the legal ability to prescribe medications and medical diagnostic studies. However, if the Ph.D. or other provider works in conjunction with a licensed physician, this problem can be minimized.

The physician's personal characteristics and medical knowledge are of paramount importance; the specialty training becomes a secondary issue. The physician in charge should be able to work well with the other members of the team and should be empathetic in understanding patients with chronic pain. Therefore, a compassionate neurologist, a psychiatrist with a knowledge of medicine, or a neurosurgeon or orthopedic surgeon who is willing to make time to take a careful history and listen to patients is an ideal selection. Important characteristics of a center's leader include the following:

- Organizational skills
- People skills
- Knowledge of pharmacology and psychopharmacology
- Knowledge of medical testing
- Knowledge of surgical procedures
- Willingness to provide continuity of care on a daily basis
- Knowledge of insurance issues and sociologic issues
- Willingness to handle administrative details, such as report writing and giving testimony

11. **Which is better: An inpatient or an outpatient chronic pain treatment center?**
This question actually begs other questions. Both inpatient and outpatient settings have advantages and disadvantages. An outpatient center reduces costs for the insurance carrier and for the patient and probably is appropriate for the vast majority of chronic pain patients. Most chronic pain patients do not need residential treatment unless they are severely depressed or unable to manage their medications. The inpatient setting can facilitate drug withdrawal and offer testing and consultations that are not readily available in the patient's home area. A hospital-based inpatient chronic pain treatment center or a freestanding residential unit may be ideal.

12. **What psychological tests should be done on admission to a pain treatment center?**
At a minimum, assessment of the patient's psychological state should include the following:
- An inventory to determine the severity of the depression.
- Suicide Risk Test to determine the potential for suicide, which, interestingly, does not always correspond with the severity of the depression.
- The SCL-90 to assess the patient's psychological states, which vary from week to week.
- A Personality Inventory to determine the patient's personality traits; this is different from the patient's psychological state, which is measured by the SCL-90. (Note that the Millon and the Minnesota Multiphasic Personality Inventory cannot be used to assess the validity of the complaint of pain.)
- The Mensana Clinic Back Pain Test. Although not used at all centers, it has been shown to correlate with the presence or absence of demonstrable organic pathology.

13. **How do you spot a malingerer?**
True malingering is unusual. It represents a conscious effort to deceive, not a psychiatric illness. One of the hallmarks of a malingerer is refusal to participate in diagnostic studies. Obviously, if the patient is malingering, he or she is concerned that studies will reveal the absence of organic pathology. Most chronic pain patients emphatically state that they will do anything to get rid of their pain. A patient who is unwilling to participate in testing or treatment becomes suspect.

The major exception to this rule is a patient who strongly objects to surgical intervention. It is perfectly reasonable not to do additional diagnostic studies in search of a surgical lesion in an individual who has already stated an unwillingness to participate in surgery. An unwillingness to have surgery is a realistic concern, and the need for diagnostic studies in this individual may then become a medical/legal issue; that is, when the patient needs to prove that there is an organic basis for the complaint even though he or she will not agree to surgery. That raises the ethical issue of providing testing with potential morbidity to a patient who may not act on the results of that testing.

14. **What percentage of patients at a chronic pain treatment center are "fakers"?**
   The incidence of malingering (see Question 14) is very small, as is the incidence of hysterical conversion reaction, which is an unconscious attempt to protect against a distressful psychological event. Physicians involved in diagnosing and treating patients with chronic pain should treat all patients as though they have organic pathology. Trying to dichotomize between "organic" and "physical" is not rewarding. Both factors are almost invariably at play. Patients who are "somatizers" are suffering, and their problems must be addressed.

15. **How are chronic pain treatment centers certified?**
   The Committee on Accreditation of Rehabilitation Facilities (CARF) has a certification program for both inpatient and outpatient chronic pain treatment centers, as well as monomodality and multidisciplinary chronic pain treatment centers. Although CARF accreditation is no guarantee of quality, certification does, at least, indicate an effort on the part of the center to reach certain minimum standards. The American Academy of Pain Management also offers certification for chronic pain treatment centers.

16. **How do multidisciplinary pain treatment centers differ from other types?**
   Multidisciplinary chronic pain treatment centers offer a broad range of treatment and diagnostic evaluations, unlike monomodality centers, which focus on a single technique, or disease-specific centers that deal with only a single entity. Examples of disease-specific centers include headache clinics, cancer pain treatment centers, back pain clinics, facial pain clinics, pelvic pain clinics, and a host of others that focus on a single complaint of disease entity. Monomodality clinics may offer only acupuncture, physical therapy, relaxation training, biofeedback, chiropractic care, or psychiatric services.

   No single modality will treat all types of pain, but there is a tendency in monomodality clinics to try to treat more types of pain than can be effectively treated by their single modality. Also, there is a tendency to bias diagnoses toward the type of medical problem that is amenable to the type of treatment that the monomodality clinic offers: "When all you have is a hammer, everything looks like a nail." Interestingly, there are now a number of pain clinics that do not have a physician or psychologist as the primary person, allowing for a broader spectrum of therapies.

17. **What is the cost of the multidisciplinary pain treatment center?**
   Costs vary from center to center, depending on the approach used. They can be as low as a single, outpatient consultation fee or as high as full hospital per diem rate.

18. **What is the ideal result of multidisciplinary pain treatment center clinic evaluations?**
   The ideal result of multidisciplinary pain treatment center clinic evaluations is to establish an accurate diagnosis and a treatment plan that is appropriate for the diagnosis. The treatment plan may be carried out within the center or referred back to physicians in the patient's area.

19. **Which multidisciplinary pain treatment center is the best?**
   Which multidisciplinary pain treatment center is best for a particular patient depends on the results that are sought. If the diagnosis is in doubt, a multidisciplinary pain diagnostic and treatment center that determines the appropriate diagnosis is best. If the diagnosis is already firmly established, a center with particular expertise in that area may be indicated. Under these circumstances, a disease-specific clinic may be ideal.

20. **How should a pain center be chosen?**
   Ideally, a pain center should be chosen by comparing published outcome data. Unfortunately, they are not readily available. Lacking that criterion, local or national reputation and representation in peer-reviewed journals should be sought.

21. **Where can I get a list of multidisciplinary pain treatment centers?**

The International Association for the Study of Pain, the American Pain Society, the American Academy of Pain Medicine, the American Academy of Pain Management, and CARF should be able to provide any interested physician with a list of the multidisciplinary chronic pain treatment centers.

22. **What are the pitfalls in interpreting outcome studies?**

This is probably the most important question in this chapter. Outcome study results can be distorted and biased by both patient selection and reporting practices. Patient selection is a critical determining factor in assessing the accuracy of a published outcome study. If patients are preselected by their ability to complete a rigorous program, the success rate will be skewed to the higher end. If "all presenters" are taken, the rate may be low. Another bias that occurs in patient selection is age of the injury. Insurance companies report that if an injured worker has been out of work for 2 years or more, the return-to-work rate is less than 1%. However, they also report that if an injured worker has been out of work for less than 1 year, the return-to-work rate is 85%.

Reporting practices depend on "the definition of success." There are different criteria required for different groups. Some of the criteria commonly used are return to work (not valid in many older patients), decreased pain intensity (often of little value if there is no functional improvement), decreased drug intake (not valid if medications produce better function), or increased functional ability.

23. **What is the aim of pain clinic treatment?**

Naturally the aim of attendance at a pain clinic is reduction in suffering. This may involve pharmacologic or nonpharmacologic intervention. However, because only a small proportion of pain sufferers actually end up in a pain clinic, there may be an educative role for pain clinics as well. They can act as centers where interested professionals can gain insight into the understanding, diagnosis, and treatment of pain, which they can then apply to their own practices outside a pain clinic setting. Furthermore, particularly with pharmacologic treatment, pain clinics can act as centers where new treatments are evaluated, and if proven to be successful advocated for others outside pain clinics to use. Therefore they should have an educational as well as treatment role.

KEY POINTS

1. Members of a multidisciplinary pain management clinic should share a common philosophy.

2. It is desirable for pain management clinics to be certified by, for example, the Committee of Accreditation of Rehabilitation Facilities or the American Academy of Pain Medicine.

3. The aim of pain clinic treatment is reduction in suffering, which may be physical, mental, or more often both.

BIBLIOGRAPHY

1. Anooshian J, Stretzler J, Goebert D: Effectiveness of a psychiatric pain clinic, *Psychosomatics* 40(3):226-232, 1999.

2. Davies HT, Crombie IK, Brown JH, Martin C: Diminishing returns or appropriate treatment strategy? An analysis of short-term outcomes after pain clinic treatment, *Pain* 70(2-3):203-208, 1997.

3. Hendler N: Validating the complaint of chronic back pain: the Mensana Clinic approach, *Clin Neurosurg* 35:385-397, 1989.

4. Hendler N, Talo S: Role of the pain clinic. In Foley KM, Payne RM, editors: *Current therapy of pain*, Philadelphia, 1989, B.C. Decker, pp 22-23.

5. Kay NR, Morris-Jones H: Pain clinic management of medico-legal ligands, *Injury* 29(4):305-308, 1998.

6. McGarrity TJ, Peters DJ, Thompson C, McGarrity SJ: Outcome of patients with chronic abdominal pain referred to chronic pain clinic, *Am J Gastroenterol* 95(7):1812-1816, 2000.

7. Pilowsky I, Katsikitis M: A classification of illness behaviour in pain clinic patients, *Pain* 57(1):91-94, 1994.

8. Skouen JS, Gradsdal AL, Haldorsen EM, Ursin H: Relative cost-effectiveness of extensive and light multidisciplinary treatment programs versus treatment as usual for patients with chronic low back pain on the long-term sick leave: randomized controlled study, *Spine* 27(9):901-909, 2002.

9. Sullivan MD, Loeser JD: The diagnosis of disability: treating and rating disability in a pain clinic, *Arch Intern Med* 152(9):1829-1835, 1992.

10. Talo S, Hendler N, Brodie J: Effects of active and completed litigation on treatment results: workers' compensation patients compared with other litigation patients, *J Occup Med* 31(3):265-269, 1989.

11. Weir R, Browne GB, Tunks E, et al: A profile of users of specialty pain clinic services: predictors of use and cost estimates, *J Clin Epidemiol* 45(12):1399-1415, 1992.

CHAPTER 46

INTERVENTIONAL PAIN MANAGEMENT

Charles E. Argoff, MD, and Gary McCleane, MD

1. **What is "interventional pain management"?**

   Interventional pain management refers to a group of minor or major surgical procedures that can be used to control acute or chronic painful conditions. These include, but are not limited to, trigger point injections, different nerve blocks, intravenous infusions, radiofrequency lesioning, botulinum toxin injections, intraspinal analgesics, and spinal or deep brain stimulation techniques. Specific training is required to perform each of these types of procedures not only with respect to the procedure itself but also with respect to the management of potential complications of the intervention. Interventional pain management procedures are often an important component of a comprehensive pain treatment program.

2. **What are trigger point injections?**

   The management of myofascial pain is dependent on the elimination of painful myofascial trigger points. Trigger point injections involve the placement of a needle into the trigger point and the subsequent injection into the trigger point of a local anesthetic, a corticosteroid, or saline. Some clinicians have advocated the use of dry needling techniques in which nothing is injected, and the needle is moved around to deactivate the trigger point; however, although success with dry needling has been reported, it is clear that patients are initially more comfortable when local anesthetics are used during the injection. Various local anesthetics can be used, including 0.5% procaine, 1% lidocaine, or 0.25% bupivicaine. There is a very significant placebo effect and it is unclear whether or not the substance injected measurably alters the response.

3. **Describe the potential benefits of trigger point injections.**

   It is hypothesized that the painful myofascial trigger point results from a chronic, perpetual, hyperexcitable state of both peripheral and central neurons, resulting in the painful neuromuscular syndrome. Myofascial trigger point injections can interrupt this pain cycle and lead to significant relief and improvement in function. Typically, multiple trigger points are injected during each treatment session. The duration of benefit of each set of injections is often measured in days; therefore, injections need to be offered as part of an interdisciplinary treatment program that includes therapeutic exercise, pharmacotherapy, and perhaps behavioral pain management approaches as well.

4. **What is a nerve block?**

   Nerve blocks are procedures that are designed to interfere with neural conduction to prevent or dampen pain. Afferent as well as efferent conduction may be interrupted. Local anesthetics are the most commonly injected substance. There is an impression that addition of a corticosteroid prolongs the duration of effect of the nerve block when used for the treatment of chronic, but not acute, pain problems.

   Diagnostic nerve blocks can define more clearly the anatomical etiology of the pain, to better understand whether or not there is a sympathetically maintained component and to help distinguish between peripheral and central pain syndromes. Prognostic nerve blocks are performed to help to predict response to a procedure that may have a greater duration of action than a nerve block with a local anesthetic. For example, a trigeminal nerve block may be performed with a local anesthetic as a predictor of what response could be experienced with a neurolytic agent such as glycerol. Prophylactic nerve blocks or preemptive analgesia are techniques employed to prevent the development of significant pain following surgery or trauma. Therapeutic nerve blocks may be used in either acute or chronic pain syndromes to reduce pain and encourage functional restoration when combined with a therapeutic exercise program.

5. **What are some of the adverse effects of nerve blocks?**
   Adverse effects of nerve blocks include allergic reactions to the local anesthetic used, effects related to toxic blood levels of the local anesthetic, physiologic manifestations of the procedure, unintended injury to neural or nonneural structures, and anxiety-related reactions.

6. **When can nerve blocks be used for acute pain?**
   Postoperative pain relief can be achieved for 12 or more hours with injection of long-acting local anesthetic into the soft tissues of operative sites following the excision of a breast mass or hernia repair, for example. Ilioinguinal nerve block can give postoperative pain relief after inguinal hernia repair. Acute bursitis and tendonitis can be treated with the infiltration of local anesthetic combined with an antiinflammatory drug such as methylprednisolone into the affected areas. Attempts to reduce the postoperative pain of various intraarticular surgeries by injecting into the joint cavity during the operation are now common. Bupivicaine and other local anesthetics are used in this regard.

7. **What type of chronic pain syndromes can be treated with nerve blocks?**
   Myofascial pain syndromes, painful scars, neuromas, degenerative joint syndrome, spinal degenerative conditions, chronic headache, and neuropathic pain syndromes may at some point in their course be treated with nerve blocks. Nerve blocks for chronic pain generally do not "cure" the problem, but rather begin a process that, when combined with other treatments, may result in a more manageable pain level and improved function. There are numerous examples of clinical conditions that can be treated with nerve blocks. Some of these nerve blocks are described in the following questions.

8. **What is a paravertebral nerve block?**
   Paravertebral nerve blocks are used diagnostically to determine the precise nerve roots or nerve segments responsible for the pain caused by a herniated disk, osteophytes, other spinal degenerative conditions, tumor, or vascular lesion. They are performed in the cervical, thoracic, lumbar, or sacral regions. They can be used prognostically for patients who are being considered for a neurostimulatory or neurolytic procedure and therapeutically to provide temporary relief of pain in the affected region. For example, frozen shoulders, rib fractures, postthoracotomy pain, and acute herpes zoster pain can be treated with this technique.
   Regardless of where the paravertebral block is performed, there is risk of unintended epidural or subarachnoid injection of the local anesthetic, which can result in respiratory depression and other adverse effects. In the thoracic region, pneumothorax is one of the more common complications.

9. **What is an occipital nerve block?**
   Occipital nerve blocks are performed to lessen the pain associated with a variety of chronic headache syndromes, including occipital neuralgia, cervicogenic headache, and chronic migraine. The greater occipital nerve can be blocked above the superior nuchal line approximately 3 cm lateral to the external occipital protuberance. Five milliliters of local anesthetic is injected. There are few complications, and the immediate results can be quite gratifying for the patient and the physician. This procedure can easily be performed in the office.

10. **What is an intercostal nerve block?**

   Intercostal nerve blocks may be diagnostic or therapeutic. They help to define and manage the pain associated with chest and abdominal wall processes. They are particularly helpful for the relief of acute posttraumatic or postoperative pain in the thoracic or abdominal wall. In this setting, lower doses of systemic opiate analgesics may be required to maintain analgesia, resulting in reduced adverse effects from these agents in an acute setting. Continuous intercostal and intrapleural blocks also have been used for chronic pain syndromes, including postherpetic neuralgia and chronic pancreatitis.

11. **What are sympathetic nerve blocks? How are they used?**

   Sympathetic nerve blocks are an important treatment modality for patients with complex regional pain syndrome (CRPS) type 1 or 2 (reflex sympathetic dystrophy or causalgia, respectively). Both conditions are associated with hyperalgesia, allodynia, burning pain, and varying degrees of vasomotor and sudomotor abnormalities. For patients with CRPS whose pain is sympathetically maintained, sympathetic nerve blocks can be an effective therapeutic modality. Other conditions that have been treated with sympathetic nerve blocks include postamputation pain, peripheral vascular disease, visceral pain syndromes, acute herpetic neuralgia, and postherpetic neuralgia. Various cancer pain syndromes have also been treated with this modality.

   Cervicothoracic (stellate ganglion), thoracic, celiac plexus, splanchnic, and lumbar sympathetic blocks can be performed. Measuring the effect of a sympathetic block mandates that measures of sympathetic function be used, including changes in skin temperature, changes in the skin conductance response, or sweat tests (see Chapter 40, Sympathetic Neural Blockade).

12. **When are intravenous nerve blocks used?**

   Isolating a limb from the systemic circulation using a tourniquet and subsequently administering various phrarmacotherapeutic agents used for pain relief can result in significant analgesia. This technique, known as a Bier block, is frequently used as a sympathetic block. Guanethidine, a drug that depletes norepinephrine from presynaptic storage vesicles, may be injected during a Bier block, resulting in sympathetic blockade. Sweating is not affected in this type of sympathetic block because cholinergic fibers are unaffected. Some suggest that intravenous phentolamine administration is effective not only as a diagnostic agent for CRPS, but also as a treatment. Intravenous or subcutaneous lidocaine administered either once or on an ongoing basis can be helpful for a wide variety of chronic pain syndromes, including CRPS, postherpetic neuralgia, central neuropathic pain, and chronic soft tissue pain such as myofascial pain or fibromyalgia.

13. **What are epidural steroid injections?**

   Epidural steroid injections involve the injection of a steroid into the epidural space at any level. Steroids have potent antiinflammatory and analgesic properties. Many advocate the use of a series of three injections as a full treatment; however, no good data exist to confirm that three is better than two or five. Although many pain specialists perform this procedure without radiologic guidance, reports of needle placement errors within the epidural space have demonstrated that, for some patients, the use of fluoroscopic guidance and contrast material may be appropriate.

14. **How are epidural steroid injections used?**

   Most often, epidural steroid injections are performed in the lumbar level to treat low back pain. Patients with diverse etiologies for their back pain, ranging from spinal stenosis to bulging disks to herniated disks to simple back sprain, have received such treatment. Many areas of the spine, including nerve roots, spinal nerves, osseous elements, and connective tissue, may be subjected to prolonged inflammatory states, stretch, or ischemia.

Orthopedists and neurosurgeons often rely on epidural steroid injections to help reduce the spine-related pain of patients who they do not believe are clear surgical candidates. Short-term benefit from these injections is commonly observed.

Complications of the procedure include epidural hematoma, infection, postprocedure headache, and adverse effects of the steroids including hypertension, congestive heart failure, abnormal menses, and fluid retention.

15. **What is the role of botulinum toxin in pain management?**

The botulinum toxins are potent agents that temporarily prevent the release of acetylcholine at the neuromuscular junction and at other cholinergic synapses. Two types of botulinum toxin are currently available in the United States: type A (Botox) and type B (Myobloc). In addition to their effect on acetylcholine, recent research suggests that the toxins may also act on other neurotransmitters, including substance P, glutamate, and calcitonin gene related peptide (CGRP), and that these effects may in part explain some of their analgesic benefit. Botulinum toxins are used for an increasing number of painful conditions including cervical dystonia, spasticity, chronic myofascial pain, chronic low back pain, whiplash-associated pain, temporomandibular joint dysfunction, and chronic headache.

16. **What is neurolytic blockade? When is it used in pain management?**

Neurolytic blockade refers to the process by which neurons are damaged to produce a desired clinical effect. Neurolysis can be achieved through injected chemicals (phenol, glycerol, or alcohol), the use of cold (cryotherapy), or the use of heat (radiofrequency lesioning). The use of chemical agents often produces nonselective, significant nerve damage, which cannot be controlled; therefore, the risk of deafferentation pain is clear. Neurolytic blocks with chemical agents are most often reserved for use in intractable states or in terminal illnesses (see Chapter 39, Permanent Neural Blockade and Chemical Ablation).

17. **Describe cryotherapy.**

Cooling is known to produce a reversible conduction block in nerves; A-delta fibers and C fibers are particularly susceptible to cold-induced damage. The term "cryoanalgesia" refers to the destruction of peripheral nerves by cold, performed to accomplish pain control. This process has been used for intractable cancer pain, facial pain, postthoracotomy pain, and other instances of chest pain. The duration of pain relief following cryoanalgesia may range from 2 days to 7 months.

18. **What is radiofrequency lesioning? When is it used in pain management?**

Radiofrequency ablation procedures employ a thermal probe and a radiofrequency generator to selectively injure A-delta fibers and C fibers for pain control. Currently, radiofrequency ablation is commonly used for various spinal pain disorders, including pain of facet or discogenic origin as well as sympathetically maintained pain and trigeminal neuralgia. Because there is a more selective destructive effect, the risk of deafferentation pain is less than with chemical neurolysis.

19. **What is intradiscal electrothermal annuloplasty?**

Intradiscal electrothermal annuloplasty (IDET) is a minimally invasive procedure currently being used most commonly for the management of chronic low back pain caused by lumbar degenerative disc disease. This procedure requires clear technical expertise, because a wire needs to be percutaneously placed around a disc so that heat can be used to treat the injured disc. Efficacy and cost-analysis studies are currently being completed to help define the role of this relatively new procedure.

20. **Describe peripheral nerve stimulation (PNS).**

    In the PNS, electrical stimulation has been shown to block nociceptive afferents. Central effects of peripheral nerve stimulation (PNS) have also been reported. Studies have reported benefits of PNS in pain related to nerve injury, CRPS type 2, and postoperative low back and radicular pain. The indication for considering PNS is peripheral neuropathic pain experienced within the territory of a single sensory or mixed motor/sensory nerve. A preoperative assessment of potential benefit must be carried out before permanent implantation is completed.

21. **What is spinal cord stimulation? When is it used in pain management?**

    Spinal stimulation techniques require the placement of epidural electrical leads designed to stimulate the spinal cord such that an area of pain is "covered" or replaced by a nonpainful, tingling, or other sensation. The exact mechanism of action of spinal cord stimulation is not known, but it clearly involves the facilitation of pain-modulating effects that dampen pain transmission. Prospective patients must be able to understand how to regulate the stimulation, because treatment success involves active participation by the patient.

    Pain caused by nerve injury, including spinal and nonspinal etiologies, remains the most common reason for using spinal stimulation. It has also been used in axial low back pain and neck and thoracic spine pain, as well as to control the dysesthesia of multiple sclerosis—all with mixed results. There is significant interest in the potential benefit of this modality for the management of pain in peripheral vascular disease and for the management of intractable angina pectoris (see Chapter 42, Neurostimulatory and Neuroablative Procedures).

22. **Describe deep brain stimulation.**

    Deep brain stimulation refers to the direct electrical stimulation of the brain with various intracerebral targets noted. Stereotactic surgical techniques are used. No large controlled studies exist to document its role in pain control. However, motor cortex stimulation appears to be a possible treatment for patients suffering from severe central or trigeminal neuropathic pain who have not benefited from other more conservative techniques.

23. **What is the role of intraspinal analgesic therapy in pain management?**

    Intraspinal opiates have been used in the management of cancer-related pain for several decades; more recently, their use in the management of chronic, non–cancer-related pain has been established as well. According to cost-benefit analysis, implanted infusion systems for cancer pain are most practical when survival times exceed 3 months. Intraspinal infusion systems are appropriate for patients who have not benefited from other systemic, interventional, and noninterventional therapies, either because of lack of efficacy or adverse effects or both.

    System types include constant flow and programmable infusion. Each requires proper patient selection, a trial of intraspinal analgesia prior to implantation, and long-term follow-up. Catheter and pump failures, although not common, are not rare either.

    Analgesics that have been used in such infusion systems include morphine, hydromorphone, sufentanil, fentanyl, meperidine, methadone, local anesthetics, and clonidine. Intraspinal baclofen is used for intractable spasticity. The use of various combinations of agents, such as an opiate and a local anesthetic together, is quite common in clinical practice.

24. **What other pharmacological agents can be injected into painful areas apart from corticosteroids?**

    It is common to add a corticosteroid to a local anesthetic when injecting it into a painful area. The corticosteroid can prolong the duration of pain relief produced by the local anesthetic. However, there may be anxiety about repeatedly injecting corticosteroid both because of local effects (e.g., telangectasia, lip atrophy) and systemic side effects (e.g., osteoporosis, hypertension, Cushing's syndrome). Some evidence exists for the use of 5-HT3 antagonists such as ondansetron, granisetron, or tropisetron, in place of corticosteroid. This may cause a temporary pain flare after injection, which can be lessened if a long-acting local anesthetic, such as bupivicaine, is coadministered; after that, useful pain relief can result. An alternative is the coadministration of the alpha-adrenoreceptor agonist clonidine, which has been shown to substantially prolong the duration of the effect of local anesthetics by a peripheral, not central, mode of action.

25. **How can a nerve block reduce joint pain?**
Injection of a local anesthetic around a nerve causes a temporary interuption of the neural activity of that nerve. The duration of anesthesia that results is directly proportional to the duration of action of the local anesthetic used. However, when a joint is chronically inflamed the supplying nerve becomes overactive, causing hyperaesthesia in that joint. Under these circumstances, deposition of a local anesthetic around that supplying nerve can cause a reduction in that neural hyperactivity that far outlives the duration of effect of the local anesthetic; thus joint pain can be usefully reduced. Further, if corticosteroid is coadministered, this effect can be further prolonged. This may be because corticosteroids have other effects apart from reduction in inflammtion. They can reduce discharge from damaged neurons, have a weak local anesthetic effect (which may be prolonged if a long-acting corticosteroid is used), and also reduce dorsal root ganglion activity at the reference level.

26. **What aids can be used to ensure correct placement of nerve blocks?**
A number of strategies can be used to increase the likelihood of correct placement of a nerve block. For example, when a nerve passes by or through an anatomical landmark, the landmark can be used to guide correct placement of a nerve block, e.g., the suprascapular nerve passes through the suprascapular notch, which can be easily identified by "walking" the needle tip along the upper scapula. Performing the nerve block under fluoroscopic control also helps to ensure correct placement. Alternatively, a nerve stimulator can be used to identify when the needle tip is touching the required nerve.

KEY POINTS

1. Numerous interventional pain management procedures are commonly used in the pain management setting.

2. One must balance the benefits with the risks of interventional pain procedures when considering these for individual patients.

3. Most often pain management interventions provide neither complete nor permanent pain relief; therefore, patient's expectations must be realistic, including the potential for continuation and integration of noninterventional therapies.

BIBLIOGRAPHY

1. Armon C, Argoff CE, Samuels J, Backonja MM: Assessment: use of epidural steroid injections to treat radicular lumbosacral pain: report of the Therapeutics Technology Assessment Subcommittee of the American Academy of Neurology, *Neurology* 68(10):723-729, 2007.

2. Carette S, Leclaire R, Marcoux S, et al: Epidural corticosteroid injections for sciatica due to herniated nucleus pulposus, *N Engl J Med* 336:1634-1640, 1997.

3. Childers MK: *Use of botulinum toxin type A in pain management*, Columbia, MO, 1999, Academic Information Systems.

4. Cummings TM, White AR: Needling therapies in the management of myofascial trigger point pain: a systemic review, *Arch Phys Med Rehabil* 82(7):986-992, 2001.

5. Kapural L, Mekhail N: Radiofrequency ablation for chronic pain control, *Curr Pain Headache* Rep 5(6):517-525, 2001.

6. Lema MJ: Invasive analgesia techniques for advanced cancer pain, *Surg Oncol Clin North Am* 10(1):127-136, 2001.

7. Loeser JD, editor: *Bonica's management of pain*, 3rd ed, Philadelphia, 2001, Lippincott, Williams & Wilkins.

8. Saal JA, Saal JS: Intradiscal electrothermal therapy for the treatment of chronic discogenic low back pain, *Clin Sports Med* 21(1):67-87, 2002.

CHAPTER 47

COMPLEMENTARY AND ALTERNATIVE MEDICINE

Robert A. Duarte, MD, and Charles E. Argoff, MD

1. **What is the definition of complementary and alternative medicine?**
   There is no one prototype definition of complementary and alternative medicine (CAM), because the therapies keep changing, as well as moving from alternative to mainstream. At present, the term applies to a number of modalities that are not routinely taught in medical schools and are not generally part of conventional medicine. Presumably, as some of these modalities are shown to be useful, they will enter mainstream teaching and no longer be "alternative," much as use of nitroglycerine and digitalis did. Chiropractic, osteopathy, and biofeedback have already entered the mainstream and are no longer considered strictly alternative. However, the general philosophy of complementary and alternative medicine is that your body has the ability to heal itself and that prevention of disease, above all, is most important.

2. **How prevalent is the use of CAM in the United States?**
   Most surveys show that about 40% of the U.S. population use one type or another of complementary medicine during a given year. Over 65% use at least one type of CAM therapy in their lifetime. About 70% of younger patients report having used some type of CAM therapy by age 33.

3. **What are the major types of CAM therapies?**
   The National Center for Complementary and Alternative Medicine (NCCAM) divides CAM into the following five categories:
   - Alternative medicine systems
   - Mind-body interventions
   - Biologically based techniques
   - Manipulative and body-based methods
   - Energy therapies

4. **What are the major precepts of Traditional Chinese Medicine?**
   Traditional Chinese Medicine (TCM) is a holistic approach to health and disease that views both states as part of a continuum. The body is a system of balance, with a primary vital energy called "qi" (pronounced chee) that needs to circulate properly through the body, along lines called "meridians." There is a complex system of these channels, and most techniques are aimed at establishing appropriate flow and movement of qi. TCM formulates a diagnosis based on eight principles: internal/external, yin/yang, hot/cold, excess/deficiency.

5. **What are the major modalities used in TCM?**
   The most commonly used techniques in TCM involve the insertion of acupuncture needles, diet through proper nutrition, preparing and ingesting Chinese herbs, and massage. Exercising the body through such activities as qigong and tai chi (movement exercises) are also thought to be vital.

6. **How is acupuncture applied?**
   Acupuncture is literally translated into *acus* = needle and *punctare* = penetration. Medically, it refers to skin puncture with needles to produce a given effect. The selection of puncture points varies depending on the underlying pathology. Acupuncture is one of the oldest forms of recorded medical therapy, with documented cases going back more than 4000 years. It is applied by the simple insertion of metal needles along the meridians (i.e., channels) and at local points known as *ah shi* points. There are different types of acupuncture stimulation, including manual, application of heat, electrical stimulation, moxa (gum wort), or laser. It is unclear that any specific type of acupuncture is superior to another, although anecdotal evidence suggests that electroacupuncture may be useful for myofascial pain syndromes and auriculotherapy for drug addiction.

7. **What are some of the variants of acupuncture currently employed for pain management?**
   TCM acupuncture focuses on meridians or channels and intervention at specific sites—depending on the goal, e.g., surgical anesthesia, relief of pain, therapeutic purposes—is presumed to reestablish appropriate energy flow. Other schools support the use of trigger point manipulation with needles, or use of the ear, hand, and scalp as representative points.

8. **What are the proposed mechanisms of action for acupuncture analgesia?**
   TCM holds that the mechanism of action for acupuncture analgesia is release of stagnation of qi (the vital force). Needling also produces an increase in blood flow and a decrease of local prostaglandin and histamine release. Many studies reveal that electrostimulation produces effects on the spinal cord, midbrain, and pituitary. Following insertion of an acupuncture needle, there is a release of enkephalin, endorphins, and possibly gammaaminobutyric acid (GABA) at the spinal site; a release of enkephalin, serotonin, and norepinephrine at the midbrain site; and a release of endorphins at the pituitary site. At least three studies have shown that naloxone, an opioid antagonist, can partially reverse the analgesia caused by acupuncture, advocating the strong possibility that at least some of the analgesia is mediated by endogenous opioids. There continues to remain a few skeptics that believe acupuncture works through a placebo effect.

9. **What were the conclusions from the U.S. National Institute for Health Acupuncture Consensus Panel meeting in 1997?**
   The U.S. National Institute for Health Acupuncture Consensus Panel's statement in 1997 held that evidence supported acupuncture for adult postoperative pain (including dental pain), myofascial pain, and low back pain. There was reasonable or promising evidence for acupuncture as a treatment for pain caused by menstrual cramps, tennis elbow, fibromyalgia, osteoarthritis, carpal tunnel syndrome, and headache. There was no evidence to support acupuncture for weight reduction or smoking cessation.

10. **True or false: The scientific evidence that acupuncture is effective for fibromyalgia is convincing.**
    False. In 2005, a randomized controlled trial of acupuncture in fibromyalgia showed no difference compared to sham acupuncture. In 1988, a systematic review reported three randomized, controlled studies and four cohort studies involving 300 subjects. Although the overall quality of the studies was considered highly variable, it was felt that there was enough data to analyze. In one of the randomized, controlled studies, acupuncture was effective for relieving pain in five out of eight measures. However, the other studies were inconclusive, and the long-term benefits of acupuncture for fibromyalgia remain unknown.

11. **Is there any scientific evidence supporting acupuncture for other chronic pain conditions?**

Yes. Recent studies suggest that acupuncture may be as effective as any active therapy for patients with osteoarthritis of the knee and low back pain. In addition, evidence is emerging that acupuncture may be equally effective with less adverse events in preventing migraines compared to some pharmacological migraine agents.

12. **List the contraindications and precautions to be taken in acupuncture.**

Acupuncture complications are uncommon in trained hands. Of particular importance is appropriate placement of needles near the chest, to avoid the possibility of a pneumothorax. Obviously, infection is a concern, and only disposable needles should be used to avoid transmission of hepatitis B or C or HIV. A transient increase in pain, euphoria, or sedation is not uncommon, but this usually resolves within a day. Anticoagulation therapy is a relative contraindication, although gentle needling can be performed by a skilled practitioner with an acceptable side-effect profile. Patients with a pacemaker should not receive electroacupuncture.

13. **Does magnetic therapy have a place in pain management?**

As with many other CAM therapies, a definitive answer is not available as to whether magnetic therapy is useful in pain management. There are anecdotal reports of efficacy for magnets aimed at diabetic neuropathy, burning feet syndrome, carpal tunnel syndrome, and headaches. There have also been some negative studies in low back pain. Magnetic therapy is considered a relatively safe alternative, without significant side effects. The placebo effect may also be significant. However, it is probably better to avoid magnetic therapy in patients with an implanted pacemaker or other electronic device.

14. **What is meant by "bioenergetic therapy"?**

Also called polarity therapy, bioenergetic therapy is a combination of Ayurveda, TCM, and Western medicine that attempts to produce balance of all systems. Some bioenergetic therapies, such as reiki, qigong, tai chi, and therapeutic touch, are specifically used for painful conditions. Reiki proposes that energy flows from the practitioner's hands into the patient's body, over 12 body locations, with the patient fully clothed. Qigong and tai chi are structured, choreographed, slow movements that are designed to reestablish proper circulation of qi (energy). Therapeutic touch is another modality in which the goal is an energy flow between the patient and the practitioner, without actual contact. One recent double-blind study of therapeutic touch found no evidence of effectiveness.

15. **What is Ayurveda?**

The term Ayurveda is a Sanskrit word that translates into "knowledge" (veda) of "life" (ayur). In its truest sense, it is meant to promote health, rather than fight disease. An original text on Ayurveda, which appeared between 1500 and 1000 B.C., addressed arthritis, rheumatism, and disorders of the nervous system. Chopra quoted one of the original texts that described pain treatment: "The patient lying on the bed moistened with the dews of moonrays covered with flax and Lotus leaves and fanned with breeze cooled by contact of sandy beach should be attended by the love and sweet-spoken women with their breasts and hands pasted with sandal and with cold and pleasing touch who remove burning sensation, pain, and exhaustion." Ayurveda combines diet, exercise, spiritual activities, and herbal medicines in a holistic healing system. Its focus in on cleansing to remove toxins and balancing influences on the body to ensure a long life.

16. **Which bioenergetic therapies are in common use in western medicine?**

Thermal therapies are very common in Western medicine. However, despite the enormous sales of heating pads, there are relatively few studies that show any clear benefit of heat for pain. However, anyone with a sore muscle will tell you that a hot bath or a vigorous shower provides some pain relief. Cryotherapy (icing an injured muscle) also is popularly accepted, but there is little support in the literature for beneficial effects. Transcutaneous electrical nerve stimulation (TENS) has enjoyed enormous popularity, but metaanalysis has not been uniformly positive. Ultrasound is widely used but similarly unsupported by good studies.

17. **What is the role of spinal manipulation in treating back pain and headache?**
Systematic reviews related to the role of spinal manipulation in treating back pain and headache are inconclusive. However, in uncomplicated acute neck and back pain, spinal manipulation has been shown to provide significant temporary relief. The picture is far less clear in chronic conditions. Patient satisfaction is higher after manipulative therapy than after most other contacts with practitioners. Although neurological and vascular complications are cited by practitioners of allopathic medicine, they are quite rare.

18. **What are some of the "mind-body" modalities that are used to treat pain?**
Biofeedback is very popular for the treatment of headache and back pain. However, there is no evidence to show that it is any better than simple relaxation techniques. Biofeedback has been used successfully to treat headache, complex regional pain syndrome, and low back pain. Guided imagery may be effective to help patients cope with stress and pain. Progressive relaxation techniques are also used to relieve muscle tension and headache. Music therapy, breathing techniques, cognitive-behavioral therapy, visualization, hypnosis, and psychotherapy all have a role in chronic pain management.

19. **True or false: A few vitamin and supplement therapies have shown promise for treating headaches.**
True. A randomized, placebo-controlled study using vitamin B2 (riboflavin) at 400 mg per day (recommended daily dose is 1.8 mg per day) was more effective than placebo in migraine and tension-headache control over a 3-month period. Although statistically valid, these results have not been widely replicated. Intravenously administered magnesium can be an effective abortive agent in patients with acute migraine. Chronic magnesium replacement has also been recommended for recurrent migraine, although well-controlled studies have not supported its use as a prophylactic agent. Any patient taking a magnesium supplement should probably also take calcium.

20. **What is the role of feverfew and butterbur in headaches?**
Tanacetum parthenium (feverfew) is a plant cultivated throughout Europe and the United States. Its principal activity is the creation of parthenolide, which is thought to have an effect on platelets and the inhibition of proinflammatory compounds. Controlled studies have yielded mixed results. Feverfew is combined with magnesium and vitamin B2 in products known as Migreleve and Migrehealth. In 2004, *Petasites hybridus* root (butterbur) was shown to be more effective than placebo in a randomized, placebo-controlled study for chronic headache.

21. **List potential interactions between herbs and analgesics.**
    - NSAIDs—ginger, willowbark, feverfew, horse chestnut
    - Opioids—valerian root, kava, chamomile

22. **To what scientific standards should CAM techniques be held?**
Keep in mind that many "standard" practices have not been established through truly evidence-based medicine. Truly randomized trials for surgery in low back pain are lacking; epidural steroid injections remain controversial; and the appropriate primary preventive treatments for stroke (with the exception of blood pressure reduction) are still being worked out. Practitioners of Traditional Chinese Medicine may well wonder why their 4000-year-old therapies are being questioned and held to the standards of Western medicine,

which has a history of only a few hundred years. The fact that something is standard in one place and considered alternative in another does not mean that either side has the correct answer.

23. **How can a clinician minimize clinical and legal risk when treating a patient with CAM?**
Cohen and Eisenberg proposed a framework that classifies therapies according to the strands of evidence regarding safety and efficacy. Clinicians are advised to determine the clinical risk level, document the literature supporting the therapeutic choice, provide adequate informed consent, continue to monitor the patient conventionally, and inquire about the confidence of other practitioners in the particular modality.

KEY POINTS

1. The general philosophy of complementary and alternative medicine (CAM) is that your body has the ability to heal itself and that prevention of disease is of the greatest importance.

2. Numerous CAM therapies are currently used with varying degrees of medical evidence to support their use.

3. Potentially significant herb-drug interactions may occur with concurrent use; therefore, all health care practitioners must take an adequate medication history so that these can be avoided.

BIBLIOGRAPHY

1. Allais G, DeLorenzo C: Acupuncture as a prophylactic treatment of migraine without aura: a comparison with flunarizine, *Headache* 44(9):855-861, 2002.
2. Berman BM, Lao L, et al : The effectiveness of acupuncture as an adjunctive therapy in OA of the knee, *Annals of Internal Medicine* 141(12): 901-910, 2005.
3. Birch S, Hesselink JK: Clinical research on acupuncture. Part 1. What have the reviews on the efficacy and safety of acupuncture told us so far? *J Altern Complement Med* 10(3):468-480, 2004.
4. Chopra A, Doiphode VV: Ayurvedic medicine: core concept, therapeutic principles, and current relevance, *Med Clin North Am* 86(1):75-89, 2002.
5. Cohen MH, Eisenberg DM: Potential physicial malpractice liability associated with complementary and integrative medical therapies, *Ann Int Med* 136:596-603, 2002.
6. Cohen MH, Hrbek A, et al: Emerging credentials practices, malpractice liability policies, and guidelines governing complementary and alternative practices and dietary supplement recommendations, *Arch Int Med* 165(3):289-295, 2005.
7. Eccles NK: A critical review of randomized controlled trials of static magnets for pain relief, *J Altern Complement Med* 11(3):495-509, 2005.
8. Ernst E, Pittler MH: The efficacy and safety of feverfew (*Tenacetum parthenium L.*): an update of a systemic review, *Public Health Nutr* 3(4A):509-514, 2000.
9. Kaptchuk TJ, Eisenberg DM: Varieties of healing. 2: A taxonomy of unconventional healing practices, *Ann Intern Med* 135(3):196-204, 2001.
10. Khadikar A, Milne S, Brosseau L, et al: Transelectrical nerve stimulation (TENS) for chronic low back pain, *Cochrane Database Syst Rev* 3:CD003008, 2005.
11. Lipton RB, Gobel H: *Petasites hybridus* root (butterbur) is an effective preventative treatment for migraine, *Neurology* 63(12):2240-2244, 2004.
12. Maizels M, Blumenfeld A, et al: A combination of riboflavin, magnesium feverfew for migraine prophylaxis: a randomized controlled trial, *Headache* 44(9)885-890, 2004.

13. Mazzata G, Sarchielli P, Alberti A, Gallai V: Electromyographical ischemic test and intracellular and extracellular magnesium concentration in migraine and tension type headache patients, *Headache* 36(6):357-361, 1996.

14. Montazeri K, Farahnakian M: The effect of acupuncture on the acute withdrawal symptoms from rapid detoxification, *Acta Anaesthesiol* 40(4):173-175, 2002.

15. Nestler G: Traditional Chinese Medicine, *Med Clin N Am* 86(1):63-73, 2002.

16. Park J, Ernst E: Ayurvedic medicine for rheumatoid arthritis, *Semin Arthritis Rheum* 34(5):705-713, 2005.

17. Schoenen J, Jacquy J, Lenaerts M: Effectiveness of high dose riboflavin in migraine prophylaxis, *Neurology* 50(2):466-470, 1998.

18. Tindle HA, Davis RB, et al: Trends in the use of complementary and alternative medicine by US adults, *Altern Ther Health Med* 11(1):42-49, 2005.

19. Tsui MLK, Cheing GLY: The effectiveness of electroacupuncture in the management of chronic low back pain, *J Altern Compl Med* 10:803-809, 2004.

20. Vickers AJ: Statistical reanalysis of four recent randomized trials of acupuncture for pain using analysis of covariance, *Clin J Pain* 20:319-323, 2004.

INDEX

Page numbers followed by *t* indicate tables; *f,* figures.

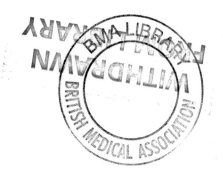
WITHDRAWN
BMA LIBRARY
BRITISH MEDICAL ASSOCIATION